Comprehensive Endocrinology

Comprehensive Endocrinology

Editor-in-Chief: Luciano Martini

Endocrine Rhythms. *Dorothy T. Krieger, Editor. 1979.*

Endocrine Control of Sexual Behavior. *Carlos Beyer, Editor. 1979.*

The Adrenal Gland. *Vivian H. James, Editor. 1979.*

Gastrointestinal Hormones. *George B. Jerzy Glass, Editor, 1980.*

The Thyroid Gland. *M. de Visscher, Editor, 1980.*

The Endocrine Functions of the Brain. *Marcella Motta, Editor, 1980.*

The Testis. *Henry Burger and David de Kretser, Editors, 1981.*

Volumes in Preparation:

Calcium Metabolism. *John A. Parsons, Editor.*

Fertility Control. *G. Benagiano and E. Diczfalusy, Editors.*

Pediatric Endocrinology. *Robert Collu et al., Editors.*

The Ovary

The Pituitary

Diabetes

Comprehensive Endocrinology

The Testis

Editors

Henry Burger, M.D., F.R.A.C.P.
Director, Medical Research Centre
Prince Henry's Hospital
Melbourne, Australia

David de Kretser, M.D., F.R.A.C.P.
Chairman, Department of Anatomy
Monash University
Clayton, Victoria, Australia

Raven Press ■ New York

Raven Press, 1140 Avenue of the Americas, New York, New York 10036

Made in the United States of America

Great care has been taken to maintain the accuracy of the information contained in the volume. However, Raven Press cannot be held responsible for errors or for any consequences arising from the use of the information contained herein.

Library of Congress Cataloging in Publication Data

Main entry under title:

The Testis.

(Comprehensive endocrinology)
Includes bibliographical references and index.
1. Testis. 2. Testis—Diseases. I. Burger,
Henry. II. de Kretser, David. III. Series.
[DNLM: 1. Testis—Physiology. WJ 830 T3421]
QP255.T48   616.6′8   76–58749
ISBN 0–89004–247–0

Preface

In recent years there has been a considerable increase in our understanding of male reproductive physiology and this knowledge is rapidly being applied to clinical situations. In keeping with the other books in the Comprehensive Endocrinology set, the aim of the present volume is to provide a balanced account of the current state of knowledge concerning testicular function, particularly with regard to man. The first part of the volume covers historical and comparative aspects, embryology and histology of the testis, together with the endocrine control in the fetus, child, and adult. Recent advances in knowledge of the functions of the Sertoli and Leydig cells are reviewed, as are the influences of the testis on its accessory structures and seasonal variations in male reproductive function. The second section is devoted to clinical aspects of testicular function before and after puberty and includes reviews of the important topics of semen analysis, cytogenetics, and varicocele.

This volume should be a valuable reference work for a wide audience: medical historians, comparative endocrinologists, embryologists, endocrinologists both at research and clinical levels, urologists, pediatricians, gynecologists, and those engaged in family planning programs. It will provide a wealth of knowledge for the medical undergraduate and postgraduate student. The editors have followed a deliberate policy of inviting contributions on an internationally representative basis—thus of the 18 chapters, 7 have been contributed from the United States and Canada, 7 from Western Europe, and 2 each from the United Kingdom and Australia.

Bremner has provided an introductory perspective on the testis in history starting with recordings on Assyrian rock tablets from the 15th century B.C., and has emphasized the importance of Berthold's demonstration of testicular endocrine function. Pilsworth and Setchell provide a comprehensive account of testicular structure and function in invertebrates and vertebrates, showing the fundamental relationship between the germ cells and specialized somatic cells and the somewhat more variable relationship between the endocrine and spermatogenic tissues. Wartenberg, describing the differentiation of this gonad, emphasizes the primary regulatory role of the mesonephros, and describes the function of the H-Y antigen in the determination of gonadal sex. He adduces evidence in support of the hypothesis that two types of Sertoli cells exist, one that stimulates and another that inhibits the meiotic process, concepts that could have implications for the development of spermatogenic disorders. His chapters are complemented by the account of the endocrine activities of the fetal testis by Faiman, Winter, and Reyes, who emphasize the requirements for testicular secretion of both testosterone and Mullerian inhibitory factor for normal male genital differentiation, while the gonadotropins appear necessary for germ cell proliferation and testicular descent. Perturbations of this system could lead to disorders of the kind described in subsequent chapters.

The further development of testicular function and its endocrine regulation from birth to puberty are described by Swerdloff and Heber who underline the multiple levels in the reproductive hormonal process at which maturational events occur. The regulation of Leydig cell and seminiferous tubule function in the adult is concisely summarized by diZerega and Sherins, who consider the regulation of gonadotropin secretion and the recent evidence for interactions between the Leydig and Sertoli cells. The growth of knowledge of the gonadal hormone inhibin is also mentioned. A detailed description of the light and electron microscopic structural features of these cells and of the spermatogenic epithelium is provided by Kerr and de Kretser, while Ritzen, Hansson, and French give a detailed account of the large body of recently acquired evidence for the central role of the Sertoli cell and its secretions in providing a milieu suitable for spermatogenesis. de Kretser, Risbridger, and Hodgson review the extensive data on the action of the gonadotropic hormones on the testes including aspects of receptor down-regulation.

The pathways of testicular steroidogenesis and their regulation are described by van der Molen and Rommerts, while Orgebin-Crist considers the important inductive and morphogenetic influence of the testicular hormones on the sex accessory glands, together with their roles in the adult. Seasonal variations in testicular function provide many insights into the control of reproductive processes in the male, and Lincoln provides a comprehensive and comparative account of the large body of data currently available.

Clinical aspects of testicular function are described in the second part of this volume. Sizonenko, Schindler, and Cuendet review the features of testicular tumors in childhood, and discuss their approach to precocious puberty and cryptorchidism. Santen and Kulin review normal and delayed puberty and the features of hypo- and hypergonadotropic hypogonadism. Baker provides a practical guide to the assessment of adult testicular function and to the management of male infertility, describing the situation where no treatment is available, where a basis exists for rational therapy, and the large group where current methods of treatment are empirical rather than clearly defined and logical. The clinical section concludes with three chapters discussing specific and important topics related to infertility, diagnosis and management, the analysis of semen with an emphasis on the appropriate nomenclature to be used in describing results thereof (Eliasson), the role of cytogenetic factors and their assessment in counselling infertile men (Skakkebaek), and the problem of variocedele including new methods of diagnosis and treatment (Comhaire).

The editors feel that this volume will provide the reader with a clearer understanding of testicular function and the value of the recent advances in this field in developing a logical approach to patients with reproductive disorders.

Henry Burger
David de Kretser

Contents

Contributors

H. W. G. Baker
Research Fellow
Howard Florey Institute of Experimental
*   Physiology and Medicine*
University of Melbourne
Parkville, Victoria, Australia 3052
and
Infertility Clinic
Prince Henry's Hospital
Melbourne, Australia 3004

W. J. Bremner
Division of Endocrinology
Department of Medicine
University of Washington
Seattle, Washington 98108

F. Comhaire
Department of Internal Medicine
Section of Endocrinology and Metabolic
*   Diseases*
Academisch Ziekenhuis
State University of Ghent
B-9000 Ghent, Belgium

A. Cuendet
Division of Pediatric Surgery
Department of Pediatrics and Genetics
Clinique Universitaire de Chirurgie Pédi-
*   atrique*
1211 Geneva 4, Switzerland

D. M. de Kretser
Department of Anatomy
Monash University
Clayton, Victoria, Australia 3168

G. S. diZerega
Developmental Endocrinology Section
Endocrinology and Reproduction Re-
*   search Branch*
National Institute of Child Health and
*   Human Development*
Bethesda, Maryland 20205

R. Eliasson
Reproductive Physiology Unit
Department of Physiology
Faculty of Medicine
Karolinska Institutet
Stockholm, Sweden

C. Faiman
Department of Physiology
and
Department of Medicine
University of Manitoba
Health Sciences Centre
Winnipeg, Manitoba, Canada

F. S. French
Department of Pediatrics
School of Medicine
University of North Carolina
Chapel Hill, North Carolina

V. Hansson
Institute of Pathology
Rikshospitalet
Oslo, Norway

D. Heber
Department of Medicine
Harbor General Hospital Campus
UCLA School of Medicine
Torrance, California 90509

Y. M. Hodgson
Department of Anatomy
Monash University
Melbourne, Victoria 3168 Australia

J. B. Kerr
Department of Anatomy
Monash University
Clayton, Victoria, Australia 3168

H. E. Kulin
Division of Pediatric Endocrinology
The Milton S. Hershey Medical Center
The Pennsylvania State University
College of Medicine
Hershey, Pennsylvania 17033

G. A. Lincoln
M.R.C. Unit of Reproductive Biology
Centre for Reproductive Biology
Edinburgh, Scotland

M.-C. Orgebin-Crist
Department of Obstetrics and Gynecology
Vanderbilt University
Nashville, Tennessee 37232

L. M. Pilsworth
Agriculture Research Council
Institute of Animal Physiology
Babraham, Cambridge CB2 4AT, United
Kingdom

F. I. Reyes
Departments of Obstetrics, Gynaecology,
and Physiology
University of Manitoba
Health Sciences Centre
Winnipeg, Manitoba, Canada

G. P. Risbridger
Department of Anatomy
Monash University
Melbourne, Victoria 3168, Australia

E. M. Ritzén
Pediatric Endocrinology Unit
Karolinska Sjukhuset
Stockholm, Sweden

F. F. G. Rommerts
Department of Biochemistry
Division of Chemical Endocrinology
Faculty of Medicine
Erasmus University
Rotterdam, The Netherlands

R. J. Santen
Division of Endocrinology
The Milton S. Hershey Medical Center
The Pennsylvania State University
Hershey, Pennsylvania 17033

A.-M. Schindler
Centre de Cytologie et de Dépistage du
Cancer
1205 Geneva, Switzerland

B. P. Setchell
Agriculture Research Council
Institute of Animal Physiology
Babraham, Cambridge CB2 4AT, United
Kingdom

R. J. Sherins
Developmental Endocrinology Section
Endocrinology and Reproduction Re-
search Branch
National Institute of Child Health and
Human Development
Bethesda, Maryland 20205

P. C. Sizonenko
Biology of Growth and Reproduction
Department of Pediatrics and Genetics
Clinique Universitaire de Pédiatrie
1211 Geneva 4, Switzerland

N. E. Skakkebaek
Laboratory of Reproductive Biology
University Departments of Obstetrics and
Gynaecology and Paediatrics YA
Righospitalet
and
University Department of Obstetrics and
Gynaecology
Herlev Hospital
DK-2100 Copenhagen, Denmark

R. S. Swerdloff
Department of Medicine
Harbor General Hospital Campus
UCLA School of Medicine
Los Angeles, California 90509

H. J. van der Molen
Department of Biochemistry
Division of Chemical Endocrinology
Faculty of Medicine
Erasmus University
Rotterdam, The Netherlands

H. Wartenberg
Institute of Anatomy
University of Bonn
5300 Bonn, West Germany

J. S. D. Winter
Department of Paediatrics
University of Manitoba
Health Sciences Centre
Winnipeg, Manitoba, Canada

The Testis, edited by H. Burger and D. de Kretser.
Raven Press, New York © 1981.

1

Historical Aspects of the Study of the Testis

William J. Bremner

*Division of Endocrinology, Department of Medicine, University of Washington, and
Veterans Administration Medical Center, Seattle Washington 98108*

The study of the structure and function of the testis historically has been
an important aspect of human and animal biology. Because of the exposed
position of the testes in most mammalian species and the fact that testicular
removal is ordinarily not life-threatening, many of the effects of orchiectomy
on reproductive function were recognized very early.

It was recorded on rock tablets from Assyria some 15 centuries B.C. that
castration of men was used as punishment for sexual offenses (1). This implies
that the effect of castration on libido and potency was recognized at least by
this time. Indeed, castration may vie with trephination of the skull for the
distinction of being the earliest surgery intentionally performed in human beings
(2). Castration as punishment for adultery is described in the Babylonian Code
of Hammurabi (ca. 2000 B.C.), in Egyptian law of the 20th Dynasty (1200–
1085 B.C.), and somewhat later in China (3).

The creation of eunuchs (prepubertal castrates) for social purposes such as
stewards, slaves, and harem attendants is an ancient practice (3). The word
"eunuch" derives from the Greek *eune* bed, and *echein,* to hold or keep (4),
i.e., bed-keeper or harem attendants. Removal of the testes for these social
purposes, with or without removal of the penis as well, probably originated in
the Near East but was widely used in China, India, and North Africa. Eunuchs
are mentioned repeatedly in both the Old and New Testaments of the Bible.
Mosaic law prohibited eunuchs from the temple:

> He that is wounded in the stones, or hath his privy member cut off, shall
> not enter into the congregation of the Lord. (5)

Eunuchs occasionally became trusted advisors to rulers, both in Moslem countries and in China. The keeping of eunuchs in China reached a peak in the
Manchu Dynasty (1644–1912) when law prescribed the number of eunuchs
that could be held by each person within the ruling hierarchy: 3,000 for the
emperor, 30 for princes, 10 for the emperor's grandsons, and so on (3). Many

primitive civilizations also practiced castration. Among the cannibalistic Caribs of the Antilles and northeast Brazil, human war captives were castrated to increase their weight and the tenderness of their flesh (3).

Although the early Christian church condemned eunuchs and the Church Council of Nicaea in 325 A.D. forbade the priesthood to eunuchs (3), prepubertal castration was practiced extensively by the later church for the production of male soprano singers. Since female singing was forbidden in the Catholic Church and the demand for soprano voices was strong, by 1600 boys were castrated specifically for this purpose. These castrati were considered by some musical authorities to be the greatest singers of any age (6–8) and as many as 4,000 to 5,000 such surgeries may have been performed annually (6). This practice was finally terminated by Pope Leo XIII in 1878, and the last castrato, Alessandro Moreschi, died in 1922.

Knowledge of the effects of castration in animals is also very ancient, probably dating at least to the Neolithic age (ca. 7000 B.C.) when animals were first domesticated (9). These effects were well understood by the time of Aristotle (400 B.C.), who provided very clear and detailed descriptions of testicular anatomy and function. The illustrations of the anatomy of the testis, efferent ducts, epididymis, and vas deferens taken from his work look surprisingly modern (Fig. 1). Aristotle (10) clearly differentiated the effects of prepubertal as opposed to postpubertal castration. He reported that if castration occurred in roosters:

> . . . after they are full grown, the comb turns yellow and they cease to crow and no longer desire sexual intercourse. If they are not full grown, these parts never reach perfection. The same is the case with human subjects, for if a boy is castrated, the hair that is produced after birth never appears, nor does his voice change; but if a full grown man is castrated, all the hair produced after birth falls off except that on the pubes, this becomes weaker, but still remains. In the eunuch, the hair present at birth does not fall off, for the eunuch never becomes bald.

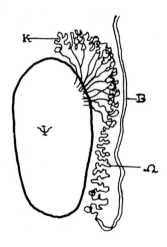

FIG. 1. Illustration of testicular and seminal duct anatomy taken from the Thompson translation of the works of Aristotle (400 B.C.) (10).

In spite of his generally accurate observations, Aristotle maintained that the testes were not necessary for fertility. One of his reasons for this belief was the fact that a bull could impregnate a cow during the first ejaculations after castration. The necessity of the testes for fertility was debated for the succeeding 2,000 years.

A very readable and interesting account of testicular and penile anatomy and function was written by Regnier de Graaf in 1668 (11). de Graaf's pungent observations concerning the history of investigation of testicular anatomy and function from ancient times to his own are well worth the brief time required to read this work. de Graaf's own careful observations clearly established the existence of seminiferous tubules and that the production of the fertilizing portion of semen occurred in the testes, not in the seminal vesicles, prostate, or other parts of the genital tract. Shortly thereafter van Leuwenhoek (1667) demonstrated the existence of spermatozoa in seminal fluid (12).

An interesting story of the work of R. van Koelliker has been recounted by E. C. Roosen-Runge (13). In 1840, Koelliker, then a 23-year-old medical student, spent his holidays studying marine invertebrates around two islands in the North Sea. He was strongly influenced by the new cell theory of tissue organization and, using recent improvements in microscope construction, looked for the cell origin of the spermatozoa that he found in the species he studied. His main conclusion was that spermatozoa develop within testicular tubules through processes analogous to the development of cells. Thus, spermatozoa were not young-developing animals as held by van Leuwenhoek and many others, but were the result of a variation on ordinary cell production.

The first clear demonstration of an endocrine role of any gland was by Berthold in 1849 (see appendix to this chapter) using the testes of birds (14). Berthold castrated fowl, demonstrating the subsequent loss of comb size and crowing. However, the loss of these male characteristics could be prevented if the testes were transplanted to an abnormal site, although nervous connections were severed. His conclusion was that something must be transmitted from the testes through the bloodstream to affect other tissues. This conclusion was reached over 50 years before the terms "hormone" and "endocrine" were coined.

Brown-Séquard, a well-known French experimental physiologist, reported in 1889 from studies on himself that injections of aqueous extracts from animal testes could produce rejuvenation (15). Brown-Séquard, then in his seventies, reported dramatic increases in well-being, including physical, mental, and sexual activity following self-injection of extracts of animal testes. This work had a large impact on experimental physiology, in particular the replacement of glandular extracts in various deficiency diseases. Although Brown-Séquard's work was soon discredited (eventually, even he stated that it had probably been a placebo effect), the use of appropriate endocrine gland extracts found therapeutic usefulness for the thyroid by 1920 and for the adrenals and gonads by 1940.

A variation on the theme of Brown-Séquard was initiated by Steinach, a Viennese surgeon, in 1920 (9). He ligated the vasa deferentia of aged rats and reported a return of youthfulness, including thickening of body hair, increase in body weight, regeneration of the seminal vesicles and prostate, and an increase in sexual activity. He reported similar results even if only one vas was ligated; in this case fertility could be returned or preserved since one vas was left open. These results seemed to confirm the opinion of Aretaeus of Cappadocia (150 A.D.):

> For it is the semen, when possessed of vitality which makes us to be men, hot, well-braced in limbs, well-voiced, spirited, strong to think and act. (16)

Steinach's results were confirmed by others in the dog and led to a large series of vas ligations in humans (17,18). In general, these early reports in humans confirmed that vas ligation did lead to partial rejuvenation. However, with studies on some of the millions of vas ligations done in recent years for contraceptive purposes, it seems well established that no consistent effect on libido or other evidence of rejuvenation is produced (19).

The testis has played an interesting role in the development of legal customs and word derivations as well as in general biology and medicine. Legal prescription of castration for certain offenses has been mentioned. The word "testis" derives from the Latin word "testis," meaning "witness," which is also the origin of the words "testify" and "testament." The reason for this derivation is unclear, but could be either because the testes bore witness of virility or because among Romans a legal witness was required to be an adult male with testes. Boys, eunuchs, and women could not be witnesses. Indeed, in certain civilizations, the witness was required to place his hand on his or someone else's testes while testifying. For example, in the Bible, where the euphemism for testes was thigh, we read:

> And Abraham said unto his eldest servant of his house, that ruled over all that he had. Put, I pray thee, thy hand under my thigh: And I will make thee swear by the Lord, the God of heaven and the God of earth. (20)

Among the Greeks, testes were called "didymi," i.e. "twins" because they were normally paired in the scrotum; thus the origin of the word "epididymis."

In addition to being of historical interest, study of the older literature may occasionally be of immediate clinical or investigational relevance. For example, the development of definite gynecomastia is described as common among men castrated prepubertally in Europe to produce castrato singers (6,8). Although initially recognized to be common in Klinefelter's syndrome, gynecomastia was not thought to be typical of other types of clinical eunuchoidism (21). However, with more recent accumulation of observations in Kallman's syndrome (hypogonadotrophic eunuchoidism) it has become apparent that gynecomastia is more common than previously realized (22). Study of older literature may occasionally be a source of information, particularly concerning human castration, not presently obtainable in any other way.

REFERENCES

1. Pritchard, J. B., editor. (1955): *Ancient Near Eastern Texts,* 2nd Ed. Princeton University Press, Princeton, New Jersey.
2. Majiro, G. (1975): *The Healing Hand: Man and Wound in the Ancient World.* Harvard University Press, Cambridge, Massachusetts.
3. Spencer, R. F. (1946): The cultural aspects of eunuchism. *Ciba Symposium,* Vol. 8, No. 7, pp. 406–420.
4. Derbes, V. J. (1970): The keepers of the bed; Castration and religion. *JAMA,* 212:97–100.
5. Deuteronomy 23:1.
6. Melicow, M. M., and Pulrang, S. (1974): Castrati choir and opera singers. *Urology,* 3:663–670.
7. Heriot, C. (1956): *The Castrati in Opera.* Secker and Warburg, London.
8. Schonberg, H. C. (1970): *The Lives of the Great Composers,* W. W. Norton and Company, New York.
9. Steinach, E. (1940): *Sex and Life: Forty Years of Biological and Medical Experiments.* Viking Press, New York.
10. Aristotle. Historia Animalium. In: *The Works of Aristotle,* Vol. IV., translated by D. W. Thompson. Clarendon Press, Oxford, 1910.
11. de Graaf, Regnier. On the human reproductive organs. Translated by H. D. Jocelyn and B. P. Setchell (1972): *J. Reprod. Fertil.,* Suppl. 17.
12. Bodemer, C. (1973): The microscope in early embryological investigation. *Gynecol. Invest.,* 4:188–209.
13. Roosen-Runge, E. C. (1977): *The Process of Spermatogenesis in Animals.* Cambridge University Press, Cambridge, England.
14. Berthold, A. A. (1849): Transplantation der Hoden. *Arch. Anat. Physiol. Wiss. Med.,* 16:42–46.
15. Brown-Séquard, C. E. (1889): Experience demontrant la puissance dynamogenique chez l'homme d'un liquide extrait de testicules d'animaux. *Arch. Phys. Norm. Pathol.,* 21:651.
16. Rolleston, H. D. (1963): *The Endocrine Glands in Health and Disease.* Oxford University Press, London. *(Quote)*
17. Benjamin, H. (1922): The Steinach operation; Report of 22 cases with endocrine interpretation. *Endocrinology,* 6:776–786.
18. Kammerer, P. (1923): *Rejuvenation and the Prolongation of Human Efficiency: Experiences with the Steinach Operation on Man and Animals.* Boni and Liveright, New York.
19. Hackett, R. C., and Waterhouse, K. (1973): Vasectomy-reviewed. *Am. J. Obstet. Gynecol.* 116:438–455.
20. Genesis 24:2–3.
21. Paulsen, C. A. (1974): The testes. In: *Textbook of Endocrinology,* 5th Ed. R. H. Williams, editor, W. B. Saunders Co., Philadelphia.
22. Bremner, W. J., Fernando, N. N., and Paulsen, C. A., (1977): The effect of luteinizing hormone-releasing hormone in hypogonadotrophic eunuchoidism. *Acta Endocrinol.,* 86:1–14.

Appendix: Transplantation of Testes[1]

On the second of August last year I caponized six cockerels. A, B, and C were 3 months old; D, E, and F were 2 months old. None of the animals had his wattle, comb, or spurs removed. Cockerels A and D had both testes removed; these animals later showed the characteristics of capons, that is, they were cowardly, fought with other cockerels only rarely and half-heartedly, and had the well-known monotonous voice of capons. Their combs and wattles became pale and developed only slightly; their heads remained small.

On the twentieth of December, when the animals were killed, only an insignificant, hardly visible scar could be found in the place where the testes had been. The spermatic cords could be recognized as thin, fragile threads.

Cockerels B and E were castrated in a similar manner except that only one testis was removed from the body and the other remained isolated in the body cavity.[2] In cockerels C and F, however, both testes were removed and then one testis of cockerel C was put into the abdominal cavity in between the intestines of cockerel F, and one testis of cockerel F was put into cockerel C in the same manner. These four cockerels (B,E,C,F) showed in general the behavior of uncastrated animals, they crowed lustily, often fought amongst each other and with other cockerels, and expressed the usual inclination toward hens. Their combs and wattles developed as in normal cocks.

Cockerel B was killed on the fourth of October. The remaining testis was attached and healed in its original site, increased more than half in its circumference, had good vascularization, and clearly showed sperm ducts. Upon cutting through it, a whitish liquid with many large and small cells but no spermatozoa was observed.

On the same day, cockerels C, E, and F had their well-developed combs and wattles cut off and their body cavities opened for examination of the testis. In cockerel E, I found the testis in the usual place, as in killed cockerel B; I dissected it, removed it from the cavity, and found it to be identical to the one from cockerel B. The abdominal wound, comb, and wattle soon healed, but the comb and wattle did not regenerate. The fowl began to emit the typical capon voice, it did not bother with hens anymore, nor did it engage in fights with other cocks; rather, it stayed clear from them and exhibited typical behavior of a true capon.

---

[1] By Professor Berthold of Göttingen (translated by B. Raess and W. Bremner), *Arch. Anat. Physiol. Wiss. Med.*, 16:42–46, 1849.

[2] *Translator's note:* apparently this testis was freed of its nervous and vascular connections but left approximately in its original site.

In cockerels C and F there were no signs of the testes in the usual site. Combs and wattles regenerated, the animals retained cock behavior, crowed as usual, and behaved normally toward hens and other cocks. These cocks were killed on the thirtieth of January, 1849. No sign of the testes was found in the usual site. Instead, in cockerel C the testis was found grown onto the side of the colon that is away from the back and bordered by the intestines without having become attached to the latter. The same was true for cockerel F, however, the place of coalescence was more posterior. In both individuals the testicle had an oval shape, a length of 15, a width of 8, and a thickness of 6 lines.[3] Well-developed arterial branches led toward the testis, penetrated it, and could be followed to the seminiferous tubules. When I cut the testicle open, a whitish milky liquid gushed out which had the consistency and odor of normal cock semen. Under the microscope in this liquid I could observe numerous smaller and larger cells of 1/450–1/150 lines in diameter and numerous spermatozoa with beautiful flagellar motility that upon mixing in a drop of water increased vividly.

These experiments yield the following results for physiology:

1. The testes belong to the organs that can be transplanted; they will reattach and heal after they have been removed from the body; the testis even permits transplantation from one individual into another and reattachment may occur at the original site of removal or in an entirely foreign location, for example, on the walls of the intestines.

2. Spermatogenesis continues even when the testis is in a foreign site; the tubules enlarge and function normally, producing semen containing spermatozoa. We find the same relationship as in plants, where the graft develops with its specific characteristics and produces its own fruit, not those of the stock.

3. It is a known fact that severed nerves can be rejoined and that in parts where nerves have been cut, sensation and mobility may be regained after healing. But in healing such as this, the nerve strands that belong together are not always reunited, as is evident from skin transplants. From the fact that a removed testis can attach itself to a very different part of the body, namely the intestine, and continue to develop and produce sperm, it is evident that there are no spermatic nerves. This is the main argument against the assumption of specific trophic nerves. The sympathetic nervous system has until recently been thought to be such a trophic system.

4. The remarkable sensual and antagonistic relationship between individual and community life as it is first seen in puberty and continues to advanced age is not affected by removing the testes from their original sites, severing them from their innervation, and allowing them to reattach in an entirely different part of the body. With respect to voice, sexual instinct, fighting, and development of combs and wattles, these animals remain true cockerels. However, since these

---

[3] *Translator's note:* 1 line ≃ $\frac{1}{12}$ inch or 0.21 cm.

transplanted testicles cannot remain in communication with their original nerves, and since as indicated in the third paragraph, there are no specific nerves underlying secretion, it follows that the results are due to the productive function of the testis. That is, the testes affect the blood and then by corresponding effects of the blood they can affect the entire organism of which, it is true, the nervous system makes up a considerable part.

The Testis, edited by H. Burger and D. de Kretser.
Raven Press, New York © 1981.

2

Spermatogenic and Endocrine Functions of the Testes of Invertebrate and Vertebrate Animals

L. M. Pilsworth and B. P. Setchell

A.R.C. Institute of Animal Physiology, Babraham, Cambridge CB2 4AT, United Kingdom

INVERTEBRATES

The term 'testis' is difficult to apply meaningfully to the diverse forms of reproductive and gametogenic architecture found among the invertebrate phyla. Roosen-Runge (114) has described the testis as "that circumscribed or demarcated tissue in which the earliest phases of spermatogenesis take place"; this is the definition used here, as in invertebrates it is sometimes impossible to describe the spermatogenic tissues in terms of definite organs.

The germ cells are the only cells in the body which possess the ability to divide meiotically. As the soma becomes increasingly complex through phylogeny, so the presumptive germinal tissue becomes more restricted embryonically. In the developing mouse for example, the primordial germ cells have been traced by histochemical methods to a localized area of the endodermal epithelium of the yolk sac in the region of the allantoic stalk, and their destruction by X-irradiation leads to permanent sterility in the individual (99). These cells represent the only cells in the body capable of differentiating into gametes. In the more lowly animals, the germ cells are derived from relatively undifferentiated cells persistent in the adult, such as the interstitial cells of Hydra, the archaeocytes of sponges, or the parenchymatous cells of the Platyhelminthes. Under certain conditions, these cells may aggregate and embark upon spermatogenesis, usually in association with specialized somatic cells, and the testis as defined thus first appears in phylogeny.

The characteristics of the testes of invertebrate animals are summarized in Table 1. In the lower animals where distinct permanent testes are uncommon, asexual reproduction is rife (Porifera, Ctenophora, and the primitive orders of both Platyhelminthes and Annelida). As gonads occur which are highly differentiated and reduced in number, the ability of somatic cells to reproduce asexually by fission, regeneration, and budding is gradually lost. This vegetative reproduction depends upon the presence in the adult body of relatively undifferentiated

9

TABLE 1. *Characteristics of the testes of invertebrate animals*

Animal	Type/number of testes	Accessory or 'nurse' cells
Porifera	Many, spherical testes containing germ cells derived from archaeocytes or choanocytes (104,120)	Yes (38)
Ctenophora	Testes are formed of thickenings of the wall of the meridinal canal (4)	Uncertain (109)
Cnidaria		
1. Hydrazoa	Interstitial cells form clusters of germ cells between the mesoglea and the epidermis. The testes are subdivided into "follicles." Germ cells develop synchronously. Four testes in Obelia sp. many in Hydra sp. (4,18)	Yes (115)
2. Anthazoa	Testes are on the mesenteries gastrodermal (18).	No (114)
3. Scyphozoa	Testes form longitudinal bands in gastrodermis. Four in Aurelia (4,18)	
Platyhelminthes		
1. Turbellaria	Diffuse germinal tissue or many separate testes, e.g. Afronta, Convoluta, Actinodactylella (4). Germ cells derived from 'wandering amoebocytes' (53)	Yes (114)
2. Trematoda	Two testes, germ cells derived from 'wandering amoebocytes'	Yes (4)
3. Cestoda	Numerous testes in each proglottid (4)	
Aschelminthes		
1. Rotifera	Single saclike testis. Germ cells derived from embryonic germ plasm (5) and spermatogenesis takes place during embryonic development (131)	
2. Gastrotricha	Diffuse testis tissue or one or two testes midbody (62)	
3. Echinoderida	One pair (55)	
4. Nematoda	Single or double longitudinal, tubular gonad. Germ cells derived from germ plasm (5,59)	No; germ cells arranged around a cytoplasmic core (142)
Nemertina	Simple saclike testis divided into follicles (61,112)	No (112)
Annelida		
1. Polychaeta	Testes in all segments of the worm, derived from peritoneal epithelium. Differentiation of gametes is completed in the coelom. Germ cells derived from embryonic germ plasm (5,105,119)	No; Germ cells grouped around cytophore formed from germ cell cytoplasm (105,119)

Group	Description	
2. Oligochaeta	Distinct gonads present in the reproductive segments (1 or 2) only. Maturation of gametes is coelomic (78)	No; as polychaeta (78)
3. Hirudinea	Distinct gonads 4–10 pairs. Gametes mature in the testicular lumen (78)	No; as polychaeta (78)
Echiura	Single testis in ventral mesentery just above nerve cord (46). Development of germ cells in clusters floating freely in coelom	Larger central cell among developing sperm in *Bonellia*. No accessory cell in Urechis (46)
Mollusca		
1. Gastropoda	Single gonad next to the digestive gland (9,135)	Yes (72)
2. Lamellibranchia	Paired gonads close to intestine (4). Anastomosing tubules in Californian Oyster (114)	Yes (114)
3. Cephalopoda	Saccular single testis (3,136).	
4. Nautiloidea	Single gonad occupying most of posterior portion of living chamber	Yes (2,51)
Echinodermata		
1. Holothuroidea	Single gonad of cluster of simple, branched tubules (4,37a)	
2. Echinoidea	Five gonads, one on each ambulacrum. Germinal epithelium surrounded by peritoneal epithelium (4,37a)	
3. Asteroidea	Masses of follicles form the testes, one pair hanging into the coelom in each interradial canal (4,37a)	
4. Ophiuroidea	Testes single, paired or numerous (4,37a)	
Arthropoda (Subphylum Chelicerata)		
1. Merostomata e.g., Limulus	Testis is a symmetrical network of tissue with sperm sacs and ductules, subadjacent to the intestine (4,36a)	
2. Arachnida (Subphylum Mandibulata)	Two tubes located ventrally in the abdomen, extending into the legs. X-, U-shaped or ladder like. Full of cysts (4,36a,114)	Yes; cyst cells surround synchronous germ cells (114)
3. Crustacea	Testes are elongate, paired organs in the hemocoel. Consist of lobulated sacs (36a). Germ cells are derived from embryonic germ plasm (5)	In Notodromas monacha (48), a continuum of 4 sustentacular cells in each testis in association with germ cells
4. Insecta	Sometimes single, often paired groups of follicles, containing cysts (36a). Only one follicle per testis in Diptera (114). Germ cells are derived from germ plasm (5)	Cyst cells surround germ cells. In the locust, a blood-germ cell barrier is present (94,129)

cells which may be drawn upon in the formation of new organisms (3a), and is never found among the Gastropoda or the many Arthropod orders where the testes are well-defined organs. So it seems that as the body becomes increasingly specialized by the centralization of tissues into localized organs, the ability to reproduce vegetatively is lost.

Although sexual reproduction affords a species the means of more rapid change, and therefore a greater chance of survival in a changing environment, the dependence on sexual reproduction imposes restrictions in the necessity of the close proximity of two organisms. These have been surmounted in various ways by animals. Hermaphroditism is common among the invertebrates (15), and as cross fertilization is the general rule, every individual is a potential mate. The evolution of the genetic trick of parthenogenesis (embryogenesis from an unfertilized egg) has been a boon to many animals which are solitary, e.g., benthic fish, or which need to reproduce rapidly where conditions are favorable (aphids, termites, and bees) (103a).

In *Hydra,* growth and reproduction seem to be antagonistic processes. Growth hormone causes the development of interstitial cells into nematoblasts; in its absence, these cells undergo meiosis and gametes are formed. The formation of gametes and the inhibition of growth can also be induced by a number of conditions such as reduction in temperature, starvation, increase in carbon dioxide tension, or stagnation in the culture medium (56).

The testes of the Cnidaria (*Hydra,* jellyfish, etc.) are formed by aggregations of interstitial cells between the ectoderm and the mesoglea. In the Hydrazoa they can form anywhere on the body surface, but in the medusae of the Scyphozoa (jellyfish) they take up permanent positions (18). These may vary in number according to the species, *Phialidium* having four, each situated around the gastrodermis in the distal half of one of the four radial canals. The testes of this species demonstrate a high degree of order, with synchronous germ cell maturation, spermatogonia situated centrally with successive stages of spermatogenesis occupying successively peripheral positions. Of particular interest are the supporting cells which are derived from the ectoderm, and which send long processes reaching between the spermatogenic cells, regularly spaced to give the testis a radially-striated appearance. These cells provide supporting columns closely applied to groups of germ cells which are developing in synchrony. One generation of spermatozoa takes 12 hr to mature. At spermiation, at which about one and a half million spermatozoa are released, the surface of the testis ruptures and the sperm are swept away from the germinal epithelium, the immature germ cells being retained by the supporting cells (115).

These supporting cells fulfill a role required in almost all metazoan animals, that of providing a microenvironment for certain stages of spermatogenesis. Although the analogous cells of different phyla often have different embryological origins (mesenchymal in the Platyhelminthes, ectodermal in Cnidaria) (114) they represent an association which evolved eventually into the intimate relationship demonstrated by the germ cells and Sertoli cells of the higher vertebrates.

Studies of the testis of *Nautilus pompilius* have demonstrated such a relationship. The testis inside the tunic is granular and consists of several blind-ending tubules which anastomose and enter a vestibule, the whole lined with epithelium continuous with the general coelom (70). Recently it has been shown that the Sertoli cells in these animals are large, branching structures in connection with a group of synchronously dividing germ cells which are themselves connected by cytoplasmic bridges. Between the Sertoli cells and developing spermatids are specialized junctional complexes reminiscent of "ball and socket joints," the Sertoli cell providing the "ball" which interdigitates with each spermatid (2). Further, the Sertoli cell extension contains a large, multivesiculate body, while small irregular vesicles can be seen in the spermatid cytoplasm immediately surrounding the junctional complexes. Similar junctional complexes may also be found between Sertoli cells and primary spermatocytes at the wall of the seminiferous tubule. The whole arrangement suggests transfer of materials from the Sertoli cells to the germ cells, as well as firm mechanical support. *Nautilus* is the last representative of the class Nautiloidea (a relative of the squid and octopus), which has been in existence since the Cambrian period, about 450 million years ago, again suggesting that the intimacy between germ cells and supporting cells is very ancient indeed.

Thus it would appear that the testis as a complex and well-ordered organ is encountered very early in phylogeny and, furthermore, that the synchronous, clonal development of germ cells and their close association with supporting, trophic, somatic elements has been observed throughout the animal kingdom (35,71,90–92,114,123).

Although any generalization in zoology is hazardous, there is a trend for the spermatogenic tissue to be confined to definite areas of the body as animal form becomes more complex. These areas evolve to form sacs which show varying degrees of specialization and eventually they are provided with ducts to convey their products to the outside. This may be observed within the phylum Platyhelminthes, where the primitive group, the Acoela (such as *Afronta*) have no true gonads, but a diffuse germinal tissue. The Polyclads (e.g., *Actinodactylella*) contain the germinal tissue within many testes situated throughout the body, but in the flukes (Trematoda) only two testes are present. Within the phylum Annelida, the germ cells in the most evolutionarily primitive class, the Polychaetes (such as *Nereis*), are produced in swellings of the peritoneum in every segment of the worm. In the more advanced Oligochaetes *(Arenicola, Tubifex)* the number of segments capable of elaborating germ cells is much reduced. [The aberrant Oligochaete *Chaetogaster orientalis* has no testes, the male germ cells being produced in various parts of the body. This condition is considered to be "a regression and not the persistence of a primitive state" (128).] *Lumbricus* possesses two reproductive segments, while some aquatic Oligochaetes have only one (4). In both these classes, the developing germ cells are shed into the coelom or specialized coelomic pouches where spermatogenesis is completed. In the still more phylogenetically advanced Hirudinea (leeches),

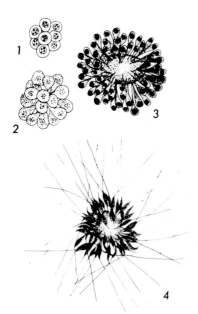

FIG. 1. Development of a cytophore in the Oligochaete *Marionina weilli.* **1:** 8-cell group of spermatogonia; **2:** 16-cell morula of spermatogonia; **3:** 64-cell morula of spermatocytes at metaphase; **4:** 64-cell morula of pedunculate spermatocytes. (From ref. 78.)

where four to ten pairs of distinct gonads are found, spermatogenesis is completed within the testicular lumen (4). Wherever they complete development, the germ cells of Annelids and Echiura form syncytial clones of cells around a central mass of cytoplasm (78,105,119). These structures are termed 'rosettes' or cytophores (Fig. 1). No nurse or supporting cells have been described in these cytophores (except for *Bonellia,* an Echiuran). Therefore these animals appear to be exceptions to the rule that the development of the male gametes takes place in close association with specialized somatic cells, but they do conform to the generalization that clones of germ cells develop synchronously with their cytoplasm still joined.

In the nematode *Caenorhabditis elegans,* the meiotic divisions take place in a localized area of the cylindrical testis. The germ cells are arranged around a central cytoplasmic core, and as there are frequent gaps in the cell membranes, the cytoplasm of the peripheral cells is continuous with the core cytoplasm. This morphological arrangement is similar to that seen in the gonad of the hermaphrodite of this species, but in the hermaphrodite there is a cellular sheath and basal lamina around the gonad at this level, whereas a cellular sheath is found only further along the testis in the male (142). Thus in these animals, spermatogenesis apparently proceeds in the absence of a direct association between germ cells and somatic cells.

In the ovotestis of the gastropod *Lymnaea,* the germinal epithelium includes both oocytes and spermatocytes but both are surrounded by somatic cells, follicle cells, and Sertoli cells, respectively (Fig. 2). The duration of spermatogenesis

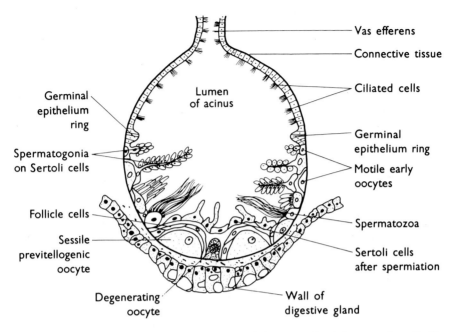

FIG. 2. Diagrammatic section through an acinus of the ovotestis of *Lymnea stagnalis*. The germinal epithelium ring gives rise to both oocytes and spermatocytes with their associated follicle and Sertoli cells. The spermatogenic zone forms a broad band adjacent to the germinal epithelium ring, whereas the young oocytes migrate to a region close to the digestive gland where they become sessile and vitellogenic. (From ref. 56; after ref. 68.)

(from spermatocyte to mature sperm) has been estimated as 10 days in the Echiuran *Urechis* (31) and in the gastropod *Phyllaplysia* (7).

It is among the Arthropods that the most advanced forms of invertebrate testes are to be found. In the shrimp, *Notodromas monacha,* a strongly PAS-positive basement membrane bounds the testis (114) and a chronological sequence of germ cells is present in the testicular tubes. Each testis has four sustentacular cells, interconnected by junctional complexes which serve to isolate the generations of germ cells from each other. The relationship between these cells and the germ cells has been compared to that between the germ cells and Sertoli cells of mammals, and in the Copepod *Diaptomus,* ultrastructural characteristics of steroid-producing cells have been reported in the sustentacular elements (47).

Perhaps one way for the male to solve the problems of spermatogenesis is to avoid them altogether, and the Rhizocephala, which are a parasitic group of Cirrepedes (the group which includes the barnacles), have managed to achieve this. They deposit immature germ cells, possibly with accompanying somatic cells, into the reproductive tract of the female where spermatogenesis is completed in "seminal receptacles" (65).

The most highly advanced, and intensively studied, invertebrate testes are found in the insects. Germ cells develop within cysts, closely applied to one or more cyst cells. Several cysts are contained within a follicle and groups of follicles constitute the testis. In some groups, for example, the Lepidoptera, these groups are surrounded by a thick wall. In Diptera, only one follicle is present. The follicle is club shaped, the wide apex containing cysts with germ cells in early stages of spermatogenesis. As the germ cells mature, the cyst migrates towards the base of the follicle so that a chronological sequence of stages is evident (Fig. 3). Cytoplasmic bridges between germinal cells have been reported in *Bombyx* (71), the honey bee *Apis* (91), and *Drosophila* (92).

A feature peculiar to the insect testis is the presence of apical cells in every follicle which may play a part in controlling the timing of spermatogenesis (143) and which demonstrate a high rate of RNA synthesis while spermatogenesis is in progress (100,114).

The germ cells are separated from the surrounding hemolymph by the cyst wall and the follicle wall. In the locusts, a further inner parietal layer is present in the basal region of the follicle, beginning at the level of cysts which contain meiotic germ cells. This layer has been shown to be impermeable to tracers such as horseradish peroxidase and lanthanum chloride in the locusts and forms a blood-testis barrier (94,129). Cellular junctions have been observed with the electron microscope in the inner parietal layer, and in *Locusta migratoria* these are in the form of desmosomes and "extensive septate junctions," the latter providing the major barrier to the tracers used (67,129) (Fig. 3).

The blood-testis barrier is probably involved in the process of spermatogenesis, by controlling the environment within the closed compartment of the follicle. The fluid in the testicular tubes of the silkworm differs in ionic composition from hemolymph, being rich in K^+ (98a). An analysis of the spermathecal fluid in the female queen bee (which probably reflects conditions within the testis follicles) has shown that the spermathecal fluid is considerably higher in potassium ion concentration (137.8 mEq/liter) than hemolymph (18.1 mEq/liter). The corresponding values for sodium are 15.7 mEq/liter inside and 31.6 mEq/liter outside; while chloride concentrations are 24 mEq/liter inside and 61 mEq/liter in the surrounding hemolymph (44). The action of the blood-testis barrier in providing a stable microenvironment for spermatogenesis here is clearly analogous to that found in the higher vertebrates. The concentrations of potassium and chloride ions in the seminiferous tubules of rats are higher than the concentrations in blood plasma, while the sodium ion concentration is higher in the plasma than inside the tubules (see 123).

The timing of spermatogenesis has been studied in several insects. The spermatocytic stage (the time from leptotene to the meiotic diakinesis) ranges from 4 to 12 days; the maturation of spermatids takes from 5 to 18 days (see 114). These times are, on the whole, shorter than the equivalent values for mammals but there is some overlap of values between the two phyla. Observations on more species are needed before any generalization is justified.

The insects are a highly evolved class, their physiological competence enabling

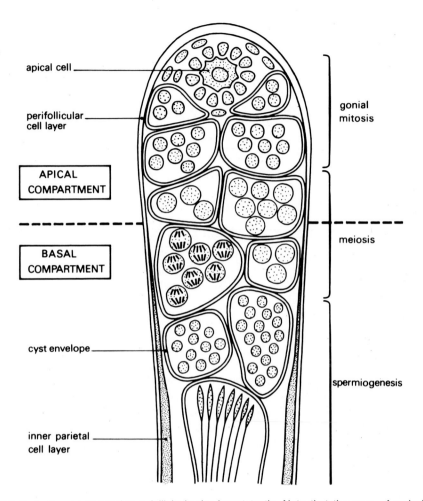

apical cell

perifollicular
cell layer

APICAL
COMPARTMENT

BASAL
COMPARTMENT

cyst envelope

inner parietal
cell layer

gonial
mitosis

meiosis

spermiogenesis

FIG. 3. A diagram illustrating a follicle in the locust testis. Note that the zone of meiosis extends into both compartments, and initiation of the meiotic process takes place in the apical compartment. (From ref. 129.)

them to become among the most successful of living animals. It is not surprising, therefore, to encounter a testis so closely analogous to that of the higher vertebrates among this advanced and successful group.

Hormones

In *Arenicola marina,* a Polychaete, it appears that the number of mature germ cells present in the coelom regulates the rate of spermatogonial proliferation in the testes. The number of spermatogonial mitoses are reduced as the coelom fills with maturing gametes prior to spawning, so that when spawning occurs, the germ cells which are available for release are all mature, with no immature stages present. Spermatogonial mitoses continue unchecked if the worms are experimentally decerebrated, and it can be reinitiated by injecting suspensions of brain homogenates taken from worms whose body cavities had been emptied of gametes a few days previously (60).

Secretions from the supraoesophageal ganglion in *Arenicola,* and the actions of a hormone involved in metamorphosis, a juvenile hormone, are both necessary for normal sexual development and gametogenesis (105). Spermatogenesis in *Nereis diversicolor* is also controlled by a gradual decrease in the secretion of an inhibitory hormone from the brain (34).

In leeches, the number of α neurosecretory cells in the brain decreases as spermatogenesis declines. In decerebrate leeches, the production of gametes is much reduced and can be restored by the injection of homogenates of brain (50). When the gonads of gastropods are cultured *in vitro,* they transform into ovaries unless the culture medium includes hemolymph or cerebral ganglia from individuals in the male phase. The transformation from male to female phase can be effected *in vivo* by removal of the optic tentacles and spermatogenesis is influenced by the injection of extracts of these organs, although the changes are not consistent in different species (see 56).

It is among the Arthropods that the effects and origins of hormones are best documented in invertebrates. At the base of the antennae or in the maxillae in the Malacostraca (crabs, lobsters, and shrimps) are masses of secretory cells which have been termed the Y-organ, and whose removal in the juvenile animal leads to impairment of gonadal maturation (57). The cause is not completely clear and may simply reflect a general metabolic defect brought about by ablation of these cells. In these animals, the development of male secondary sexual characteristics is controlled by the androgenic gland which is situated at the end of the vas deferens. In the amphipod *Orchestia gammarella,* removal of this gland causes loss of male characteristics and the transformation of the testis into an ovary. Its effect when implanted into a female is to cause formation of infertile testes and the development of male characteristics (45,118). The gland may have arisen from the same source as the interstitial cells of the testis as it demonstrates a definite androgenic role in these nonvertebrate animals. In the order Isopoda, male hormone is produced within the testis itself and the interstitial cells show cyclic changes related to spermatogenesis (19,118).

Naisse (101) has suggested that the apical tissue in the beetle *Lampyris noctiluca* produces an androgenic hormone which stimulates the formation of a male gonad, although differentiation of sex in insects is thought not to be usually under hormonal control (79). Menon (98) observed that apical cells resemble, ultrastructurally, the crustacean androgenic gland, so perhaps hormonal control here should not be ruled out (see ref. 41 for a review).

Hormones play an important role in the reproduction of insects. Germ cell multiplication is stimulated by the actions of median neurosecretory brain cells in the fruit fly *(Drosophila melanogaster)* (42), and the involvement of hormones in the development of the blood-testis barrier and meiosis in the locust *(Schisto-cerca gregaria)* had been discussed by Jones (67). She showed that ecdysone (molting hormone) and juvenile hormone (the hormone preventing the development of an adult stage) are involved, providing a delicate control mechanism which allows the blood-testis barrier to be set up in the third larval instar and meiosis to be completed during the fifth instar, ready for the last molt into adulthood.

Previous experiments using the pupae of Saturnid moths (69) showed that in these animals, ecdysone seems to play a permissive role in spermatogenesis by altering the permeability of the external, thick walls to allow entry of a "macromolecular factor" necessary for completion of meiosis.

VERTEBRATES

Morphology

The testes of vertebrates have their phylogenetic origin in coelomic pouches arranged in a row down each side of the body, discharging their products into the coelom. As phylogeny proceeds, the gonad becomes reduced to a short, fertile region in close proximity to the kidneys whose excretory ducts originally provided the germ cells with an exit from the body. In the Cyclostomes (hagfish and lampreys), germ cells find their way into the mesonephric (Wolffian) duct through pores in the duct (8), but in more advanced vertebrates, the testis and the mesonephric duct have a more intimate relationship. In the primitive fish (Dipnoi, Holosteans), the testis is connected to the anterior part of the mesonephros by the efferent ducts which are elaborated by the whole length of the testis (Fig. 4).

This pattern is also present in the Amphibia, where there is a tendency for

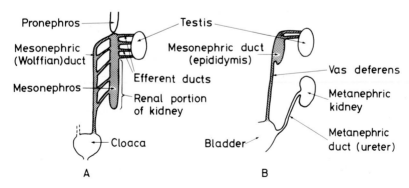

FIG. 4. Diagram of the testis and its relationship with the mesonephric duct in various animals. **A:** Primitive fish and amphibia (*Rana,* apoda, urodeles). **B:** Amniota (reptiles, birds, and mammals).

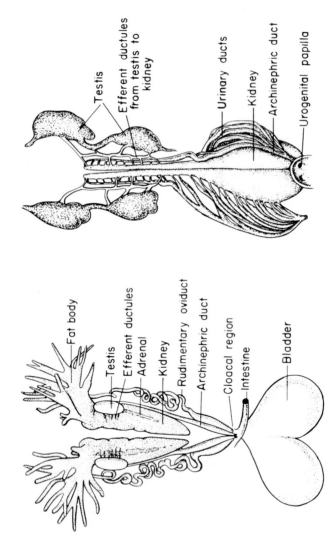

FIG. 5. Urogenital system of two amphibia. **A:** *Rana*, an anuran. **B:** *Salamandra*, a urodele. (From ref. 113.)

Fat body

Testis

Efferent ductules

Adrenal

Kidney

Rudimentary oviduct

Archinephric duct

Cloacal region

Intestine

Bladder

Testis

Efferent ductules from testis to kidney

Urinary ducts

Kidney

Archinephric duct

Urogenital papilla

the number of efferent ducts to be reduced from an extensive system in the Apoda and Urodeles to a more localized one in Anura. The gametes still pass through the kidney and are conveyed to the outside by the mesonephric duct. In the more advanced fish and Amphibia, the pattern is complicated by the development of ancillary ducts to take over either the role of sperm transport (as in Teleosts) or to convey urine to the cloaca and to leave the Wolffian duct for genital products (Elasmobranchs and some Amphibia) (see 113).

In the Amniota, the innovation of the metanephros as the functional kidney, drained by the metanephric duct, frees the mesonephros altogether of its renal function. In the reptiles, birds, and mammals, the Wolffian duct serves solely to convey male gametes, and has become modified into the epididymis (Fig. 4B), where sperm maturation and storage take place.

The role of the epididymis is fulfilled in Anura by specialized outpocketings of the mesonephric duct, termed "seminal vesicles," which provide a fluid environment rich in glycoproteins and low in concentrations of sodium and chloride ions (93). These seminal vesicles are strongly androgen-dependent and regress after castration.

In Cyclostomes, the testis is reduced to a single, elongate organ (32), but in most fishes, and in anuran amphibians, the paired testes are ovoid or elongate. In some urodele amphibia (e.g., *Salamandra maculosa*) they are distinctly lobed because of localized development of stem cells (Fig. 5). The lobulation is not constant since the inactive cells in the narrow "necks" between the active areas may become active at a later stage (63,64,83). In the Apoda (caecilian amphibians), each testis consists of a series of oval lobes of nearly equal size, each containing a number of locules or "subunits." The lobes are connected to each other by a central duct and bear a series of transverse ducts that carry the spermatozoa to the kidney tubules (133).

In reptiles and birds, the testes are paired ovoid organs, except in the burrowing blind snakes (*Typhlops* and *Leptotyphlops*) in which each testis consists of a spindle-shaped string of four to six closely abutting small lobules (cf. urodele amphibians). The testes lie in the abdominal cavity, approximately level with the last rib (see 39,75,86,95) and close to the aorta and posterior vena cava; their blood supply is uncomplicated (121) (Figs. 6–8). They lie cranial to the true kidney or metanephros, but this is in part owing to the fact that the latter does not migrate as far cranially in these animals as it does in mammals (141).

In the adults of all mammals, including the monotremes, the kidneys lie cranial to the testes whose position is very variable. In some, such as the Monotremata, Proboscidea, Hyracoidea, Sirenia, Macroscelididae, Chrysochloridae, and Tenrecinae, the testes migrate very little and remain close to the caudal borders of the kidneys (Type 1). In *Notoryctes* Edentata, Cetacea, Oryzorictinae, and Solenodontidae, the testes migrate to the caudal end of the abdominal cavity (Type 2). In *Erinaceus, Manis, Orycteropus*, Phocidae, Microchiroptera, Tapiridae, and Rhinocerotidae, they migrate to or just through the ventral abdominal wall without producing any external swelling; in the Phocidae they are covered

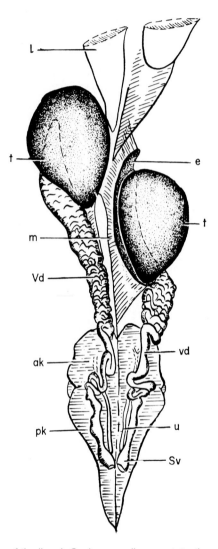

FIG. 6. Urogenital system of the lizard, *Sceloporus olivaceus*. t, testis; e, epididymis; Vd, ductus deferens; Sv, seminal vesicles; u, ureter; l, lung; m, mesorchium; ak and pk, anterior and posterior kidney. (From ref. 39.)

by several inches of blubber (Type 3). In Soricidae and Talpidae, a cremasteric sac is formed near the base of the tail but again no external swelling is obvious (Type 4). In Rodentia, Lagomorpha, Carnivora, Otariidae, Megachiroptera, *Tupaia,* Equidae, Suiformes, and Camelidae, a nonpendulous scrotum is formed ventral to the anus (Type 5). The most extreme form of testicular migration is seen in Marsupialia (except *Notoryctes*), Primates, and Ruminantia, in which

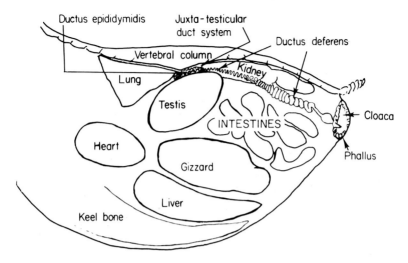

FIG. 7. Diagrammatic sagittal section through the thorax and abdomen of the male fowl, showing the relationship of the various body organs to the reproductive tract. (From ref. 75.)

a prominent pendulous scrotum is formed (Type 6) (21,126). The reason for this migration is still not known and it has even been suggested that the cause is not testicular, but epididymal (6,52). The testes are certainly not migrating to a cooler environment in those mammals with higher body temperatures, as suggested by Wislocki (138, see also 29). There is no particular relationship between body temperature and position of the testes, although it is true that *some* species with Type 1, 2, and 3 testes do seem to have lower body temperatures than mammals in general (21). In any case, the body temperature of birds is considerably higher than any mammal, and there is no foundation (54,77) in the suggestion made by Cowles (29) and that the testes are cooled by the nearby air-sacs. However, one feature which is related to the degree of migration of the testis is the complexity of its vasculature, culminating in the eutherian mammals with pendulous scrota in the formation of a spermatic cord consisting of an elongated, coiled artery surrounded by the multiple venous branches of the pampiniform plexus. In the Marsupialia, there is an analogous arrangement of an arterial rete of up to 200 parallel branches interspersed amongst a similar number of parallel venous branches (121,122). The full importance of these vascular arrangements is not yet understood, but both systems serve to dampen the arterial pulse and to precool the arterial blood by countercurrent heat exchange (134). Substances may also pass from vein to artery in the cord or vice versa (40), but this appears to be quantitatively insignificant for testosterone, which is the only substance studied in any detail (see 123). Although the testis probably does not migrate to find a cooler environment, there is no doubt that if a scrotal testis is heated to deep body temperature spermatogenesis is disrupted, although androgen production is not so severely affected (see 123).

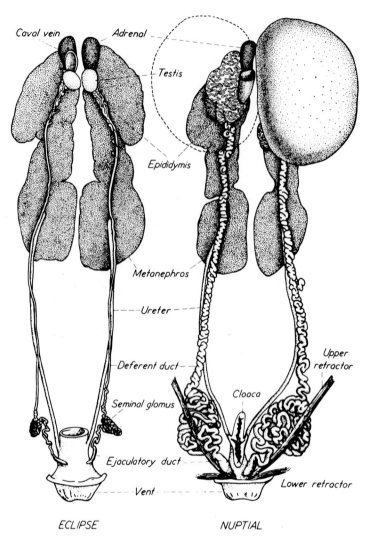

FIG. 8. The urogenital organs of the house sparrow during maximum and minimum sexual activity. (From ref. 141.)

Spermatogenesis

The gametes of the primitive vertebrates, the Cyclostomes, develop in cysts, in clones surrounded by cyst cells and are simply shed into the body cavity. More highly evolved fish also show cystic spermatogenesis with various arrangements of the cysts, but the male gametes are never released into the coelom;

instead they are conveyed by a closed system of ducts from the testis to the outside.

In Selachians, the testis is lobed and made up of follicles which in *Scyliorhinus* move away from the germinal zone, which is at the rostral end of the testis, to the caudal region where sperm are released and where the follicle subsequently degenerates (Figs. 9 and 10). In the germinal zone, spermatogonia become associated with sustentacular cells. These have also been termed Sertoli cells and their cytoplasm isolates the developing germ cells from the blood supply. A lumen develops in the follicle, and the nuclei become arranged in two layers with the spermatogonial nuclei around the outside. All the germ cells inside the follicle develop synchronously, and as meiosis approaches the Sertoli cell nuclei migrate to the periphery of the follicles. At meiosis, each Sertoli cell forms a single hollow pocket containing about 64 spermatids. This group is termed a spermatocyst and the lumen of the spermatocyst pocket opens centrally into the lumen of the follicle. Each follicle contains a large number of spermatozoa, about 32,000 in *Scyliorhinus* and about 16,000 in *Torpedo*. When development of the spermatozoa is complete, the follicle forms an opening into the collecting duct system, and the spermatozoa are expelled from the follicles which, along with the supporting cells, then degenerate (127). Although the Sertoli cells have been compared to those of mammals in that they enwrap the developing germ cells and isolate them from the blood supply, they differ in two important respects. In the Selachians, each "Sertoli" cell contains germ cells which are all at the same stage of development, and at spermiation the Sertoli cell degenerates.

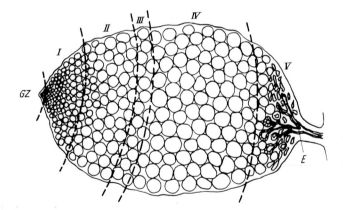

FIG. 9. Diagram showing the zonation of the testis of the dogfish *Scyliorhinus caniculus,* as seen in transverse section. The germinal zone (GZ) is where the seminiferous follicles are continuously formed. I to V indicate the zones where follicles of progressively later development are found. I: spermatogonia; II: primary spermatocytes; III: secondary spermatocytes; IV: spermatids; V: zone of follicular degeneration and release of the spermatozoa; E: efferent ductule. (From ref. 127.)

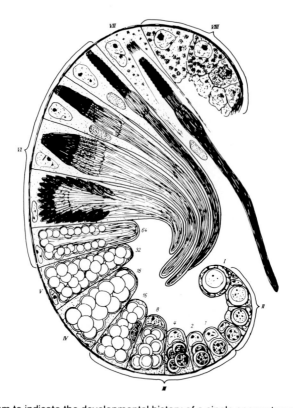

FIG. 10. Diagram to indicate the developmental history of a single spermatocyst of the dogfish. Development proceeds from lower right (I) round to the upper right (VIII). I shows a newly formed seminiferous follicle consisting of a spermatogonium surrounded by follicle cells. This is the only section of the diagram showing a whole follicle. The rest shows parts of the epithelium extending from the wall to the lumen. The segment marked II illustrates the stage of mitotic proliferation of spermatogonia and of follicle cells and the formation of the follicle lumen. III shows the stage during which spermatogonial mitoses continue after engulfment of a single spermatogonium by a single follicle cell. The arabic numerals at the inner end of each spermatocyst indicate the number of germ cells contained within each follicle cell. When the spermatocyst contains 16 spermatogonia they transform into 16 primary spermatocytes (IV), then into 32 secondary spermatocytes (V) and 64 spermatids (VI) and at this stage each spermatocyst develops a hollow pocket. Spermiogenesis (VI) is followed by spermiation (VII) and progressive degeneration of the retained somatic elements of the spent follicle (VIII). Note: This diagram represents successive stages in time. At any moment the follicle contains spermatocysts which are all at the same stage of development. (From ref. 127.)

The Teleost testis is also lobed, and in seasonally breeding fish, each lobule is lined either with Sertoli cells and resting germ cells, or with cysts containing spermatogonia, spermatocytes, or spermatids. The cysts eventually discharge the spermatozoa into the lumen of the lobule (Fig. 11B and C) (14). In *Poecilia*, a nonseasonal breeder, each lobe consists of a central cavity with radiating tubules which end blindly in close proximity to blood vessels (Fig. 11A). The youngest spermatogenic stages are found here, where they become enclosed in cysts. The cysts, containing synchronously developing germ cells, migrate down the tubule and discharge sperm into the central canal (11). As spermatogenesis proceeds, 50% of the contacts between adjacent Sertoli cells become specific. Desmosomes have been observed, and zonulae occludentes between Sertoli cells have been noted at the beginning of spermiogenesis (13). [Key references to teleost spermatogenesis may be found in Roosen-Runge (114).]

The duration of the various parts of spermatogenesis has been estimated in a few Teleost fishes. In *Poecilia reticulata* kept at 25°C, the spermatogonial divisions last about 22 days and it takes 14 days for the leptotene spermatocytes to develop into spermatozoa ready to be shed (10,11). In *Oryzias latipes* kept at 25°C this latter period can be divided into a time of 5 days for the spermatocytes to reach meiosis and a further 7 days for the spermatids to mature. These times are increased to 12 and 8 days, respectively, if the fish are kept at 15°C (36).

In the Urodeles, testis morphology is similar to that of the Teleosts. A series of locules are drained by a single ductule, and spermatogenesis takes place within cysts or ampullae which migrate caudally as differentiation proceeds (63,64,66,83). In the Apoda, ducts join the spermatogenic locules as the sperm mature, but a variety of developmental stages can be found in adjacent areas of the same locule (133). Tubules are present in Anura, containing the spermatogenic cysts in which synchronous maturation of early germ cell stages occurs. As spermiogenesis begins, the cyst wall ruptures to form a cup-shaped structure into which the heads of the developing spermatids are embedded, their tails floating in the lumen of the tubules. Spermiation then takes place into the lumen (114,139,140). Van Dongen et al. (33) showed that a rapid depolymerization of intratubular acid mucopolysaccharides leads to an increase in colloid osmotic pressure within the tubule. The resulting rapid intake of water flushes the sperm out. The ultrastructure of spermiation in the toad has been described by Burgos and Vitale-Calpe (16). The presence of smooth-muscle-like cells around the tubules in some Anura has been reported (132), but these are thought not to be involved in sperm transport.

Spermatogenesis in most amphibia is intermittent and usually occurs immediately *after* the copulatory period, so-called "postnuptial spermatogenesis": the spermatozoa are stored until the next mating period which may be almost 12 months later (82,83). Very little information is available on the timing of spermatogenesis in Amphibia but spermatocyte development takes at least 3 days (17). Bridges between germinal cells have been reported in the urodele *Amphiuma* (90).

In the Reptilian testis, the transformation to the pattern found eventually in mammals is complete. The parenchyma is composed of seminiferous tubules which house the germ cells and Sertoli cells and the whole is enclosed by a fibrous tunica albuginea. No cysts are present and spermatogenesis follows the mammalian plan (see 22,39,137). Spermatogenesis is usually seasonal, but there are some tropical species in which spermatogenesis is continuous. Both postnup-

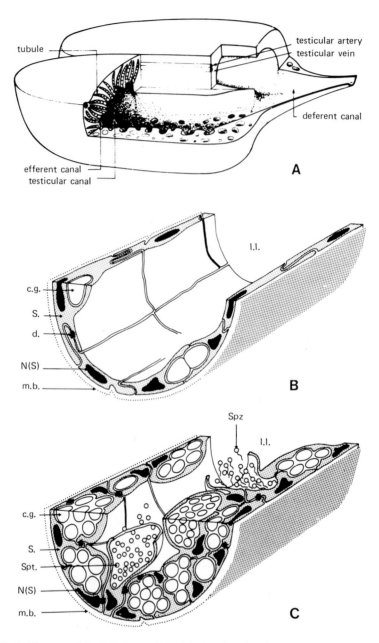

FIG. 11. A. Diagram of the structure of the lobulated testis of a teleost fish *(Poecilia)* with no clear breeding season. Each lobule consists of a number of tubules radiating from a central cavity. The ends of the tubules are blind and are oriented towards the periphery, and particularly towards the blood vessels. Each of the approximately 250 tubules communicates with the central cavity (or testicular canal) by a short efferent canal. At the blind end of each tubule is a cluster of dividing spermatogonia. From this cluster, single spermatogonia are enclosed

tial and prenuptial patterns can be found (39,84). No information appears to be available on the timing of spermatogenesis in reptiles.

In birds, the seminiferous tubules are extensively branched (74,97) but the general features of spermatogenesis are similar to those in mammals (25). The ultrastructure of the Sertoli cells (28), the boundary tissue of the seminiferous tubules (117) and the Leydig cells (103,116) is essentially similar to that of equivalent cells in mammals. Spermatogenesis is seasonal in most birds with virtual collapse of the testis at the end of the breeding season, and even a new tunica albuginea reforms at the beginning of each new season. However, some birds produce spermatozoa throughout the year (86,95). The timing of spermatogenesis appears to be appreciably faster in birds (5.5 days for the meiotic prophase, 7 days for spermiogenesis) (110) than in mammals. Functional evidence has been obtained for a blood-testis barrier in birds. A lower value for relative blood flow was obtained in rooster and drake testes with ^{86}Rb-rubidium, than with iodoantipyrine (Setchell, *unpublished observations*), as in the testes and brain but not other organs of rats (125). There is also morphological evidence that this barrier is located in roosters at the junctions between Sertoli cells as in mammals [B. Rothwell, and E. J. Cooksey, *unpublished observations,* see Setchell and Waites (125, Fig. 32).]

The subject of spermatogenesis in mammals has been very thoroughly reviewed (see 27,114,123). All that need be said here is that the timing of spermatogenesis is similar in the few species (rat, mouse, hamster, rabbit, vole, dog, ferret, ram, bull, boar, monkey, horse, man, hedgehog, mole, shrew, brush-tailed possum, and wallaby) in which it has been determined. Furthermore, in these species and in the African and Indian elephants, there is a similar ratio of the time from shedding the spermatozoa from the epithelium to the meiotic division, to the time from meiosis to sperm release; the duration of meiosis is also a similar fraction of one spermatogenic cycle in the various species. Unfortunately very few measurements of parameters of spermatogenesis have been made on mammals with nonscrotal testes and, in particular, no estimates have been made of rates of sperm production in these species, so it is not yet possible to say whether the evolution of a scrotum confers any reproductive advantage on the

---

by single Sertoli cells and form spermatocysts which increase in size as they proceed along the tubule, while the germ cells become spermatocytes and then spermatids. Eventually spermatozoa are released into the testicular canal. The number of Sertoli cells enclosing each cyst increases with the size of the cysts. **B and C:** Diagram of the structure of the wall of one lobule of the testis of a teleost fish with a well-defined breeding season. **B:** During the sexually inactive period. The Sertoli cells (S) and their nuclei [N(S)] are located at the periphery of the lobules, close to the basement membrane (mb). The inactive germinal cells (c.g) are completely enclosed by the Sertoli cells. The central lumen of the lobule (l.l.) usually contains some spermatozoa left behind from the previous breeding season, but eventually becomes empty during the nonbreeding season. d: desmosome. **C:** During the sexually active period. Spermatogonial divisions, meiosis, and finally spermiogenesis take place inside cysts. At the end of spermatogenesis, the spermatozoa (spz) and sometimes even the spermatids (spt) are discharged into the lumen of the lobule (l.l.) (From refs. 11 and 14.)

species. However, it is interesting that the daily sperm production per gram of testis is approximately ten times higher in birds (1.6×10^8 sperm/g/day) (111), and fish (1.5×10^8 sperm/g/day) (12), than in mammals (1.3–4.0×10^7 sperm/g/day) (1).

Spermatogenesis is seasonal in many mammals, but is normally uninterrupted in a number of species including man, rat, and several domestic animals. However, even in the seasonal breeders during the breeding season, spermatogenesis is continuous with spermatozoa leaving the testis at a steady rate (124). Whole areas of the individual tubules are at the same stage of spermatogenesis. The extent of these areas varies with species; they occupy considerable lengths of tubule in the rat (81) and bull (58), but are much smaller in the baboon (24). In man, they are so small that a single cross-section of a tubule usually cuts across several stages (26). However, it is curious that adjacent areas of the tubule are always at consecutive stages and in rat and bull, at least, the stages are usually arranged in "waves" of complete sets of areas at consecutive stages (Fig. 12). Furthermore there is, in general, a progression from more advanced to less advanced stages as one moves along the tubule away from the rete (58,108). The significance or origin of this arrangement is not known, but it

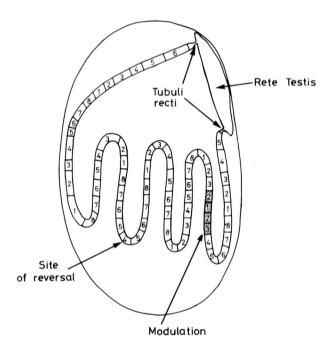

FIG. 12. A diagram of the stages of spermatogenesis in a seminiferous tubule of a rat testis. Note that in general the stages are arranged in descending order from both ends at the rete, forming waves proceeding to a "site of reversal." The wave is interrupted by a variable number of "modulations."

is conceivable that each area or each "wave" is a sort of open-ended cyst with a continuous current of fluid flowing through the lumen. Each tubule could then be considered as a string of cysts linked to one another.

Hormones

Evidence for Testicular Hormones

The effects of castration or androgen administration have been studied in a variety of vertebrates including amphibians, fishes, reptiles, birds, and mammals. In all these animals, castration is followed by regression of various secondary sexual characteristics, and these can be restored in castrated or hypophysectomized and induced in immature animals by injections of androgens (23,32,37, 107,141).

Morphology of Hormone-Producing Cells

In many nonmammalian vertebrates including the anuran amphibians, many teleost fish, and most reptiles, steroid-producing cells can be demonstrated between the seminiferous tubules or lobules (82,83,85) in much the same position as Leydig cells in mammals. However in some animals, particularly the urodele amphibians and some fresh water teleosts, the endocrine cells are found in the lobule or tubule wall, the so-called tubule boundary cells (82,96). Tubule boundary cells with an endocrine function are also found in the Algerian water turtle (82). In the Teiid lizard *Cnemidophorus,* the Leydig cells are mostly found just beneath the testicular tunica with very few in the intertubular spaces (30, 89,102). The enzymes 3β-hydroxysteroid and 17β-hydroxysteroid dehydrogenase have been demonstrated in the interstitial cells of a number of species (80,86,88) and this has been taken to indicate a steroid-producing role for these cells. These enzymes can also be found in the Sertoli cells in many animals, but as they are involved in transforming steroids rather than in *de novo* synthesis, the significance of their distribution is rather uncertain.

A "lipid cycle" in the Leydig cells has been described. In immature or sexually quiescent birds, the Leydig cells are small with very little lipid. There is a build-up of obvious lipid and cholesterol as the sexual season approaches, depletion of this material at the height of the season, and as the cells become exhausted they become strongly fuchsinophilic. This cycle correlates well with a seasonal variation in function of these cells, particularly as this cycle is synchronized in many species with seasonal changes in the androgen-dependent secondary sex organs and spermatogenesis (82,85). These authors have also reported a "lipid cycle" in the Sertoli cells of a number of species with an accumulation of cholesterol-rich lipoidal material following the ejection of the spermatozoa. Lipid also accumulates in these cells in rats after hypophysectomy or locally heating the testes (73). These observations have been interpreted as evidence that the Sertoli cells have a steroidogenic function. It seems more likely that the accumulated lipid represents material which is salvaged by the Sertoli cells from shed or damaged germinal cells and which is reused for the next generation of spermatozoa. Furthermore, most authors agree that Sertoli cells may transform steroids but probably do not synthesize them *de novo* from cholesterol (see 123).

Steroids Produced by the Testis

Testosterone has been measured in the testes of a number of species of non-mammalian vertebrates and has also been shown to be present in peripheral blood plasma in concentrations which, except for the birds, are generally higher than those in mammals (49,76,106). In many fish, 11-keto-testosterone has been shown to be an important androgenic steroid in blood, often exceeding testosterone in concentration (106).

However, actual production of testosterone by the testes (i.e., a higher concentration of the steroid in testicular venous than arterial blood) has been demonstrated only in one nonmammal, the Pekin duck (43). The concentrations found (3.4–15.8 ng/ml) in the internal spermatic venous plasma are at the lower end of the mammalian values (123), but as the blood flow per unit weight of testis is probably higher in birds than in mammals (121), production rates may be quite similar.

In mammals, including the platypus and several marsupials, testosterone appears to be the principal androgen secreted (20,122,123). However, very low concentrations of testosterone were found in blood from the internal spermatic vein of the marsupials *Pseudocheirus* and *Perameles* although the accessory organs were well developed and spermatogenesis was proceeding, suggesting that other androgens may be secreted in these species (20).

A considerable amount of effort has been directed towards studies involving the incubation of testes with radioactively labelled precursors of testosterone (84,87,130). These studies are of doubtful relevance to the situation in the intact animal as the precursors used are beyond the stages normally controlled by trophic hormones (see 123) and therefore the measurements are of enzymic potential rather than physiological rates of hormone production.

CONCLUSION

It would appear that the interrelationship between germ cells and somatic cells is a very long-standing one in phylogeny and that the basic cellular changes seen in the germ cells are also very similar in a wide range of species. Continuous spermatogenesis is a more recent development, but the transition from the cystic type of spermatogenesis may not be as abrupt as appears at first sight. From the small amount of evidence available, the testes of mammals do not appear to be as efficient as those of birds or fish in the production of spermatozoa per unit weight of testis. Androgens are also quite ancient phylogenetically, although the morphological relationships between the endocrine and spermatogenic tissues seem to be rather variable. The most recently evolved part of the male reproductive tract, the scrotum, is confined to mammals, but its significance still remains obscure.

ACKNOWLEDGMENT

The authors wish to thank Dr. Annette Szöllözi for reading the manuscript and for her helpful suggestions.

REFERENCES

1. Amann, R. P. (1970): Sperm production rates. In: *The Testis,* Vol. I, edited by A. D. Johnson, W. R. Gomes, and N. L. Van Demark, pp. 433–482. Academic Press, New York.
2. Arnold, J. M. (1978): Spermiogenesis in *Nautilus pompilius.* II. Sertoli-cell-spermatid junctional complexes. *Anat. Rec.,* 191:261–268.
3. Arnold, J. M., and Williams-Arnold, L. D. (1977): Cephalopoda: Decapoda. In: *Reproduction of Marine Invertebrates,* Vol. IV, edited by A. C. Giese and J. S. Pearse, pp. 243–290. Academic Press, New York.
3a. Balinsky, B. I. (1970): *An Introduction to Embryology.* Saunders, Philadelphia.
4. Barnes, R. D. (1963): *Invertebrate Zoology.* Saunders, Philadelphia.
5. Beams, H. W., and Kessel, R. G. (1974): The problem of germ cell determinants. *Int. Rev. Cytol.,* 39:413–479.
6. Bedford, J. M. (1977): Evolution of the scrotum: The epididymis as the prime mover? In: *Reproduction and Evolution,* edited by J. H. Calaby and C. H. Tyndale-Biscoe, pp. 171–182. Australian Academy of Science, Canberra.
7. Beeman, R. D. (1977): Gastropoda: Opisthobranchia. In: *Reproduction of Marine Invertebrates,* Vol. IV, edited by A. C. Giese and J. S. Pearse, pp. 115–179. Academic Press, New York.
8. Beer, G. R. De (1951): *Vertebrate Zoology.* Sidgwick and Jackson, London.
9. Berry, A. J. (1977): Gastropoda: Pulmonata. In: *Reproduction of Marine Invertebrates,* Vol. IV, edited by A. C. Giese and J. S. Pearse, pp. 181–226. Academic Press, New York.
10. Billard, R. (1968): Influence de la temperature sur la durée et l'efficacité de la spermatogénèse du guppy *Poecilia reticulata. C. R. Scand. Acad. Sci.,* 266:2287–2290.
11. Billard, R. (1969*a*): La spermatogénèse de *Poecilia reticulata* I. Estimation du nombre de générations goniales et rendement de la spermatogénèse. *Ann. Biol. Anim. Biochim. Biophys.,* 9:251–271.
12. Billard, R. (1969*b*): La spermatogénèse de *Poecilia reticulata.* II. La production spermatogénétique. *Ann. Biol. Anim. Biochim. Biophys.,* 9:307–313.
13. Billard, R. (1970): La spermatogénèse de *Poecilia reticulata.* III. Ultrastructure des cellules de Sertoli. *Ann. Biol. Anim. Biochim. Biophys.,* 10:37–50.
14. Billard, R., Jalabert, B., and Breton, B. (1972): Les cellules de Sertoli des poissons tetostéens. I. Etude ultrastructurale. *Ann. Biol. Anim. Biochim. Biophys.,* 12:19–32.
15. Blum, M. S. (1970): Invertebrate Testes. In: *The Testis,* Vol. II, edited by A. D. Johnson, W. R. Gomes, and N. L. Van Demark, pp. 393–438. Academic Press, New York.
16. Burgos, M. H., and Vitale-Calpe, R. (1967): The mechanism of spermation in the toad. *Am. J. Anat.,* 120:227–252.
17. Bustos, E., and Cubillos, M. (1967): Ciclo celular en la e spermatogenesis de *Bufo spinolosus* Wiegman. Estudio radioautografico preliminar. *Biologica,* 40:62–68.
18. Campbell, R. D. (1974): Cnidaria. In: *Reproduction of Marine Invertebrates,* Vol. I, edited by A. C. Giese and J. S. Pearse, pp. 133–199. Academic Press, New York.
19. Carlisle, D. B., and Knowles, F. (1959): *Endocrine Control in Crustaceans.* Cambridge University Press, Cambridge.
20. Carrick, F. N., and Cox, R. I. (1977): Testicular endocrinology of marsupials and monotremes.

In: *Reproduction and Evolution,* edited by J. H. Calaby and C. H. Tyndale-Biscoe, pp. 137–141. Australian Academy of Science, Canberra.
21. Carrick, F. N., and Setchell, B. P. (1977): The evolution of the scrotum. In: *Reproduction and Evolution,* edited by J. H. Calaby and C. H. Tyndale-Biscoe, pp. 165–170. Australian Academy of Science, Canberra.
22. Cavazos, L. F. (1951): Spermatogenesis in the horned lizard, *Phrynosoma cornutum. Am. Nat.,* 85:373–379.
23. Chester Jones, I., Bellamy, D., Chan, D. K. O., Follett, B. K., Henderson, I. W., Phillips, J. G., and Snart, R. S. (1972): Biological actions of steroid hormones in non-mammalian vertebrates. In: *Steroids in Non-mammalian Vertebrates,* edited by D. K. Idler, pp. 414–480. Academic Press, New York.
24. Chowdhury, A. K., Marshall, G., and Steinberger, E. (1977): Comparative aspects of spermatogenesis in man and baboon *(Papio anubis).* In: *Reproduction and Evolution,* edited by J. H. Calaby and C. H. Tyndale-Biscoe, pp. 143–156. Australian Academy of Science, Canberra.
25. Clermont, Y. (1958): Structure de l'épithélium seminal et mode de renouvellement des spermatogonies chez le canard. *Arch. Anat. Microsc. Morphol. Exp.,* 47:47–66.
26. Clermont, Y. (1963): The cycle of the seminiferous epithelium in man. *Am. J. Anat.,* 112:35–45.
27. Clermont, Y. (1972): Kinetics of spermatogenesis in mammals: Seminiferous epithelium cycle and spermatogonial renewal. *Physiol. Rev.,* 52:198–236.
28. Cooksey, E. J., and Rothwell, B. (1973): The ultrastructure of the Sertoli cell and its differentiation in the domestic fowl *(Gallus domesticus). J. Anat.,* 114:329–345.
29. Cowles, R. B. (1965): Hyperthermia, aspermia, mutation rates and evolution. *Q. Rev. Biol.,* 40:341–367.
30. Currie, C., and Taylor, H. L. (1970): A histochemical study of the circumtesticular Leydig cells of a teiid lizard, *Cnemidophorus tigris. J. Morphol.,* 132:101–108.
31. Das, N. K. (1968): Developmental features and synthetic patterns of male germ cells of *Urechis caupo. Arch. Entwicklungsmech. Organ.,* 161:325–335.
32. Dodd, J. M. (1960): Gonadal and gonadotrophic hormones in lower vertebrates. In: *Marshall's Physiology of Reproduction,* Vol. I, Part II, edited by A. S. Parkes, pp. 417–482. Longmans, London.
33. Dongen, W. J. van., Bailleux, R. E., Geursen, H. J., and Offermans, T. (1960): Spermiation in the common frog *(Rana temporaria).* III. Histochemical and chemical investigations. *Proc. Kon. Ned. Acad. Wet.,* C63:257–263.
34. Durchon, M., and Porchet, M. (1971): Premieres données quantitative sur l'activité endocrine du cerveau des Nereidiens au cours de leur cycle sexuel. *Gen. Comp. Endocrinol.,* 16:555–565.
35. Dym, M., and Fawcett, D. W. (1971): Further observations on the numbers of spermatogonia, spermatocytes and spermatids connected by intercellular bridges in the mammalian testis. *Biol. Reprod.,* 4:195–215.
36. Egami, N., and Hyodo-Taguchi, V. (1967): An autoradiographic examination of the rate of spermatogenesis at different temperatures in the fish, *Oryzias latipes. Exp. Cell Res.,* 47:665–667.
36a. Ettershank, G., Main, B. Y., Williams, W. D., Blower, J. G., and Ghent, R. L. (1972): Phylum Arthropoda. In: *Textbook of Zoology. Invertebrates,* edited by A. J. Marshall and W. D. Williams, pp. 392–613. Macmillan, London.
37. Evennet, P. J., Dodd, J. M. (1963): Endocrinology of reproduction in the river lamprey. *Nature (Lond.),* 197:715.
37a. Fell, H. B. (1972): Phylum Echinodermata. In: *Textbook of Zoology. Invertebrates,* edited by A. J. Marshall, and W. D. Williams, pp. 776–837. Macmillan, London.
38. Fell, P. E. (1974): Porifera. In: *Reproduction of Marine Invertebrates,* Vol. I, edited by A. C. Giese and J. S. Pearse, pp. 51–132. Academic Press, New York.
39. Fox, H. (1977): The urogenital system of reptiles. In: *Biology of the Reptilia,* Vol. 6, edited by C. Gans and T. S. Parsons, pp. 1–157. Academic Press, London.
40. Free, M. J. (1977): Blood supply to the testis and its role in local exchange and transport of hormones in the male reproductive tract. In: *The Testis,* Vol. IV, edited by A. D. Johnson and W. R. Gomes, pp. 39–90. Academic Press, New York.
41. Gallien, L. (1967): Developments in sexual organogenesis. *Adv. Morphol.,* 6:259–318.

42. Garcia–Billido, A. (1964): Analyse der physiologischin Bedingungen des Vermehrungswachstums männlicher Keimzellen von *Drosophila melanogaster. Roux' Arch. Entwickel,* 155:611–631.
43. Garnier, D. H., and Attal, J., (1970): Variations de la testosterone du plasma testiculaire et des cellules interstitielles chez le canard Pekin an cours du cycle annuel. *C. R. Scand. Acad. Sci. D.,* 270:2472–2475.
44. Gessner, B., and Gessner, K. (1975): Analysis of the inorganic ions in the spermathecal fluid and their transport across the spermathecal membrane of the honey bee queen *Apis Mellifica Carnica.* Pfluegers Arch. (Suppl.), 359:253.
45. Gilbert, L. I. (1963): Hormones controlling reproduction and moulting in invertebrates. In: *Comparative Endocrinology,* edited by U. S. Von Euler and H. Heller. Academic Press, New York.
46. Gould-Somero, M. (1975): Echuira. In: *Reproduction of Marine Invertebrates,* Vol. III, edited by A. C. Giese and J. S. Pearse, pp. 277–311. Academic Press, New York.
47. Gupta, B. L. (1964): Cytological studies of the male germ cells in some freshwater ostrapods and copepods. Ph.D. Dissertation, University of Cambridge, Cambridge.
48. Gupta, B. L.: quoted by Roosen-Runge (113).
49. Gustafson, A. W., and Shemesh, M. (1976): Changes in plasma testosterone levels during the annual reproductive cycle of the hibernating bay, *Myotis lucifugus lucifugus* with a survey of plasma testosterone levels in adult male vertebrates. *Biol. Reprod.,* 15:9–24.
50. Hagadorn, I. R. (1966): Neurosecretion in the Hirudinea and its possible role in reproduction. *Am. Zool.,* 6:251–262.
51. Haven, N. (1977): Cephalopoda: Nautiloidea. In: *Reproduction of Marine Invertebrates,* Vol. IV, edited by A. C. Giese and J. S. Pearse, pp. 227–241. Academic Press, New York.
52. Heller, R. E. (1929): New evidence for the function of the scrotum. *Physiol. Zool.,* 2:9–17.
53. Henley, C. (1974): Platyhelminthes (Turbellaria). In: *Reproduction of Marine Invertebrates,* Vol. I, edited by A. C. Giese and J. S. Pearse, pp. 267–343. Academic Press, New York.
54. Herin, R. A., Booth, N. H., and Johnson, R. W. (1960): Thermoregulation effects of abdominal air sacs on spermatogenesis in domestic fowl. *Am. J. Physiol.,* 198:1343–1345.
55. Higgins, R. P. (1974): Kinorhyncha. In: *Reproduction of Marine Invertebrates,* Vol. I, edited by A. C. Giese and J. S. Pearse, pp. 507–518. Academic Press, New York.
56. Highnam, K. C., and Hill, L. (1977): *The Comparative Endocrinology of the Invertebrates.* Edward Arnold, London.
57. Hoar, W. S. (1973): *General and Comparative Physiology.* Prentice/Hall International, Englewood Cliffs.
58. Hochereau, M.-T. (1963): Etude comparée de la vague spermatogénètique chez le tareau et chez le rat. *Ann. Biol. Anim. Biochim. Biophys.,* 35:20.
59. Hope, W. D. (1974): Nematoda. In: *Reproduction of Marine Invertebrates,* Vol. I, edited by A. C. Giese and J. S. Pearse, pp. 391–469. Academic Press, New York.
60. Howie, D. I. D., and McClenaghan, C. M. (1965): Evidence for a feedback mechanism influencing spermatogonial division in the lugworm (Arenicola Marina L.). *Gen. Comp. Endocrinol.,* 5:40–44.
61. Humes, A. G. (1941): The male reproductive system in the nemertean genus *Carcinomertes. J. Morphol.,* 69:443–454.
62. Hummon, W. D. (1974): Gastrotricha. In: *Reproduction in Marine Invertebrates,* Vol. I, edited by A. C. Giese and J. S. Pearse, pp. 485–506. Academic Press, New York.
63. Humphrey, R. R. (1922): The multiple testis in urodeles. *Biol. Bull.,* 43:45–67.
64. Humphrey, R. R. (1926): The multiple testis in *Diemyctyhis. J. Morphol. Physiol.,* 41:83–309.
65. Ichikawa, A., and Yanamagichi, R. (1958): Studies on the sexual organisation of the Rhizocephala I. The nature of the "testes" of *Peltogasterella socialis Kruger. Annot. Zool. Jpn.,* 31:82–86.
66. Joly, J. (1971): Les cycles sexuels de Salamandra (L.) I. Cycle sexuel des males. *Ann. Sci. Nat. Zool. (Paris),* 13:451–504.
67. Jones, R. T. (1978): The blood/germ cell barrier in male *Schistocerca gregaria:* The time of its establishment and factors affecting its formation. *J. Cell Sci.,* 31:145–163.
68. Joose, J., and Reitz, D. (1969): Functional anatomical aspects of the ovotestis of *Lymnaea stagnalis. Malacologia,* 9:101–109.

69. Kambysellis, M. P., and Williams, C. M. (1971): In vitro development of insect tissues. I. A macromolecular factor prerequisite for silkworm spermatogenesis. *Biol. Bull.,* 141:527–540. II. The role of ecdysone in the spermatogenesis of silkworms. *Biol. Bull,* 141:541–552.
70. Kerr, G. J. (1895): On some points of the anatomy of *Nautilus pompilius. Proc. Zool. Soc. (Lond),* 664–686.
71. King, R. C., and Akai, H. (1971): Spermatogenesis in *Bombyx mori.* I. The canal system joining sister spermatocytes. *J. Morphol.,* 134:47–56.
72. Kugler, O. E. (1965): A morphological and histochemical study of the reproductive system of the slug *Philomycus carolinianus (Bosc). J. Morphol.,* 116:117–132.
73. Lacy, D., and Lofts, B. (1965): Studies on the structure and functions of the mammalian testis. I. Cytological and histochemical observations after continuous treatment with oestrogenic hormone and the effects of FSH and LH. *Proc. R. Soc. Biol.,* 162:188–197.
74. Lake, P. E. (1957): The male reproductive tract of the fowl. *J. Anat.,* 91:116–129.
75. Lake, P. E. (1971): The male in reproduction. In: *Physiology and Biochemistry of the Domestic Fowl,* Vol. 3, edited by D. J. Bell and B. M. Freeman, pp. 1411–1447. Academic Press, London.
76. Lake, P. E., and Furr, B. J. A. (1971): The endocrine testis in reproduction. In: *Physiology and Biochemistry of the Domestic Fowl,* Vol. 3, edited by D. J. Bell and B. M. Freeman, pp. 1469–1488. Academic Press, London.
77. Langford, B. B., and Howarth, B. (1972): Diurnal rhythm of testicular temperature and spermatogenic activity in the domestic fowl. *Poultry Sci.,* 51:1828.
78. Lasserre, P. (1975): Clitellata. In: *Reproduction in Marine Invertebrates,* Vol. III, edited by A. C. Giese and J. S. Pearse, pp. 215–275. Academic Press, New York.
79. Lauge, G. (1970): Problèmes posés par les insectes concernant la différentiation du sexe. *Bull. Soc. Zool. Fr.,* 95:363–377.
80. Lazard, L. (1976): Spermatogenesis and 3β-HSDH activity in the testis of the axolotl. *Nature (Lond),* 264:796–797.
81. Leblond, C. P., and Clermont, Y. (1952): Definition of the stages of the cycle of the seminiferous epithelium in the rat. *Ann. NY Acad. Sci.,* 55:548–573.
82. Lofts, B. (1968): Patterns of testicular activity. In: *Perspectives in Endocrinology. Hormones in the Lives of Lower Vertebrates,* edited by E. J. W. Barrington and C. B. Jorgensen, pp. 239–304. Academic Press, London.
83. Lofts, B. (1974): Reproduction. In: *Physiology of the Amphibia,* Vol. II, edited by B. Lofts, pp. 107–218. Academic Press, New York.
84. Lofts, B. (1977): Patterns of spermatogenesis and steroidogenesis in male reptiles. In: *Reproduction and Evolution,* edited by J. H. Calaby and C. H. Tyndale-Biscoe, pp. 127–136. Australian Academy of Science, Canberra.
85. Lofts, B., and Bern, H. A. (1972): The functional morphology of steroidogenic tissues. In: *Steroids in Non-mammalian Vertebrates,* edited by D. R. Idler, pp. 37–125. Academic Press, New York.
86. Lofts, B., and Murton, R. K. (1973): Reproduction in birds. In: *Avian Biology,* Vol. III, edited by D. S. Farner and J. R. King, pp. 1–107. Academic Press, New York.
87. Lofts, B., Phillips, J. G., and Tam, W. H. (1966): Seasonal changes in the testis of the cobra, *Naja naja* (Linn). *Gen. Comp. Endocrinol.,* 6:466–475.
88. Lofts, B., and Tsui, A. W. (1977): Histological and histochemical changes in the gonads and epididymides of the male soft-shelled turtle, *Trionyx sinensis. J. Zool. (Lond),* 181:57–68.
89. Lowe, C. H., and Goldberg, S. K. (1966): Variation in the circumtesticular Leydig cell tunic of teiid lizards *(Cnemidophorus* and *Ameiva). J. Morphol.,* 119:277–282.
90. McGregor, J. H. (1899): The spermatogenesis of *Amphiuma. J. Morphol.,* 15:57–104.
91. MacKinnon, E. A., and Bassur, P. K. (1970): Cytokinesis in the gonocysts of the drone honey bee (*Apis emllifera* L.). *Can. J. Zool.,* 48:1163–1166.
92. Mahowald, A. P. (1971): The formation of ring canals by cell furrows in *Drosophila. Z. Zellforsch. Mikrosk. Anat.,* 118:162–167.
93. Mann, T., Lutwak, C. L., and Hay, M. F. (1963): A note on the so-called seminal vesicles of the frog *Discoglossus pictus. Acta Embryol. Morphol. Exp.,* 6:21–25.
94. Marcaillou, C., and Szöllözi, A. (1975): Variations de permeabilité du follicule testiculaire

chez le Criquet Locusta migratoria (Orthoptere) au cours du dernier stade larvaire. *C. R. Acad. Sci. (Paris),* 281:2001–2004.

95. Marshall, A. J. (1961): Reproduction. In: *Biology and Comparative Physiology of Birds,* Vol. II, edited by A. J. Marshall, pp. 169–213. Academic Press, New York.

96. Marshall, A. J., and Lofts, B. (1956): The Leydig-cell homologue in certain Teleost fishes. *Nature (Lond),* 177:704.

97. Marvan, F. (1969): Postnatal development of the male genital tract of the *Gallus domesticus. Anat. Anz.,* 124:443–462.

98. Menon, M. (1969): Structure of the apical cells of the testis of the Tenebrionid beetles *Tenebrio molitor* and *Zaphobas rugipes. J. Morph.,* 127:409–430.

98a. Michejda, J. W., and Thiers, R. E. (1963): Ionic regulation in the development of males of a silkworm: *Hyalophora cecropia. Proceedings: XVIth International Congress of Zoology,* Vol. 2, edited by S. A. Moore, p. 39. International Congress of Zoology, Washington, D.C.

99. Mintz, B. (1960): Embryological phases of mammalian gametogenesis. *J. Cell. Comp. Physiol.,* 56 (Suppl. 1):31–47.

100. Muckenthaler, F. A. (1964): Autoradiographic study of nucleic acid synthesis during spermatogenesis in the grasshopper *Melanoplus differentialis. Exp. Cell Res.,* 35:531–597.

101. Naisse, J. (1970): Influence des hormones sur la différentiation sexuelle de *Lampyris noctiluca* (Coleoptere). *Bull. Soc. Zool. Fr.,* 95:377–382.

102. Neaves, W. B. (1976): Structural characterization and rapid manual isolation of a reptilian testicular tunic rich in Leydig cell. *Anat. Rec.,* 186:553–564.

103. Nicholls, T. J. and Graham, G. P. (1972): Observations on the ultrastructure and differentiation of Leydig cells in the testis of the Japanese quail *(Coturnix coturnix japonica). Biol. Reprod.,* 6:179–192.

103a. Ohno, S. (1976): The development of sexual reproduction. In: *Reproduction in Mammals,* Vol. 6, edited by C. R. Austin and R. V. Short, pp. 1–31. Cambridge University Press, Cambridge.

104. Okada, Y. (1928): On the development of a Hexactinellide sponge, *Farrea sollaisi. J. Fac. Sci. Tokyo Univ.,* 2:1–27.

105. Olive, P. J. W., and Clark, R. B. (1978): *Physiology of Annelids,* edited by P. J. Mill, pp. 271–368. Academic Press, London.

106. Ozon, R. (1972): Androgens in fishes, amphibians, reptiles and birds. In: *Steroids in Non-mammalian Vertebrates,* edited by D. R. Idler, pp. 328–389. Academic Press, New York.

107. Parkes, A. S., and Marshall, A. J. (1960): The reproductive hormones in birds. In: *Marshall's Physiology of Reproduction,* Vol. 1, Part II, edited by A. S. Parkes, pp. 583–706. Longmans, London.

108. Perey, B., Clermont, Y., and Leblond, C. B. (1961): The wave of the seminiferous epithelium in the rat. *Am. J. Anat.,* 108:47–77.

109. Pianka, H. D. (1974): Ctenophora. In: *Reproduction of Marine Invertebrates,* Vol. I, edited by A. C. Giese and J. S. Pearse, pp. 201–265. Academic Press, New York.

110. Reviers, M. de (1968): Détermination de la durée des processus spermatogénètiques chez le coq a l'aide de thymidine tritiée. *Proc. 4th Int. Congress Animal Reproduction Artif. Insem.,* 1:183–185.

111. Reviers, M. de (1975): Sperm transport and survival in male birds. *In: The Biology of Spermatozoa,* edited by E. S. E. Hafez and C. G. Thibault pp. 10–16. S. Karger, Basel.

112. Riser, N. W. (1974): Nemertinea. In: *Reproduction of Marine Invertebrates,* Vol. 1, edited by A. C. Giese and J. S. Pearse, pp. 359–389. Academic Press, New York.

113. Romer, A. S. (1966): *The Vertebrate Body.* Saunders, Philadelphia.

114. Roosen-Runge, E. C. (1977): *The Process of Spermatogenesis in Animals.* Cambridge University Press, Cambridge.

115. Roosen-Runge, E. C., and Szöllözi, D. (1965): On the biology and structure of the testis in *Phialidium Leuckhard* (Leptomedusae) *Z. Zellforsch Mikrosk. Anat.,* 68:597–610.

116. Rothwell, B. (1973): The ultrastructure of Leydig cells in the testis of the domestic fowl. *J. Anat.,* 116:245–253.

117. Rothwell, B., and Tingari, M. D. (1973): The ultrastructure of the boundary tissue of the seminiferous tubule in the testis of the domestic fowl (Gallus domesticus). *J. Anat.,* 114:321–328.

118. Scheer, B. T. (1960): The neuroendocrine system of Arthropods. *Vitam. Horm.,* 18:141–204.

119. Schroeder, P. C., and Hermans, C. O. (1975): Annelida: Polychaeta. In: *Reproduction of Marine Invertebrates,* Vol. III, edited by A. C. Giese and J. S. Pearse, pp. 1–213. Academic Press, New York.

120. Schulze, F. E. (1878): Untersuchungen über den Bau and die Entwicklung der Spongien. IV. Die Familie der Aplysinidae. *Z. Wiss. Zool.,* 30:379–420.

121. Setchell, B. P. (1978): *The Mammalian Testis.* Elek Books, London.

122. Setchell, B. P. (1970): Testicular blood supply, lymphatic drainage and secretion of fluid. In: *The Testis,* Vol. 1, edited by A. D. Johnson, W. R. Gomes, and N. L. Van Demark, pp. 101–239. Academic Press, New York.

123. Setchell, B. P. (1977): Reproduction in male marsupials. In: *The Biology of Marsupials,* edited by B. Stonehouse and D. P. Gilmore, pp. 411–457. Macmillan, London.

124. Setchell, B. P., Scott, T. W., Voglmayr, J. K., and Waites, G. M. H. (1969): Characteristics of testicular spermatozoa and the fluid which transports them into the epididymis. *Biol. Reprod.,* (Suppl. 1):40–66.

125. Setchell, B. P., and Waites, G. M. H. (1975): The blood-testis barrier. *Handbk. Physiol., Section 7, Endocrinology.* Vol. 5:143–172.

126. de Smet, W. M. A. (1977): The position of the testes in cetaceans. In: *Functional Anatomy of Marine Mammals,* Vol. 3, edited by R. J. Harrison, pp. 361–386. Academic Press, London.

127. Stanley, H. P. (1966): The structure and development of the seminiferous follicle in *Scyliorhinus caniculus* and *Torpedo marmorata* (Elasmobranchii). *Z. Zellforsch. Mikrosk. Anat.,* 75:453–468.

128. Stephenson, J. (1922): Contributions to the morphology classification and zoogeography of Indian Oligochaeta. IV: On the diffuse production of sexual cells in a species of Chaetogaster (Fam. Naididae). *Proc. Zool. Soc. (Lond),* 51:467–525.

129. Szöllözi, A., and Marcaillou, C. (1977): Electron microscope study of the blood-testis barrier in an insect *Locusta migratoria. J. Ultrastruct. Res.,* 59:158–172.

130. Tam, W. H., Phillips, J. G., and Lofts, B. (1969): Seasonal changes in the in vitro production of testicular androgens by the cobra *(Naja naja Linn). Gen. Comp. Endocrinol.,* 13:117–125.

131. Thane, A. (1974): Rotifera. In: *Reproduction of Marine Invertebrates,* Vol. 1, edited by A. C. Giese and J. S. Pearse, pp. 471–484. Academic Press, New York.

132. Unsicker, K. (1975): Fine structure of the male genital tract and kidney in the Anura *Xenopus laevis Daudin, Rana temporaria L.* and *Bufo bufo L.* under normal and experimental conditions. *Cell. Tissue Res.,* 158:215–240.

133. Wade, M. H. (1968): Evolutionary morphology of the Caecilian urogenital system. I: The gonads and the fat bodies. *J. Morphol.,* 126:291–332.

134. Waites, G. M. H. (1970): Temperature regulation and the testis. In: *The Testis,* Vol. 1, edited by A. D. Johnson, W. R. Gomes, and N. L. Van Demark, pp. 241–279. Academic Press, New York.

135. Webber, H. H. (1977): Gastropoda: Prosobranchia. In: *Reproduction of Marine Invertebrates,* Vol. IV, edited by A. C. Giese and J. S. Pearse, pp. 1–97. Academic Press, New York.

136. Wells, M. F., and Wells, J. (1977): Cephalopoda: Octopoda. In: *Reproduction of Marine Invertebrates,* Vol. IV, edited by A. C. Giese and J. S. Pearse, pp. 291–336. Academic Press, New York.

137. Wilhoft, D. C., and Reiter, E. O. (1965): Seasonal cycle of the lizard *Leiolopisma fuscum,* a tropical Australian skink. *J. Morph.,* 116:379–388.

138. Wislocki, G. B. (1933): Location of the testes and body temperature in mammals. *Q. Rev. Biol.,* 8:385–396.

139. Witschi, E. (1914): Experimentelle Untersuchung über die Entwicklungsgeschichte der Keimdrusen von *Rana Temporaria. Arch. Mikrosc. Anat.* 85:9–113.

140. Witschi, E. (1924): Die Entwicklung der Keimzellen der *Rana temporaria L.* I. Urkeimzellen und Spermatogenese. *Z. Zell. Gervebelehre,* 1:523–526.

141. Witschi, E. (1961): Sex and secondary sexual characters. In: *Biology and Comparative Physiology of Birds,* Vol. II, edited by A. J. Marshall, pp. 115–168. Academic Press, New York.

142. Wolf, N., Hirsh, D., and McIntosh, J. R. (1978): Spermatogenesis in males of the free-living Nematode, *Caenorhabditis elegans. J. Ultrastruct. Res.,* 63:155–169.

143. Zick, K. (1911): Beiträge zur Kenntnis der postembryonalen Entwicklungsgeschichte der Genitalorgane bei Lepidopteren. *Z. Wiss. Zool.,* 98:430–477.

The Testis, edited by H. Burger and D. de Kretser.
Raven Press, New York © 1981.

3

Differentiation and Development of the Testes

Hubert Wartenberg

*Anatomical Institute, University of Bonn, Nussallee 10, D-5300 Bonn 1,
Federal Republic of Germany*

The interpretation of the development of the male as well as the female gonad is extremely difficult, and consequently has given rise to quite a number of theories on this subject. The difficulties of arriving at a common picture on the developmental process are owing to the fact that considerable differences exist between mammalian species concerning the structural manifestations and the chronological sequence of steps of gonadal differentiation.

Accordingly, this review presents some comparative aspects concerning some events during early gonadal and testicular development which have been observed in single mammalian species in a more pronounced manner than in others. The content of this chapter deals mainly with the process of human testicular development.

Primarily, this presentation focuses on the morphological and cytological studies. The origin and developmental process of the nongerminal somatic tissue components will be followed together with the well-known details of the extra-gonadal origin and germ track of the primordial germ cells. Most emphasis will be placed on the morphology of the primary differentiation of the gonadal ridge, the sexual differentiation of the gonad into the male or female organ, the relationship between germ cell differentiation and supporting cells, and the role of a gonadal blastema during further testicular development. The latter refers to the question of the origin and differentiation of intratubular supporting cells (Sertoli cells) and extratubularly situated interstitial and peritubular cells (Leydig cells and boundary tissue).

PRIMARY DIFFERENTIATION AND DEVELOPMENT OF THE INDIFFERENT GONAD

Although the mammalian gonad is basically determined by the genetic sex, it runs through a sexually indifferent period of gonadal development. In human development, this period lasts approximately 7 to 10 days and the sexually indifferent gonads can be found during the 6th week of gestational age (39,103). Initial signs of differentiation in the gonadal ridge have been observed in embryos of 5 to 7 mm crown-rump length (CR) (19,39,75,92,101).

Onset of Gonadal Development

The coelomic epithelium which covers the mesonephric fold becomes thickened and attracts mesenchymal cells and primordial germ cells which both accumulate beneath the superficial epithelium forming a primary blastema. This process seems to be connected with the lack of the basal lamina between epithelium and mesenchymal core (30,39,98).

The question arises as to the influence under which the proliferation of the epithelium occurs. There is strong evidence that the primordial germ cells can be ruled out. On the other hand, it seems unlikely that plain mesenchymal cells could provide this inductive influence. Witschi (102), however, characterized these cells as originating from the mesonephros. If the very early gonadal development in different mammalian species is carefully followed, good evidence can be found for Witschi's concept. These cells are, in all probability, not mesenchymal elements. They can be easily traced back to the mesonephros (Fig. 1), as has been done in the mouse (20), rabbit (52,96), and man (95). Although the

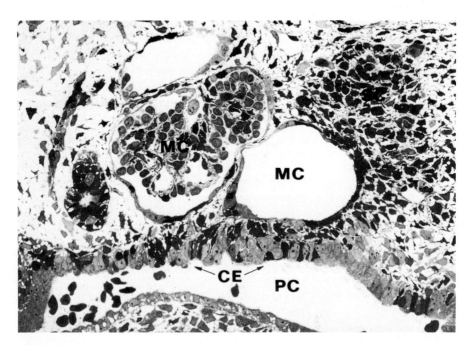

FIG. 1. Genital ridge area of a human embryo, 12 mm long (cross-section, Epon, 1 μm, toluidine blue): PC peritoneal cavity; MC mesonephric corpuscle; SC blastema of suprarenal cortex, deriving (outgrowing) from Bowman's capsules; CE proliferating coelomic epithelium: light epithelial cells are intermingled with dark cells, which derive from mesonephric sources.

blastema, concentrated beneath the coelomic epithelium, may be regarded as of mesonephric origin, it would seem likely that the epithelium proliferates under the inductive influence of this mesonephrogenic blastema. Summarizing this reasoning, one may conclude that derivatives of the mesonephros determine the gonadal anlage and regulate the primary differentiation of the indifferent gonad, inducing the coelomic epithelium to proliferate.

Structural Composition of the Sexually Indifferent Gonad

During the further development of the indifferent gonad, the genital ridge is built up by epithelial cells and mesonephrogenic cells which form a primary gonadal blastema due to their tendency to intermingle: strands of mesonephrogenic cells grow into the more compact layer of the proliferating epithelium. To most former investigators this structural composition conveyed the impression that the superficial epithelium exhibits a "first proliferation," invading the deeper "mesenchymal core" and giving rise to "primary sex cords." In the genetically male gonad, these were held to be the precursors of the definitive seminiferous tubules of the testicular medulla. In the female gonad, they were considered to represent the "first ingrowth" of the superficial epithelium, subsequently giving rise to medullary cords of the definitive ovary. This classical concept, which assumed the male medullary structures as well as the female cortical structures to be derived from the superficial epithelium, has been rejected by other workers (19,29,65). This group held the view that the male and female gonadal blastema was derived from mesenchymal cells without participation of the superficial epithelium.

Witschi (102) finally elaborated his theory of cortico-medullary antagonism (Fig. 2). On the basis of extensive comparative observations on mammalian

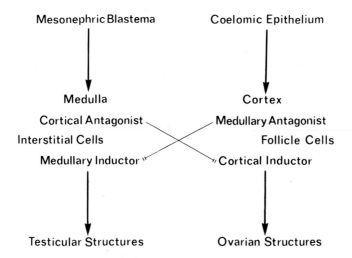

FIG. 2. Schematic representation of Witschi's theory of gonadal development on the basis of a cortico-medullary antagonism.

and nonmammalian species, he proposed that two blastemas build up the indifferent gonad: a superficial blastema—the cortex—which gives rise to the ovary (granulosa cells), and a central blastema—the medulla—which originates from the mesonephric blastema and which differentiates into the interstitial cell line (102,103,105). The main point of Witschi's concept which makes it differ from the classical theory and the "mesenchymal" theory (8) is the conclusion he draws from his observations in connection with the basic problem of sexual differentiation of the gonad. Since he assumed a clear separation of the cortical and medullary blastemas by a special gonadal cavity (albuginea), he postulated an inductor theory of sex differentiation (104). Both blastemas were conceived to influence one another by means of two hypothetical factors whereby either the cortex or the medulla were given preference in order to develop female-cortical or male-medullary structures (Fig. 2). Indeed, histological sections cut through the indifferent gonad of some mammalian species exhibit a narrow space within the common gonadal blastema which may even separate the epithelial and mesonephrogenic parts and which may be due to a vascular plexus of sinusoid capillaries. On the other hand, sections through the gonadal anlage of a rabbit embryo [day 12–13 post coitum (p.c.)] explicitly demonstrate a very important aspect of the behavior of the mesonephrogenic blastema in respect

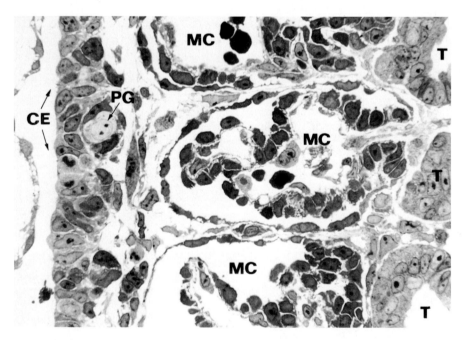

FIG. 3. Longitudinal section through the genital ridge of a 12 days old rabbit embryo demonstrating the close contact of the mesonephric corpuscle (MC) to the proliferating coelomic epithelium (CE) which consists of light epithelial and dark mesonephrogenic cells. PG primordial germ cell; T tubule of the mesonephric nephros. (From ref. 96.)

to the epithelial blastema: during the indifferent period, mesonephrogenic cells invade the superficial epithelium (Figs. 1 and 3). As mentioned before, meso-nephrogenic and epithelogenic cells intermingle; they include the migrating germ cells (for the relationship of germ and somatic cells during this period, see pages 56–57). The final composition of the genital ridge consists of a common blastema (primary blastema) which shows no separation into two distinct primor-dia. Contrary to Witschi's opinion, no individual cortex and medulla are distin-guishable throughout this early period.

SEXUAL DIFFERENTIATION DURING GONADAL DEVELOPMENT

The mechanisms which determine the differentiation of sex are multifactorial and cause sexual differentiation to occur in a stepwise fashion. In mammalian development, the sex is primarily determined at fertilization and the "genetic sex" is required for a normal development encompassing sexual differentiation of the gonad. The "gonadal sex," on the other hand, influences and regulates differentiation of the "body sex" (somatic sex) whereby the testis influences the development of the male genital system and male characteristics (45,46,48). The final step in this sequence is the differentiation of the "psychic sex" (62) which depends on the early determination of neural centers (32).

Theories on Determination of Gonadal Sex

The process of differentiation of the sexually indifferent gonad for subsequent transformation into a testis or an ovary has been the subject of many discussions and has given rise to numerous theories. Witschi's concept has already been mentioned in the preceding section (pages 41–42). Over a period of decades he sought to establish his theory of cortico-medullary antagonism (100,102–108), which aroused lively interest but did not, in the end, gain full acceptance. The concept (Fig. 2) that the cortex could serve as an inductor of female differen-tiation suppressing the male medullary structures, and that the medulla could act as an inductor of male differentiation inhibiting the cortical development, remained unsubstantiated.

During the last two decades a different theory has been developed by Jost (43–49). This theory is based on the "chronological asymmetry of gonadal differ-entiation" (51) (Fig. 4). Jost assumes a fundamental difference in testicular and ovarian development insofar as "in males, testicular organization is actively imposed, under genetic control, on a primordium which otherwise would slowly acquire an ovarian structure" (51, pp. 32–33). Sex differentiation of the gonad is guided under the influence of a masculinizing mechanism (male organizer) and results in the formation of testicular structures. On the other hand, "for a prolonged period of time, presumptive ovaries are characterized mainly by the fact that they do not become testes. They actually remain undifferentiated" (51, p. 32). Female differentiation does not need an active principle and the

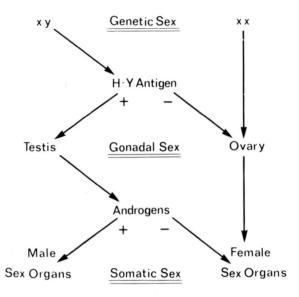

FIG. 4. Schematic representation of Jost's theory of gonadal development and sexual differenti-ation of the reproductive tract. Dependent upon the male organizer (H-Y antigen) the indifferent gonad differentiates into male organ, while absence of this organizing principle results in the differentiation of an ovary. In a similar way, androgens which are produced by the fetal testis guide the indifferent genital tract to become a male system while the failure of this activating hormonal influence results in the formation of a female tract.

genetically determined female gonad simply continues its indifferent period by growing further until ovarian follicles are formed. This concept is part of a basic comprehensive theory of sex differentiation in mammals (Fig. 4).

H-Y Antigen and Determination of the Gonadal Sex

Jost's postulate of asymmetrical development of the gonadal sex is supported by the concept of a very simple system of one regulatory gene influencing testicu-lar differentiation (54,66–69). This gene induces the expression of the so-called H-Y antigen (90,91) which in turn determines the maleness of the gonad. Re-cently Wolf (109) proposed a three-gene hypothesis, assuming the structural gene for H-Y antigen production to be autosomal. This structural gene is sus-pected to be under the activating or repressing influence of two genes linked with the Y and X chromosomes. It is assumed that H-Y antigen is a hormone-like substance, since it is actively secreted by the testis (61). Nonexistence of this H-Y antigen results in a continuation of the indifferent development and subsequently in female differentiation of the gonad. Experimental work with anti-H-Y antiserum has corroborated this concept (69,110,113). Suspensions of testicular cells of newborn rats or mice, dissociated by trypsin treatment, reorganize into folliculoid structures after an anti-H-Y antiserum has been added.

TABLE 1. *Expression of H-Y antigen, binding capacity for H-Y antigen in gonadal and nongonadal tissues of the rat*[a]

Tissues examined	H-Y antigen	H-Y receptor
Male gonadal tissue, newborn	+	+
Female gonadal tissue, newborn	−	+
Male gonadal tissue, adult	+	(+)
Female gonadal tissue, adult	−	+
Male extragonadal tissue	+	−
Female extragonadal tissue	−	−

[a] From refs. 60, 61, 110.

Control suspensions reorganize into tubule-like structures. Surprisingly, suspended ovarian cells of newborn rats reorganize into testicular structures after H-Y antigen has been added (110,112). This result substantiates the existence of a specific H-Y antigen receptor (60). Although this receptor in testicular tissues fails to work beyond the prenatal and newborn period, it can be detected in ovarian tissues even in adults (60,110). Nongonadal tissues of both sexes show no evidence of such receptor sites for H-Y antigen (Table 1). Immature germ cells are H-Y antigen-negative too (111).

Evidently, sex determination of the male gonad would seem to depend on the presence of H-Y antigen, while the distribution of H-Y antigen receptor sites is nonspecific in respect of their occurrence in male as well as in female gonads. However, this is to adjudge merely the newborn situation. How do the structural histogenic events correspond to this antigen-receptor mechanism? How do the microscopical observations on sexual differentiation correspond to this antigen-receptor mechanism which induces sexual determination?

Developmental Events During Sexual Differentiation of the Gonad

Students of sexual differentiation maintain that the realization of the maleness of the gonad expresses itself by the sudden formation of testicular cords, while onset of femaleness does not exhibit any concomitant remodelling of the basic structural situation. Careful studies on the sexual differentiation period reveal a somewhat different view of the problem. Rabbit indifferent gonads evince an alternative behavior in the male-determined anlage in comparison with the future female gonad. While the male blastemal cells continue to follow the tendency of becoming intermingled, in the female anlage an increasing segregation of the two blastemal parts becomes apparent (Figs. 5a–5c). Finally, testis and ovary are clearly distinguishable. In the testis, mesonephrogenic blastemal cells have penetrated the core of the primary blastema and now separate the superficial epithelium from the blastema, forming a primitive tunica albuginea. The core of the primary blastema, which still consists of intermingled cells of epithelial and mesonephric origin, has lost its connection to the surface of the genital ridge. It forms the medulla of the testis (Fig. 6). Primordial germ cells have

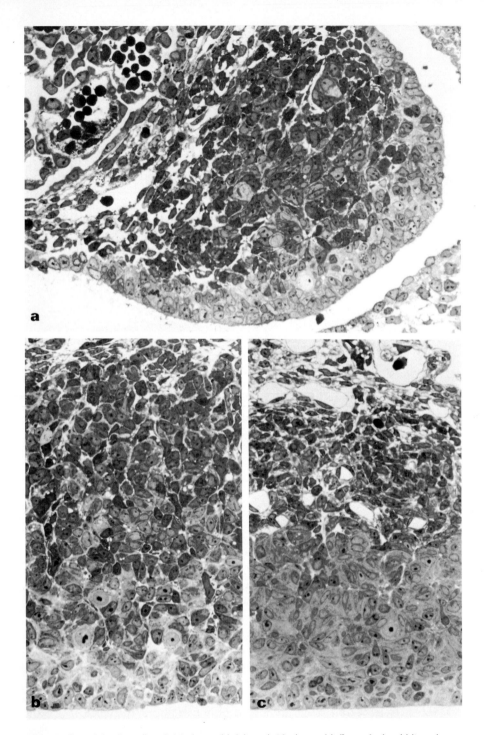

FIG. 5. Gonadal primordia of 14 days old **(a)** and 16 days old **(b and c)** rabbit embryos demonstrate the different processes of male and female gonadal differentiation, respectively. In the male **(b)** determined blastema the dark mesonephrogenic cells grow into the coelomic epithelium (compare the early situation on day 12 in Fig. 3) while in the female **(c)** the two blastemas of mesonephric and coelomic origin remain separated forming an inner and outer layer.

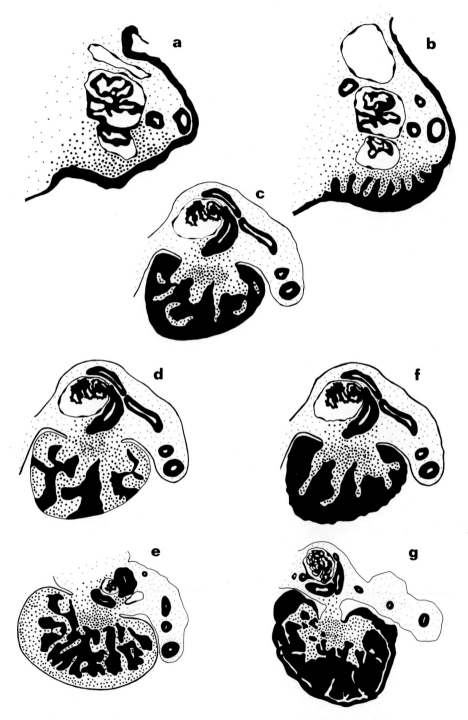

FIG. 6. Development of the indifferent human gonad **(a–c)** from 12 mm **(a)** to 21 mm long embryo **(c)** and the different growth of the mesonephrogenic (dotted) and epithelial blastema (black) in the male (left, **d–e**) and female (right, **f–g**) gonad during sexual differentiation. (From ref. 95.)

participated in this centripetal movement and become enclosed in the future seminiferous tubules. The latter begin forming by separation of the blastema into a network of plate-like strands and interstitial tissue. The female gonad, on the other hand, exhibits what amounts to a reversion to the original situation. Although both blastemal portions have proliferated, the penetration of the epithelial part by the mesonephrogenic cells has been unsuccessful and the two blastemas have become largely separated (Fig. 6). This process results in formation of the female "cortex" which, for the time being, consists of epithelial cells. Most of the primordial germ cells are enclosed in the cortical layer.

If the male or female arrangement of the two blastemas is achieved, the process of sexual differentiation is completed. The establishment of the male situation is mainly owing to the increasing amalgamation of the two blastemal parts in conjunction with the centripetal displacement of the superficial epithelial layer and formation of the medulla. Separation of the medullary blastema into cords and interstitium seems to be simply the last stage of this differentiating process.

Returning to the question of how the structural histogenetic events of sexual differentiation correspond to the H-Y antigen-receptor mechanism, one has to assume that the cause of the different behavior may be attributable to the presence or absence of H-Y antigen. On this assumption the presence of the antigen should result in an increasing invasion of the mesonephrogenic blastema into the superficial epithelial layer with subsequent displacement of the epithelial cells from their superficial position into the medulla. In addition, the separation of the blastema into testicular cords and interstitial tissue is clearly dependent on H-Y antigen positivity. Absence of the H-Y antigen prevents any merging of the two blastemas and allows them to return to their original topographical position.

TESTICULAR DIFFERENTIATION

Onset of Testicular Differentiation and Formation of Plate-like Medullary Structures

The first sign of male differentiation of the gonad that is clearly recognizable in common histological sections is the appearance of testicular cords. Differentiation of cords has been observed in embryos of from 13 to 20 mm CR length (43–50 days) (39,40). In a 21 mm embryo with an ovulation age of 42 days, the separation of testicular cords from the interstitial space is completed (89,95). Elias (15) has shown evidence, by means of stereological methods, that the initially formed medullary structures are plate-like rather than cord-like. These plates build up a three-dimensional reticulum with a preferentially radial orientation. Typical cords with circular cross-section profiles do not appear before the end of the 8th week (day 63), at which time the embryos are about 35 to

40 mm long (15). In other mammals, similar observations can be made during early testicular development.

A further important event needs to be accentuated with regard to differentiation of medullary structures; in most mammalian species additional testicular cords or plate-like structures are still being formed long after primary sexual differentiation has terminated. The length of this period depends on the duration of the entire developmental process. In mouse or rat, formation of the testicular cords is completed within some hours. In rabbit, however, it lasts from day 16 to day 22. In the human testis, the formation of testicular cords is an extensive repetitive process requiring a period of some weeks; it corresponds to the differentiation process of female cortical structures.

The Gonadal Blastema and Its Role in Medullary Differentiation

The source of this new formation of medullary plates (precursors of testicular cords) is a common blastema (central gonadal blastema) which serves as a pool for all sorts of testicular cells and is similar to the primary gonadal blastema. Size and distribution of the gonadal blastema, or of such structures that are analogous to the blastema, differs among various mammalian species. Small mammals such as mouse or rat show no real central blastema (Fig. 7a) despite some cellular connections between mesonephric and testicular tubules. The rabbit, however, exhibits a more pronounced, loose accumulation of cellular strands (Fig. 7b) which is known as "rete-blastema." Similar strands have been observed in cross-sections of human testes which most authors have classified as the future rete testis (39,89,102,105) (Fig. 7c). If one traces these "rete-strands" upwards, the reticular blastema is seen to continue into a very compact mass of blastemal cells (Fig. 8) constituting the main part of the gonadal blastema which occupies the upper pole of the testicular anlage (89,95,96). A true "central" blastema is evident in the calf fetus (Fig. 7d): it consists of an undifferentiated blastema that is in close contact with the peripherally located testicular cords. The rete blastema, which initially is enclosed in the hilar region of the central blastema, gradually augments and finally merges into the central blastema.

The Origin of the Blastemal Cells

In human embryos, the gonadal blastema consists of a mass of somatic cells which enclose single primordial germ cells. Judging by their histological appearance, the somatic elements can be divided into at least two groups: "light" and "dark" cells. Since the gonadal blastema exhibits a conspicuous contact with a limited group of the upper "degenerating" mesonephric nephrons (Fig. 8), it seems not unlikely that blastemal cells still originate from the mesonephros just as, earlier, cellular elements contributed to the indifferent gonad. The cells of the gonadal blastema are predominantly dark. Their origin from the meso-

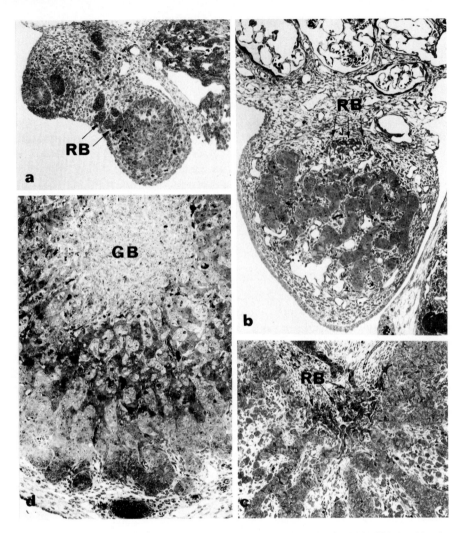

FIG. 7. Cross sections through the central region of developing testes of 13 days old spiny mouse **(a),** 17 days old rabbit **(b),** 62 days old human embryo **(c),** and approximately 61 days old cattle embryo **(d),** demonstrating the topography and extension of the gonadal blastema (GB) or the "rete blastema" (RB) respectively. (See text for explanation.)

FIG. 8. (a): Longitudinal section through the upper pole of the testis of 62-day-old human embryo demonstrating the close contact of the "degenerating" segments of the mesonephros (M) to the gonadal blastema (GB) and the "rete blastema" (RB). TC testicular cords, which are continuously formed by the gonadal blastema (A-A and B-B indicate the level of cross sections in Figs. 7c and 8b). **(b):** Cross section through the upper pole of mutual (contralateral) testis of same embryo (see level B-B in Fig. 8a). Strands of mesonephrogenic blastemal cells (arrow) connect the Bowman's capsule and the mesonephric tubule with the gonadal blastema (GB) and the testicular cords (TC). **(c):** Semischematic drawing of a longitudinal section through the testis and mesonephros of a 28 mm long (approximately 55 days old) human embryo: The upper portion of the mesonephros segregates cellular material (three arrows) which is concentrated in the gonadal blastema (dotted area). The gonadal blastema

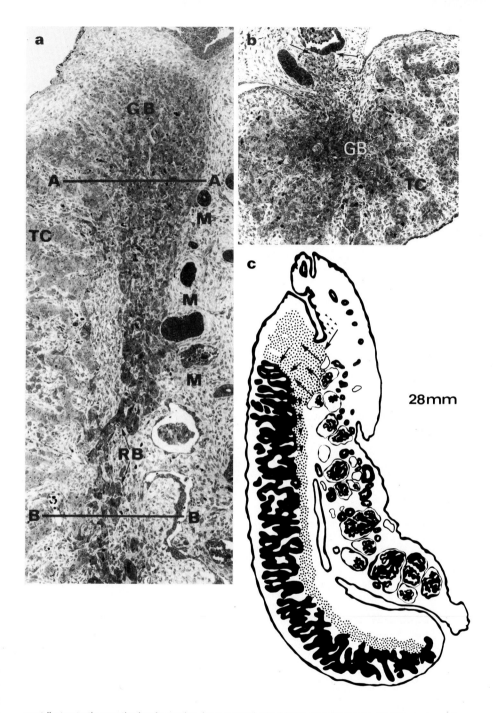

contributes to the continuing formation (two arrows) of additional testicular cords (black strands) while an axial continuation of the blastema forms the so-called "rete blastema" (four arrowheads). From the upper coelomic bay additional epithelial cells move into the gonadal blastema (small arrowheads). (From ref. 95.)

nephric nephrons can be traced back to two different structures: (a) cells of the Bowman's capsule, and (b) podocytes of the glomeruli. Malpighian corpuscles of the upper mesonephric segments (about 20%) degenerate early according to Wilson (99). Studies at cellular level, however, demonstrate that the meso-nephric nephrons cease their activity and release cells from their glomerular end. The development of the Malpighian corpuscle seems to occur in reverse. Single cells become detached from the capsule of Bowman, and partly disintegrated loops of the glomeruli become expelled through the vascular pole (Fig. 9). The podocytes "redifferentiate" by shedding their redundant processes; in their final appearance they are hard to distinguish from pure mesenchymal cells, although their cytoplasm and nuclear chromatin are denser (Fig. 10). They move into the testicular anlage, forming strands which connect the mesonephric structures and the gonadal blastema. They retain some characteristics of epithelial cells and, additionally, develop some of the features of mesenchymal cells. Although they (a) form epitheloid associations, on the other hand they (b) migrate over long distances (1); they (c) concentrate around primordial germ cells covering the latter with their thin, tongue-like processes, or (d) some of them phagocytoze extracellular material, e.g., the detritus of their former processes. This postulated morphogenetic process, which is corroborated only by histological evidence, receives more support from observations on the gonadal development of the

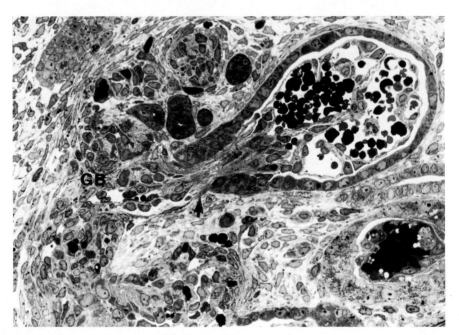

FIG. 9. Malpighian corpuscle of the rabbit mesonephros exhibiting a "degenerative" reversal of its developmental process. At the vascular pole (arrow) the corpuscle is despoiled of its glomerular content, in the course of which podocytes move into the gonadal blastema (GB).

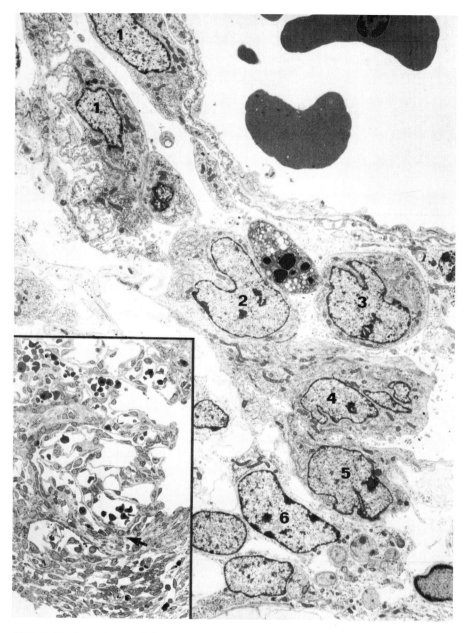

FIG. 10. Electron micrograph demonstrating the "de-differentiation" of mesonephric podocytes (1,2,3) into mesonephrogenic blastemal cells (4,5,6). (Inset: light micrograph of this area.) (From ref. 52.)

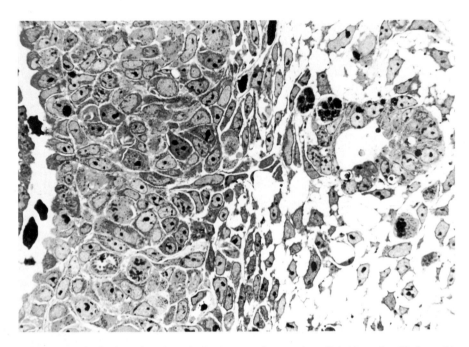

FIG. 11. Longitudinal section through the mesonephros and genital ridge of a 12 days old mouse embryo. The vesicular structure corresponds to a developing glomerulus of a mesonephric nephron whose epithelial connection shows signs of disintegration. Dark mesenchymal-like cells are detached from the glomerular vesicle and form a dense blastema close to the proliferating epithelium occupying a superficial position.

mouse. Like most of the small mammals, the mouse does not have an active mesonephros (20). The upper segments of the nephrogenic cord, however, develop some S-shaped tubuli. One end of this tubule forms a small vesicle which corresponds to the glomerulus. The vesicular tip of this nephroid structure functions in a way similar to that observed in mammals with an active mesonephros: this "glomerular" end releases mesonephrogenic cells (Fig. 11) which migrate into the testis during the early phase of testicular development (day 13–14 p.c.) (20,24); here they become incorporated, to some extent, into the testicular cords. Additional cells of the same origin form strands which connect testicular cords and mesonephric tubules and constitute the blastema of the future rete testis.

Gonadal Blastema and Rete Blastema: Their Function During Early Testicular Differentiation

Comparing the distribution of the gonadal blastema and rete blastema in different mammalian species (Figs. 7 and 8), one comes to the conclusion that both tissue concentrations fulfill similar functions with regard to early testicular differentiation. In small mammals such as mouse, rat, hamster, and even rabbit, mesonephrogenic cells form short or more extended strands ("rete blastema"), but no gonadal blastema develops. These strands primarily serve as a means for the mesonephrogenic cells to move into the testis and towards the testicular cords, where they become incorporated into them, constituting their somatic cellular content. Finally, they form the rete testis. In large mammals, including man, a gonadal blastema develops. It depends on the duration of the developmental process and the size of the final gonad whether a gonadal blastema appears that exhibits a more or less expansive pool for blastemal cells. In human testes, the gonadal blastema is eccentrically located and the "rete blastema" connects the gonadal blastema and/or the mesonephros with those parts of the testis which are already filled with testicular cords (Fig. 8). They deliver additional blastemal cells to these areas. The rete blastema consists of dark mesonephrogenic cells and a lesser amount of light cells. These cells migrate into two compartments of the developing testis: (a) into the interstitium, where they differentiate into Leydig and peritubular cells (see pages 69–73); (b) into the proximal segments of the testicular cords. In human testes, approximately 3 weeks after primary sexual differentiation, strands of the rete blastema are linked to testicular cords (about day 60–64) (95) and "dark" mesonephrogenic cells have free access to the cords (Fig. 12). Since, during this period, the number of dark sustentacular cells increases rapidly while the number of light cells becomes reduced, this

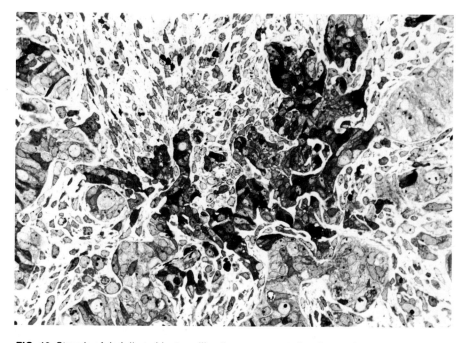

FIG. 12. Strands of dark "rete blastemal" cells are connected to the proximal end of testicular cords in a 40 mm long human embryo (approximately 63 days old). This area corresponds to cross section seen in Fig. 7c. Dark mesonephrogenic cells have free access to the intratubular as well as the interstitial space contributing to the Sertoli cell and the Leydig precursor cell content. (From ref. 96.)

mechanism seems to be indicative of how mesonephrogenic cells—via the rete blastema—may become added to the content of somatic cells within the testicular cords. In the bovine testicular anlage, the central location of the gonadal blastema enables the blastemal cells to have direct access to the testicular cords and the interstitium. The functional implication of this process will be discussed in the next section.

In the differentiating ovary, the cellular content of a gonadal blastema and a rete blastema act in a similar fashion. Blastemal cells originating from the mesonephros form part of the medulla and become concentrated close to the border of the cortex. Corresponding to the growth of the cortex, dark blastemal cells invade the cortex and intermingle with a light type of cortical cell, e.g., supporting cells, which originate from the coelomic epithelium. As in the testicular cords, light and dark supporting cells take up a close relationship to the germ cell.

THE GERM CELL DURING TESTICULAR DEVELOPMENT

Certain peculiarities characterize the germ cell during gonadal differentiation. These include the extragonadal origin of the germ cells, their ability to migrate or to become transferred from their site of origin to the germinal ridge, their aptitude to gain close contact to some kinds of somatic cells and, finally, their ability to become influenced by an inductive system in order to proliferate. It should be pointed out that male and female germ cells go through a very similar sequence of structural changes and periods of differentiation. There is only one great difference between them: while female germ cells enter the prophase of meiosis, the male germ cells, though seeming to prepare for this event, do not begin meiosis during embryogenesis (34,37,53,93,94,95).

Extragonadal Origin of Germ Cells and Their Migratory Period

The origin of the germ cell outside the site of its final destination has been, in the first instance, subject of the "Keimbahn" theory and has given rise to a long-lasting debate. The Keimbahn (germ track) theory comprises two aspects which Nussbaum, the founder of the theory (63), has precisely formulated as follows: (a) the origin of the germ cells in an extragonadal position and, subsequently, the notion of their differentiation from the endodermal germ layer, and (b) the concept of the continuity of a sexual principle (germ plasm) independent of the somatic system (germ and soma). In mammals, only the site of the first appearance of the germ cells and the track of their migration into the gonadal anlage have so far been substantiated.

In human embryos, the sites through which the primordial germ cells pass on their migrational track are well-documented (39,75,101): In the 4-somite stage (approximately 22 days old) they have been detected in the endoderm of the allantois and in the mesenchymal tissue of the connecting stalk (39); early in the fourth week they start migrating from the gut endoderm and the dorsal yolk sac epithelium via the dorsal mesentery by means of amoeboid movement, and during the fifth week they gather in the gonadal primordium (101,103). Histochemical "labelling" by using the alkaline phosphatase reaction (57,58) brought an additional proof of the migratory theory. Conclusive evidence has been achieved by experimental work on the mouse (16,17,59) and Clark and Eddy (11) described the structure of the mouse primordial germ cell during its migratory period at the submicroscopic level. The primordial germ cells show an alkaline phosphatase reactivity on their superficial cell membrane during their sojourn in the gut epithelium and their migration towards the gonadal ridge. Their ability to form pseudopodial processes (Fig. 13) and their affinity for the coelomic epithelium, which the germ cells prefer to contact during their migration, are indicative of their active movement; also revealed is a mechanism by which the germ cells become attached to the genital ridge epithelium, guided by a chemotactic substance (101). (For further details see refs. 21,31,114.)

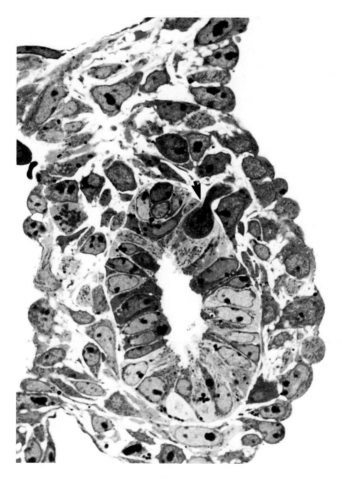

FIG. 13. Primordial germ cell (arrow) of a 10.5 day old mouse embryo which leaves the hind gut endoderm forming a pseudopodial process. (From ref. 20.)

The Proliferation of the Male Germ Cell and its Differentiation During the Prespermatogenic Period

After arrival of the primordial germ cells in the genital ridge and settlement on the gonadal primordium, these show two characteristics: (a) In respect of the supporting cells or their blastemal precursors, the germ cells prefer to become located in those areas where blastemal cells of epithelial origin are concentrated. Accordingly, the primordial germ cells gather close to the superficial coelomic epithelium during the early indifferent period of gonadal development. If the medullary blastema is formed and the epithelial cells are displaced from the surface into the medulla, germ cells join them. Subsequently, germ cells become enclosed in testicular cords and surrounded by blastemal cells, primarily those of epithelial origin. In human testes, this happens on about day 42. (b) Germ cells proliferate. This mitotic activity is different from single divisions of the primordial germ cells during migration and early settlement in the gonadal ridge. It has been demonstrated (34,36,37) that male as well as female germ cells in the rat start proliferating at the same time and enter a period of rapid multiplications which lasts about 2 days (day 14–16). The mechanism is identical to that of spermatogonial proliferation in the adult testis and results in an increasing number of fetal gonia which are linked by intercellular bridges (26, 27,93,94,97). On the basis of the synchronized and rapid multiplication of the germ cells, and because they differ structurally from primordial germ cells, Hilscher et al. (34) called these cells M-prospermatogonia (M = multiplying) (Figs. 14 and 15). In the ovary of the rat, female germ cells run through an identical period of multiplication. Oogonia proliferate as rapidly as prospermatogonia. If oogonia cease their proliferation and transform into oocytes which

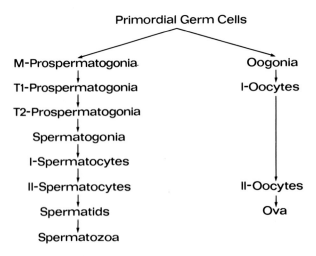

FIG. 14. Germ cell differentiation (gametogenesis) in the male and female line of small rodents using the terminology proposed by Hilscher. (From ref. 34 and 36.)

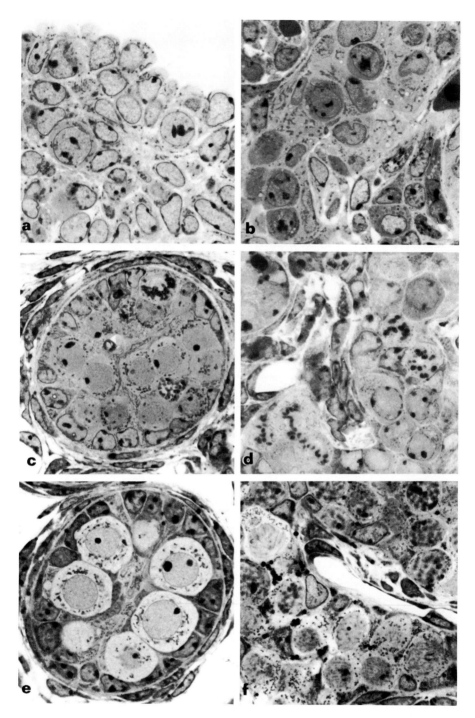

FIG. 15. Germ cell differentiation during pre- and postnatal development of the golden hamster: **(a)** Primordial germ cells in the undifferentiated gonad on day 14 post conception. **(b)** M-prospermatogonia in testicular cords on day 15 p.c. **(c and d)** M-prospermatogonia and oogonia in testis and ovary on day of birth. **(e and f)** T-prospermatogonia and premeiotic oocytes on day 4 post partum.

start meiotic prophase, the M-prospermatogonia discontinue their phase of multi-plication too, and enter a second period. The so-called T-prospermatogonia (Fig. 15) (T = transitional) (34) are germ cells which rest during the ensuing period that runs concomitantly with the meiotic prophase of the female cells. In the rat, the resting period and the meiotic prophase last from the 17th prenatal day until day 5 after birth. If oocytes have terminated their meiotic prophase and start forming follicles, the T-prospermatogonia enter a further proliferating phase [T_2-prospermatogonia, according to Hilscher et al. (34)]. These prosperma-togonia finally become transformed into the A-spermatogonia of the adult testis (34,37). This pronounced parallelism between male and female germ cell differen-tiation and stepwise development characterizes the prenatal and early postnatal period of most of the small mammals (rat, mouse, hamster) (Figs. 14–16) (24,94).

Human germ cells and those of other mammals with a prenatal development of comparatively long duration clearly do not reveal these regularities. The issue of germ cell differentiation in human fetal testes becomes indistinct due to an overlap of the single periods (Fig. 16). This probably explains why the efforts of many authors to define the male germ types during testicular develop-ment have been at variance (13,25–28,34,35,40,56,97). Comparative studies relat-

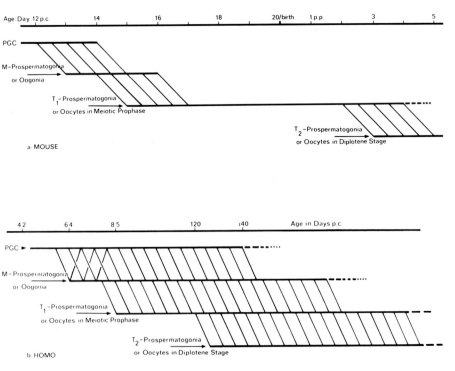

FIG. 16. Periods of male and female germ cell differentiation during prenatal development of the mouse **(a)** and human embryogenesis **(b)**. (For explanation see text.)

ing to the differential issue of the female germ cell in the prenatal human ovary indicate parallelism with that of the male germ cell in the fetal testis, the male differentiation being characterized by similar changes in structure and mitotic function. Typical landmarks in male and female gonadal development character- ize the initial appearance of proliferating prospermatogonia and oogonia as well as nonproliferating prospermatogonia and premeiotic oocytes (Fig. 16) (95).

Thus, the classification and definition of male germ cells should be undertaken, preferably on a functional basis:

Primordial germ cells include the entire group of early undifferentiated germ cells which have not yet entered the multiplication period; they migrate from the site of their original appearance to the gonadal anlage, settle in the gonadal primary blastema and finally become enclosed in the male gonadal cords or the female cortex. Gondos (26) subdivided this group into (a) primitive germ cells, which are part of the indifferent gonad; and (b) gonocytes, which—in the male gonad—have entered the testicular cords (71).

Pro- or prespermatogonia have entered the prespermatogenetic period and may be subdivided into (a) M-prospermatogonia, which multiply mitotically; and (b) T-prospermatogonia, which are cells of a transitional phase during which the gonia first rest (T_1-prospermatogonia) and finally proliferate (T_2-prosper- matogonia) in order to transform into the adult A-spermatogonial stage (34).

In human prespermatogenesis, the process of germ cell proliferation seems to be a good deal more complicated than in mouse and rat. To judge from several histological observations, there is good evidence that the male germ cell, once it has left the primordial stage, enters a 3-week period during which it repeatedly tries to proliferate. However, the multiplication process ceases abruptly after a single mitosis and the resulting prospermatogonia relapse into an intermediate stage which is unlike that of the resting T-prospermatogonia and more similar to the primordial germ cell stage (22,95). This behavior becomes more logical if one correlates the developmental process of the germ cells and the somatic cells which "support" them.

THE CONCEPT OF A DUAL SERTOLI CELL SYSTEM

A crucial problem and one of fundamental importance concerns the control of the meiotic process. While the female germ cells begin meiosis early during pre- or postnatal development, an inhibitory effect seems to prevent the male germ cell from entering meiosis. According to Jost et al. (50,51), the enclosure of the male germ cell by the fetal Sertoli cells could be responsible for the inhibition. In addition, Tsafriri and Channing (85) and Byskov and Saxén (6) have postulated a "meiosis-preventing" substance which seems to be essential for regulation of the female meiotic process as well as for the mechanism in the male gonad. On the other hand, Byskov and Saxén (6) have demonstrated, by explanting fetal mouse testes and ovaries and culturing these in pairs, that male germ cells of the fetal period may enter meiosis. The initiation of the

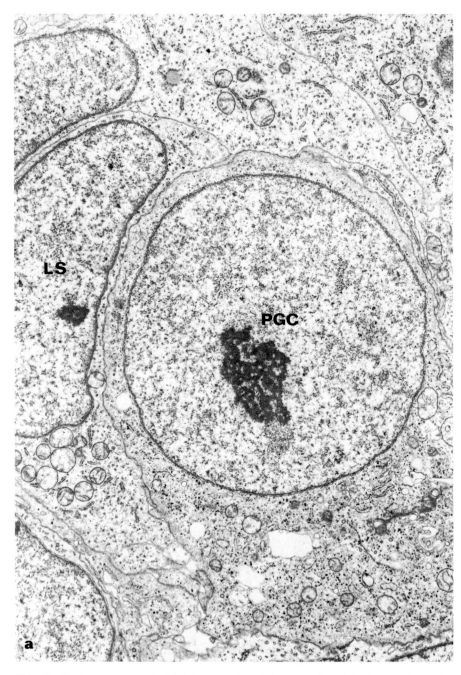

FIG. 17. Electron micrograph of **(a)** human primordial germ cell and light supporting cells (LS) and **(b)** M-prospermatogonium and dark mesonephrogenic supporting cell (DS).

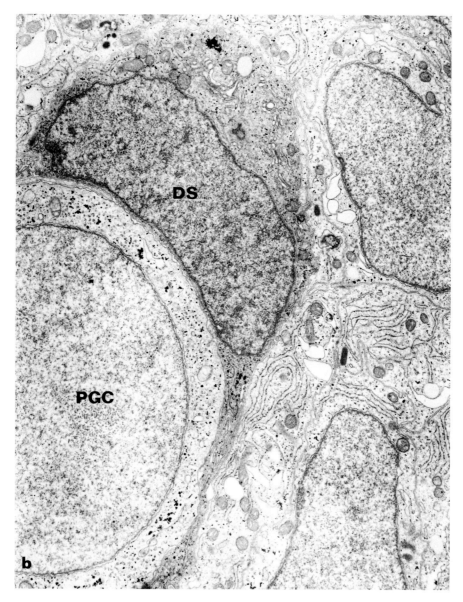

FIG. 17. *contd.*

meiotic prophase in fetal male germ cells has been observed in squash preparations in the normal cat (70) and in hamster and mouse gonads under experimental conditions (64,72). An inductive effect has been attributed to a "meiosis-inducing" substance which diffuses through millipore filters. The substance would appear to be elaborated by the fetal gonad (9), and it has been shown that cells of the rete ovarii initiate the meiotic process in the female gonad (2,3). Since it has been suggested by the same author that the rete ovarii is the source of granulosa cells (3,4,5,7,80), the speculation was expressed that fetal supporting cells might produce the stimulating factor (114).

This idea of a dualistic mechanism, enabling an activating and an inhibitory agent to induce or prevent the meiotic process, has been combined with the notion of a cellular system of two separate supporting cells (95) and transferred and adapted to the male conditions. There is convincing evidence that the dark and light supporting cells of the fetal testis represent this dualistic system, exercising either a stimulating or an inhibitory effect on the germ cells by means of immediate cellular contact and direct substantial influence. One may consider that this substantial influence acts positively on the mitotic proliferation of the prospermatogonia and, on the other hand, prevents onset of meiosis. In the fetal ovary the cellular system triggers both the onset of premeiotic proliferation and that of the meiotic prophase, while it interrupts meiosis before or when oocytes become enclosed in primordial follicles.

What are the facts that corroborate this concept of antagonistic influence mediated by a dual cellular system?

(a) During mammalian testicular development the appearance of proliferating prospermatogonia coincides with that of the dark mesonephrogenic cells, while periods characterized by the existence of primordial germ cells or resting prospermatogonia correspond with the augmentation of light supporting cells.

In human testes, for instance, if the male cords are formed between days 42 and 49, a small number of dark cells are added to numerous light cells. This minor population of dark mesonephrogenic cells even decreases during the next week, since the light supporting cells undergo a relative augmentation by numerous mitotic divisions. Under these conditions the primordial germ cells persist in their undifferentiated stage (Figs. 17a and 18a and b). At the end of this period, however, the number of dark supporting cells increases rapidly and at the beginning of the 10th week these cells are numerous and show close

FIG. 18. Stages of human germ cell differentiation associated with dark and light (inducing and inhibiting) supporting cells (Sertoli cell precursors). (a) Primordial germ cells with "light" cells in testicular primordium on day 46 (embryo 21 mm long). (b) PGC in early testicular cords with light and dark cells (day 50). (c) and (d) PGC in testicular cords on day 64 which start to proliferate (mitosis in Fig. 18d) with "dark" and some "light" cells. (e) M-prospermatogonia surrounded by "dark" cells during maximum of proliferation. (f) Postmitotic *(left)* and growing T-prospermatogonia *(right)* showing "pseudo" preleptotene condensation of chromatin. (g) T-prospermatogonium with "light" cells and prophase (h) of proliferating prospermatogonium with "dark" cells in a 28 cm embryo.

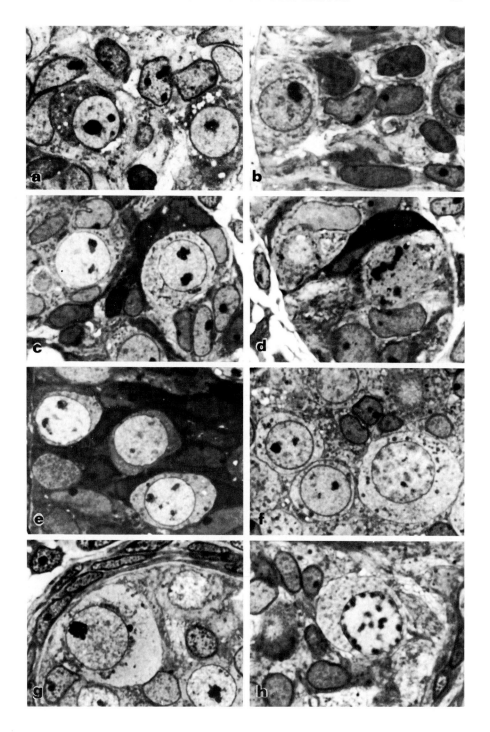

contact to the germ cells which, on their part, start proliferating (M-prospermato-gonia) (Figs. 17b and 18c–e). Histologically, the dark cells differ from the light cells by the density of their cytoplasm, the slender shape of their cell bodies and their long and thin processes which they use to separate germ cells from light supporting cells (Fig. 17b). Another 3 weeks later (13th week), in the proximal sections of the testicular cords, the (relative) amount of activating dark cells decreases and the germ cells stop proliferating (T-prospermatogonia). During this period the germ cells show a preleptotene stage of chromosome condensation (53) (Fig. 18f).

(b) The parallelism of the events in the developing testis and ovary lends additional support to the idea that the male germ cells, like the female germ cells, prepare for the onset of meiotic prophase by entering premeiotic proliferation. They do this under the activating influence of the dark mitosis- and meiosis-inducing cells. But, unlike conditions in the female gonad, the light mitosis- and meiosis-preventing cells regain dominance in the testicular cords, and meiosis is arrested before it starts.

(c) There is another observation which favors the idea of a cellular control of the germ cell proliferation or nonproliferation. Germ cells that have not yet entered the testicular cord, or germ cells that have failed to become enclosed in the cords, are induced to begin mitotic division on encountering dark meso-nephrogenic cells. Situations of this kind may occur during the early migrational period, in the mesentery, or when primordial germ cells have reached the genital ridge. Aberrant germ cells at extragonadal sites may be affected in this way, or those germ cells which can be found in the tunica albuginea contacting the superficial epithelium (Fig. 19a). Here, primordial germ cells come into contact with cells of the superficial epithelium and with mesonephrogenic cells. Under the activating influence of the latter, the germ cells start proliferating, forming clusters of prospermatogonia. Cellular groups of this kind have been observed in human fetal testes as well as in other mammalian testes during any stage of development (40,92) (Figs. 19b and c). Finally, these extratubular germ cells must degenerate, although the time and circumstances of this cell death are unknown.

(d) Some observations reported in the literature may be indicative of the existence of two types of supporting cells. Vilar (86) and Vilar et al. (87), referring to the paper of Johnsen (41), describe dark and light supporting cells in the immature human testis, especially in the postnatal period.

Summarizing the points so far discussed in this section, it may be concluded from evidence of a mainly structural nature that the germ cells are regulated, in respect of their capability of proliferating and of entering and continuing meiosis, by the numerical ratio of dark (inducing) to light (preventing) cells. Whether or not a germ cell starts proliferating depends on the grade of cellular contact elaborated by the inducing cellular system. As long as protection from the inhibiting influence of the preventing cellular system prevails, the germ cell divides mitotically and may even continue by entering meiosis provided

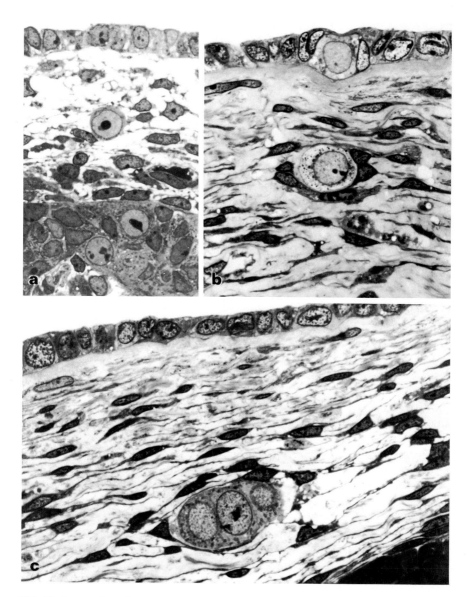

FIG. 19. Germ cells in Tunica albuginea of 64 day old **(a)** and 109 day old **(b)** and **(c)** human testes. **(a)** Germ cell is still in the primordial stage (compare with cells inside testicular cords) without much contact to mesenchymal-like cells. **(b)** Two further differentiated germ cells (similar to T-prospermatogonia), one within superficial epithelium and the other surrounded by "dark" mesenchymal-like cells of the tunica. **(c)** Group of three germ cells within tunica.

that the cellular arrangement has not changed. The special arrangement in the testicular cords, which differs from that in the ovarian cortex, could be owing to the fact that male germ cells do not enter meiosis during the prenatal or prepubertal period.

Accepting the idea of an antagonistic regulation of germ cell differentiation mediated by two somatic, supportive cell populations, some conclusions must be drawn which give rise to certain questions. If the double set of Sertoli cells continues to exist beyond pubertal differentiation, it is not unlikely that this system is relevant for the regulation of spermatogenesis. Evidence supporting this concept is scanty. In the ovary, however, the growth of the follicles seems to be correlated with an increase of a dark type of granulosa cell, while in the resting follicle a light type of granulosa cell predominates (78). Consequently the question arises, of what chemical nature are the two hypothetical substances that exert their activating or inhibiting influence on the germ cells? Androgens or estrogens are definitely available in the fetal gonads before germ cells start proliferating. In the rabbit fetus, the content of testosterone or estrogen reaches high levels in testes and ovaries, respectively, on day 22 p.c. (23), while the proliferation of prospermatogonia and oogonia starts close to day 22 p.c. Whether or not androgens or estrogens basically influence the proliferation and induction of meiosis prenatally, and whether this process depends on the concentrating effect of an androgen or estrogen binding protein remains questionable (81). Other substances could exert their activating influence on the germ cells and, in the same way, it needs to be demonstrated whether or not the testis produces an inhibiting substance that is different from the Müllerian inhibiting factor which originates in the fetal Sertoli cells (42).

Finally, the disturbed relationship of the two Sertoli cells might provide an explanation of some of the fertility disturbances and malformations. If the optimal quantitative proportion of activating and inhibiting supportive cells has not been attained during early development of testis or ovary, the regular increase in the number of germ cells or the successive phases of the differentiating gonia during the pre- and postnatal period could be disturbed. On the basis of these suppositions, the number and ratio of the two types of Sertoli cells and the number of "spermatogonia" should be methodically ascertained when studies of testicular lesions are made during prepubertal age.

DEVELOPMENT OF THE TESTICULAR CORDS UNTIL PUBERTY

During early development, the diameter of the growing testicular cords depends on the intratubular situation. Rapid proliferation of germ cells or supporting cells coincides with a rapid increase of the diameter of the cords. During late prenatal and during postnatal development, progress of growth becomes slow and steady. Hence, the mean diameter of a given number of testicular cords at a definite age can be used as a parameter for establishing whether testicular growth is regular and undisturbed. Another test correlating with the diameter of the cords is a count of germ cells in 50 or 100 circular cross-sections of tubules (33,55,79). Structurally, the composition of the testicular cords remains unchanged until initiation of puberty. In human prepubertal testes the cords show an arrangement of proliferating and nonproliferating prospermatogonia and light and dark supporting cells which does not fundamentally alter from midgestation until the age of 11. Different types of A-spermatogonia may appear in limited numbers with advancing years. These spermatogonia, however, do not continue into full spermatogenesis. Although the initiation of spermatogenesis with reference to cell maturation has been studied in some mammals (13,26), so far it has not been understood in adolescent human testes.

There is strong evidence that dark supporting cells play an important role in maintaining prepubertal germ cell proliferation, counteracting the inhibiting effect of the light supporting cells. The number of dark cells increases rapidly when the testis begins to undergo its early pubertal structural changes (Figs. 20a and b). In small mammals, concomitant with the increase in number of A-spermatogonia, the testicular cords are filled with dark supporting cells still corresponding to the premature stage of Sertoli cells. In tissue culture, Solari and Fritz (77) were able to demonstrate the structural changes which correlate with the maturation of the Sertoli cells. These cells differ from the dark pre-Sertoli cells in that they exhibit a less dense cytoplasm: "The light cell type may represent a stage of stimulation of the smooth endoplasmic reticulum elicited by FSH." (Cited after ref. 77.)

A similar differential change can be observed in tissue sections which demonstrate a chronological sequence of postnatal and early pubertal development of the testicular cords of the golden hamster (H. Wartenberg, *unpublished data*) (Fig. 20).

Finally, the Sertoli cells show a decrease in number of their mitotic divisions, an event that appears to be induced by FSH. When most germ cells have concluded their prespermatogonial stage and start spermatogenesis, Sertoli cells achieve full maturation and suspend their multiplication. "Speculatively, the total number of mitotic divisions that a Sertoli cell can undergo may have an upper limit which cannot be exceeded." (Cited after ref. 77.)

Connected with the Sertoli cell maturation is the occurrence of intercellular junctional specializations which in turn should represent the morphological correlate of the establishment of the blood-testis barrier (88).

DIFFERENTIATION OF THE EXTRATUBULAR TESTICULAR STRUCTURES: INTERSTITIAL CELL SYSTEM (LEYDIG CELLS) AND MYOID CELLS

The Leydig cell system originates from mesenchymal cells. This seems to be the most widely accepted concept (25,26), although Witschi (102) has presented evidence of a mesonephric origin of the precursor cells; he assumed "that the entire steroid-producing organs" are derivatives of the mesonephros (105).

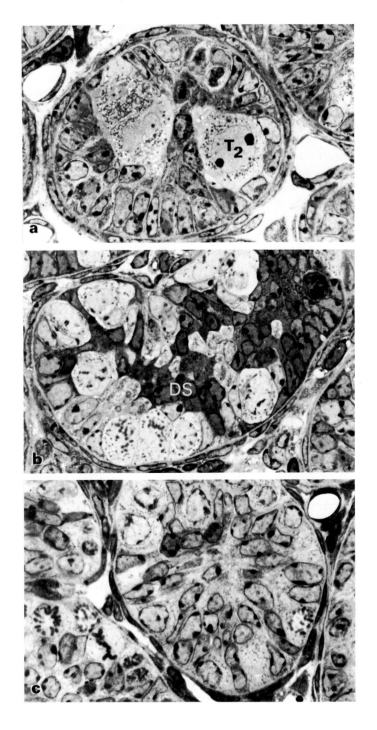

First differentiated Leydig cells appear, obviously, at some interval after onset of testicular differentiation, but this process is immediately followed by commencement of androgen synthesis (26). Leydig cell differentiation and initiation of steroidogenesis, however, precedes the period of germ cell proliferation and is concomitant with the appearance of the dark Sertoli cells within the testicular cords.

In human fetal testes, the period characterized by a highly developed interstitial cell system lasts from the 8th (Fig. 21a) to the 18th week (26,38,74,89). At about the 14th week they have reached their maximum expansion and constitute more than 50% of the testicular volume (10,38). After this period the Leydig cell system regresses slowly and a few days or weeks after birth, in most mammals, Leydig cells dedifferentiate, resulting in a "quiescent stage" (26) during the postnatal period.

During pre- and postnatal testicular development of the pig, three periods of Leydig cell differentiation can be distinguished (83). The first period corresponds to the fetal stage seen in all mammals so far; the second period is placed perinatally, viz., from 2.5 weeks before to 2.5 weeks after birth. The adult Leydig cell population develops during a third period that begins about 13 weeks postpartum.

Comparing the topographical distribution of the Leydig cells during these three periods, two distinct types of cell population can be discerned: the intertubular type, predominating during the fetal and perinatal periods, and the peritubular type, which first appears in small amounts and is still not fully differentiated when the intertubular Leydig cells of the perinatal period attain maximum development shortly after birth. Peritubular Leydig cells prevail from the prepuberal development onward, owing to a numerical increase giving rise to the adult Leydig cell population (83,84).

In postnatal human testes, a few months after birth the intertubular space is devoid of Leydig cells. The renewed differentiation of the Leydig cell during the onset of puberty at about 12 to 13 years of age again raises the question as to the origin of the interstitial cell. In addition to mesenchymal or fibroblast-like cells, one suspects peritubular myoid cells (10,14,18) or macrophages (histiocytes) (12,82) as being precursor cells of the Leydig cell system. If one extends Witschi's concept, according to which the Leydig cells originate from mesonephrogenic blastemal cells, one has to bear in mind the structural situation during early gonadal and sexual differentiation. After the mesonephrogenic

---

FIG. 20. Stages of prepubertal differentiation of the testicular cords of the golden hamster. **(a)** On day 8 post partum T-prospermatogonia increase in size and form clusters due to their mitotic activity (T_2-prospermatogonia). **(b)** Finally, on day 13, most of the T_2-prospermatogonia are contacting the basement membrane, decreasing in size while they continue to proliferate. Most of the supportive cells are "dark" (DS); others belong to the light group. Both types of Sertoli cell precursors may have contact to the germ cells. **(c)** On day 16 p.p. all germ cells are transformed to T-spermatogonia and the number of "light" supporting cells dominates in this cord.

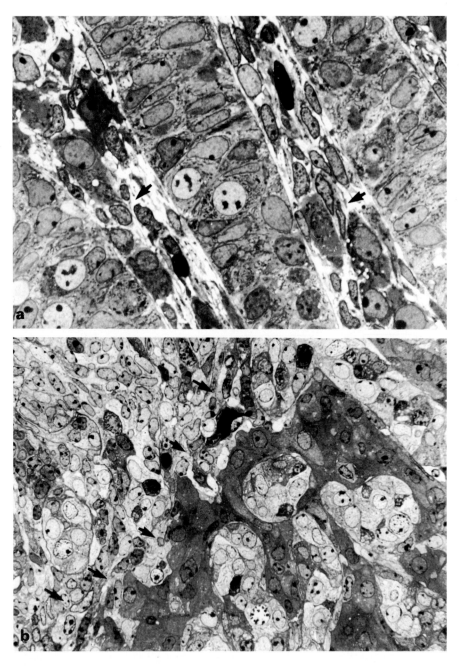

FIG. 21. (a) Interstitial (Leydig) cells between straight testicular cords in a 58 day old embryo (4.0 cm), which differentiate from mesenchymal-like cells. **(b)** Testis of a 65 mm long calf fetus demonstrating the area of the central gonadal blastema *(upper left)* and interstitial tissue *(lower right)* which is crowded with fetal Leydig cells. Intermediate stages of Leydig cell formation are visible at the border of the gonadal blastema *(arrows)*.

blastema has been confronted with, and has invaded, the superficial blastema (see pages 45–48), the mesenchyme-like cells of mesonephric origin are distributed in the interstitial space all over the testis, while others become enclosed in the testicular cords. These cells, which differ from plain mesenchymal cells, might form the stock for Leydig cell differentiation. A further supply of Leydig cell precursors comes from the gonadal blastema via the "rete blastema" (see pages 54–56) during the early testicular differential period. In fetal bovine testes, which exhibit a close contact of the central gonadal blastema to the area of cord formation (Fig. 7d), a sequence of differential steps can be followed, starting with the "fibroblast-like" undifferentiated blastemal cell and terminating in a fully developed Leydig cell (Fig. 21).

Recalling some of the characteristics which have been mentioned in connection with the blastemal cell deriving from the mesonephric structures (page 64) might explain those observations from which it has been deduced that Leydig cells stem from nonmesenchymal cellular contents. The marked capacity of the mesonephrogenic system to "trans"-differentiate from one fully developed state (podocyte of the mesonephros) into a second state of completely different significance (Sertoli cell, Leydig cell) might continue. Viewed from this aspect, it does not seem unlikely that Leydig cells, contractile elements (myoid cells of the boundary tissue), and even phagocytozing elements are derivatives of the same mesonephrogenic blastemal cell and are interchangeable by means of "transdifferentiation." The differentiation of a "peritubular" early Leydig cell aggregation during testicular development which, in the rat, finally transforms into (73), or in human cryptorchid testes may derive from, the myoid cellular system (76), supports this concept. In addition, the dependency of the Leydig cell as well as the myoid cell on the gonadotrophic influence of the pituitary would favor a close relationship of these cellular contents of the interstitial tissue.

CONCLUDING REMARKS: THE MESONEPHROS AND THE CONTROL OF GONADAL DEVELOPMENT AND GERM CELL DIFFERENTIATION

If one tries to sum up the main points on the development of the testes discussed in this chapter, the mesonephros obviously plays a fundamental role in the process of gonad formation. Cells which can be deduced to derive from the mesonephros or its precursor (nephrotom, stalks of the somites), and which "dedifferentiate," form blastemal cells. These mesonephrogenic cells first influence the neighboring cells of the coelomic epithelium in order to initiate a proliferative process (Fig. 22). The genital ridge is formed by two types of blastemal somatic cells: one of mesonephric, the other of epithelial origin. The process of sexual differentiation is based on the continuing attempt of the mesonephric blastema to maintain the close contact to the epithelial blastema. In the male gonad the two blastemal components become mixed. In the female gonad the mesonephrogenic and the epithelial blastemas remain separated, forming

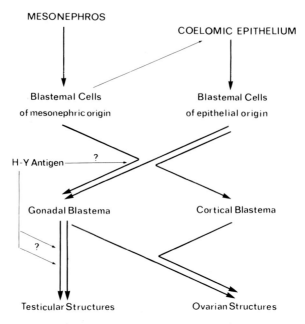

FIG. 22. Schematic representation of a concept of mammalian gonadal development and sexual differentiation.

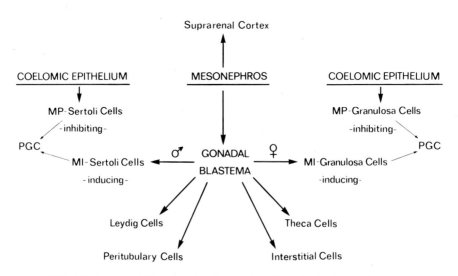

FIG. 23. Concept of histogenesis of somatic cells of the testis and the ovary.

an unmixed gonadal blastema and a cortical blastema. Further testicular development expresses itself in the differentiation of testicular structures from the mixed blastema while the female development makes up for the failure, and an ovarian cortex is formed by a similar process of combining mesonephrogenic and epithelial cells (Fig. 22).

Just as the mesonephros causes primary gonadal development to take place, cellular derivatives of the mesonephros influence the proliferation and differentiation of the germ cells. A double set of male and female supporting cells (Sertoli cells, granulosa cells) regulates the mitotic activity and the meiotic process of the germ cell by inducing or inhibiting it (Fig. 23).

Finally, attention should be drawn to the peculiar role of the mesonephrogenic cells. After losing its highly differentiated state, the blastemal cell becomes multipotential and is distinguished by the competence to differentiate into suprarenal cortex cells as well as a great variety of somatic cells of both the testis and the ovary (Fig. 23). All these cellular systems originating from the mesonephros have one characteristic in common: they produce steroids, or they have a mediating function regarding the production of these.

ACKNOWLEDGMENT

This work was supported by a grant from the Deutsche Forschungsgemeinschaft.

REFERENCES

1. Armstrong, P. B., and Armstrong, M. T. (1973): Are cells in solid tissues immobile? Mesonephric mesenchyme studied in vitro. *Dev. Biol.,* 35:187–209.
2. Byskov, A. G. (1974): Does the rete ovarii act as a trigger for the onset of meiosis? *Nature,* 252:396–397.
3. Byskov, A. G. (1975): The role of the rete ovarii in meiosis and follicle formation in the cat, mink and ferret. *J. Reprod. Fert.,* 45:201–209.
4. Byskov, A. G. (1978): The anatomy and ultrastructure of the rete system in the fetal mouse ovary. *Biol. Reprod.,* 19:720–735.
5. Byskov, A. G., and Lintern-Moore, S. (1973): Follicle formation in the immature mouse ovary: the role of the rete ovarii. *J. Anat.,* 116:207–217.
6. Byskov, A. G., and Saxén, L. (1976): Induction of meiosis in fetal mouse testis in vitro. *Dev. Biol.,* 52:193–200.
7. Byskov, A. G., Skakkebaek, N. E., Stafanger, G., and Peters, H. (1977): Influence of ovarian surface epithelium and rete ovarii on follicle formation. *J. Anat.,* 123:77–86.
8. Carlon, N., and Stahl, A. (1973): Les premiers stades du développement des gonades chez l'homme et les vertébrés supérieurs. *Pathol. et Biol. (Paris),* 21:903–914.
9. Challoner, S. (1975): Studies of oogenesis and follicular development in the golden hamster. 2. Initiation and control of meiosis in vitro. *J. Anat.,* 119:149–156.
10. Christensen, A. K. (1975): Leydig cells. In: *Handbook of Physiology,* Vol V., Sect. 7, Chapt. 3, edited by R. O. Greep, and E. B. Astwood. American Physiological Society, Washington, D.C.
11. Clark, J. M., and Eddy, E. M. (1975): Fine structural observations on the origin and associations of primordial germ cells of the mouse. *Dev. Biol.,* 47:136–155.
12. Clegg, E. J., and Macmillan, E. W. (1965): The phagocytic nature of Schiff-positive interstitial cells in the rat testis. *J. Endocrinol.,* 31:299–300.

13. Courot, M., Hochereau-de Reviers, M.-Th., and Ortavant, R. (1970): Spermatogenesis. In: *The Testis*, Vol. I, edited by A. D. Johnson, W. R. Gomes, and N. L. Vandemark. Academic Press, New York.
14. De Kretser, D. M. (1967): The fine structure of the testicular interstitial cells in men of normal androgenic status. *Z. Zellforsch.*, 80:594–609.
15. Elias, W. (1974): Frühentwicklung des Samenkanälchen beim Menschen. *Verh. Anat. Ges. (Jena)*, 68:123–131.
16. Everett, N. B. (1943): Observational and experimental evidences relating to the origin and differentiation of the definitive germ cells in mice. *J. Exp. Zool.*, 92:49–91.
17. Everett, N. B. (1945): The present status of the germ-cell problem in vertebrates. *Biol. Rev.*, 20:45–55.
18. Fawcett, D. W., and Burgos, M. H. (1960): Studies on the fine structure of the mammalian testis. II. The human interstitial tissue. *Am. J. Anat.*, 107:245–269.
19. Fischel, A. (1930): Über die Entwicklung der Keimdrüsen des Menschen. *Z. Anat. Entwicklungsgesch.*, 92:34–72.
20. Fraedrich, J. (1979): Licht- und elektronenmikroskopische Untersuchungen über den Zusammenhang der Mesonephros- und frühen Gonadenentwicklung der weißen Maus. Dissertation: Bonn, Med. Fak.
21. Franchi, L. L., Mandl, A. M., and Zuckerman, S. S. (1962): The development of the ovary and the process of oogenesis. In: *The Ovary*, Vol. I, Chapt. 1, edited by S. S. Zuckerman. Academic Press, New York.
22. Fukuda, T., Hedinger, C., and Groscurth, P. (1975): Ultrastructure of developing germ cells in the fetal human testis. *Cell Tissue Res.*, 161:55–70.
23. George, F. W., Milewich, L., and Wilson, J. D. (1978): Oestrogen content of the embryonic rabbit ovary. *Nature*, 274:172–173.
24. Gerharz, C. (1978): Histologische Untersuchungen an Semidünnschnitten über die Gonadenentwicklung der weissen Maus: Oogenese und Präspermatogenese als synchrone Prozesse. Dissertation, Bonn, Med. Fak.
25. Gondos, B. (1974): Differentiation and growth of cells in the gonads. In: *Differentiation and Growth of Cells in Vertebrate Tissues*, Chapt. 6, edited by G. Goldspink. Chapman and Hall, London.
26. Gondos, B. (1977): Testicular development. In: *The Testis*, Vol. IV, Chapt. 1, edited by A. D. Johnson and W. R. Gomes. Academic Press, New York.
27. Gondos, B., and Conner, L. A. (1973): Ultrastructure of developing germ cells in the fetal rabbit testis. *Am. J. Anat.*, 136:23–42.
28. Gondos, B., and Hobel, C. J. (1971): Ultrastructure of germ cell development in the human fetal testis. *Z. Zellforsch.*, 119:1–20.
29. Gropp, A., and Ohno, S. (1966): The presence of a common embryonic blastema for ovarian and testicular parenchymal (follicular, interstitial and tubular) cells in cattle, Bos taurus. *Z. Zellforsch.*, 74:505–528.
30. Gruenwald, P. (1942): The development of the sex cords in the gonads of man and mammals. *Am. J. Anat.*, 70:359–397.
31. Hardisty, M. W. (1967): The numbers of vertebrate primordial germ cells. *Biol. Rev.*, 42:265–287.
32. Harris, G. W. (1964): Sex hormones, brain development and brain function. *Endocrinology*, 75:627–648.
33. Hedinger, C. (1971): Über den Zeitpunkt frühest erkennbarer Hodenveränderungen beim Kryptorchismus des Kleinkindes. *Verh. Dtsch. Ges. Pathol.*, 55:172–175.
34. Hilscher, B., Hilscher, W., Bülthoff-Ohnolz, B., Krämer, U., Birke, A., Pelzer, H., and Gauss, G. (1974): Kinetics of gametogenesis. I. Comparative histological and autoradiographic studies of oocytes and transitional prospermatogonia during oogenesis and prespermatogenesis. *Cell Tissue Res.*, 154:443–470.
35. Hilscher, B., Hilscher, W., Delbrück, G., and Lerouge-Bérnard, B. (1972): Autoradiographische Bestimmung der S-Phasen-Dauer der Gonocyten bei der Wistarratte durch Einfach- und Doppelmarkierung. *Z. Zellforsch.*, 125:229–251.
36. Hilscher, W. (1974): Kinetik der Präspermatogenese und Spermatogenese. *Verh. Anat. Ges.*, 68:39–62.

37. Hilscher, W., and Hilscher, B. (1976): Kinetics of the male gametogenesis. *Andrologia,* 8:105–116.
38. Holstein, A. F., Wartenberg, H., and Vossmeyer, J. (1971): Zur Cytologie der pränatalen Gonadenentwicklung beim Menschen. III. Die Entwicklung der Leydigzellen im Hoden von Embryonen und Feten. *Z. Anat. Entwicklungsgesch.,* 135:43–66.
39. Jirásek, J. E. (1971): *Development of the Genital System and Male Pseudohermaphroditism,* edited by M. M. Cohen, Jr. Johns Hopkins Press, Baltimore.
40. Jirásek, J. E. (1976): Principles of reproductive embryology. In: *Disorders of Sexual Differentiation,* Chapt. 1, edited by J. L. Simpson. Academic Press, New York.
41. Johnsen, S. G. (1969): Two types of Sertoli cells in man. *Acta Endocrinol. (Kbh),* 61:111–116.
42. Josso, N., Picard, J.-Y., and Tran, D. (1977): The antimüllerian hormone. *Recent Prog. Horm. Res.,* 33:117–163.
43. Jost, A. (1953): Problems of fetal endocrinology: The gonadal and hypophyseal hormones. *Recent Prog. Horm. Res.,* 8:379–413.
44. Jost, A. (1965): Gonadal hormones in the sex differentiation of the mammalian fetus. In: *Organogenesis,* edited by R. L. DeHaan and H. Ursprung. Holt, Rinehart and Winston, New York.
45. Jost, A. (1970): General outline about reproductive physiology and its developmental background. In: *Mammalian Reproduction. Colloquium der Gesellschaft für biologische Chemie, Mosbach,* edited by H. Gibian and E. J. Plotz. Springer-Verlag, Berlin.
46. Jost, A. (1970): Hormonal factors in the sex differentiation of the mammalian foetus. *Philos. Trans. R. Soc. Lond. B.,* 259:119–130.
47. Jost, A. (1970): Hormonal factors in the development of the male genital system. In: *The Human Testis,* edited by E. Rosemberg and C. A. Paulsen. Plenum Press, New York.
48. Jost, A. (1971): Embryonic sexual differentiation (morphology, physiology, abnormalities). In: *Hermaphroditism, Genital Anomalies and Related Endocrine Disorders,* 2nd Ed., Chapt. 2, edited by H. W. Jones and W. W. Scott. Williams & Wilkins, Baltimore.
49. Jost, A. (1972): A new look at the mechanisms controlling sex differentiation in mammals. *Johns Hopkins Med. J.,* 130:38–53.
50. Jost, A., Magre, S., Cressent, M., and Perlman, S. (1974): Sertoli cells and early testicular differentiation. In: *Male Fertility and Sterility, Proceedings of the Serono Symposia,* Vol. 5, edited by R. E. Mancini and L. Martini. Academic Press, New York.
51. Jost, A., Vigier, B., Prépin, J., and Perchellet, J. P. (1973): Studies on sex differentiation in mammals. *Recent Prog. Horm. Res.,* 29:1–35.
52. Kinsky, I. (1979): Bildung des somatischen Gonadenblastems durch degenerierende Urnierenanteile des Kaninchens. *Verh. Anat. Ges. (Innsbruck),* 73:403–406.
53. Luciani, J. M., Devictor, M., and Stahl, A. (1977): Preleptotene chromosome condensation stage in human foetal and neonatal testes. *J. Embryol. Exp. Morphol.,* 38:175–186.
54. Lyon, M. F. (1974): Role of X and Y chromosomes in mammalian sex determination and differentiation. *Helv. Paediatr. Acta* (Suppl.), 34:7–12.
55. Mancini, R. E., Rosemberg, E., Cullen, M., Lavieri, J. C., Vilar, O., Bergada, C., and Andrada, J. A. (1965): Cryptorchid and scrotal human testes. I. Cytological, cytochemical and quantitative studies. *J. Clin. Endocrinol.,* 25:927–942.
56. Mauger, A., and Clermont, Y. (1974): Ultrastructure des gonocytes et des spermatogonies du jeune rat. *Arch. Anat. Microsc. Morphol. Exp.,* 63:133–146.
57. McKay, D. G., Hertig, A. T., Adams, E. C., and Danziger, S. (1953): Histochemical observations on the germ cells of human embryos. *Anat. Rec.,* 117:201–219.
58. McKay, D. G., Adams, E. C., Hertig, A. T., and Danziger, S. (1955): Histochemical horizons in human embryos. I. Five millimeter embryo-Streeter horizon XIII. *Anat. Rec.,* 122:125–151.
59. Mintz, B. (1959): Continuity of the female germ cell line from embryo to adult. *Arch. Anat. Microsc. Morphol. Exp.,* 48 bis:155–172.
60. Müller, U., Aschmoneit, I., Zenzes, M. T., and Wolf, U. (1978): Binding studies of H-Y antigen in rat tissues. Indications for a gonad-specific receptor. *Hum. Genet.,* 43:151–157.
61. Müller, U., Siebers, J. W., Zenzes, M. T., and Wolf, U. (1978): The testis as a secretory organ for H-Y antigen. *Hum. Genet.,* 45:209–213.

62. Neumann, F. (1977): Hormonale Regulation der Sexualdifferenzierung bei Säugetieren. In: *Vorlesungsreihe Schering,* Heft 3, edited by Pharma-Forschung der Schering AG Berlin/Bergkamen. Schering AG, Berlin, Bergkamen.
63. Nussbaum, M. (1880): Zur Differenzierung des Geschlechts im Thierreich. *Arch. Mikro. Anat.,* 18:1–120.
64. O, W.-S., and Baker, T. G. (1976): Initiation and control of meiosis in hamster gonads in vitro. *J. Reprod. Fertil.,* 48:399–401.
65. Odor, D. L., and Blandau, R. J. (1969): Ultrastructural studies on fetal and early postnatal mouse ovaries. I. Histogenesis and organogenesis. *Am. J. Anat.,* 124:163–186.
66. Ohno, S. (1971): Simplicity of mammalian regulatory systems inferred by single gene determination of sex phenotypes. *Nature,* 234:134–137.
67. Ohno, S. (1976): Major regulatory genes for mammalian sexual development. Rev. *The Cell,* 7:315–321.
68. Ohno, S. (1977): The Y-linked H-Y antigen locus and the X-linked Tfm locus as major regulatory genes of the mammalian sex determining mechanism. *J. Steroid Biochem.,* 8:585–592.
69. Ohno, S., Nagai, Y., and Ciccarese, S. (1978): Testicular cells lysostripped of H-Y antigen organize ovarian follicle-like aggregates. *Cytogenet. Cell Genet.,* 20:351–364.
70. Ohno, S., Stenius, Ch., Weiler, C. P., Trujillo, J. M., Kaplan, W. D., and Kinosita, R. (1962): Early meiosis of male germ cells in fetal testis of Felis domestica. *Exp. Cell Res.,* 27:401–404.
71. Ortavant, R., Courot, M., and Hochereau de Reviers, M. T. (1977): Spermatogenesis in domestic mammals. In: *Reproduction in Domestic Animals,* 3rd Ed., Chap. 8, edited by H. H. Cole and P. T. Cupps. Academic Press, New York.
72. Ozdzenski, W. (1972): Differentiation of the genital ridges of mouse embryos in the kidney of adult mice. *Arch. Anat. Microsc. Morphol. Exp.,* 61:267–278.
73. Passia, D., and Hahner, J. (1979): Enzymhistochemische Untersuchungen an dem inter- und peritubulären Leydigzell-System der Ratte. *Verh. Anat. Ges. (Innsbruck),* 73:699–700.
74. Pelliniemi, L. J., and Niemi, M. (1969): Fine structure of the human foetal testis. I. The interstitial tissue. *Z. Zellforsch.,* 99:507–522.
75. Politzer, G. (1933): Die Keimbahn des Menschen. *Z. Anat. Entwicklungsgesch.,* 100:331–361.
76. Schulze, C., and Holstein, A.-F. (1978): Leydig cells within the lamina propria of seminiferous tubules in four patients with azoospermia. *Andrologia,* 10:444–452.
77. Solari, A. J., and Fritz, I. B. (1978): The ultrastructure of immature Sertoli cells. Maturation-like changes during culture and the maintenance of mitotic potentiality. *Biol. Reprod.,* 18:329–345.
78. Sprumont, P. (1978): Ovarian follicles of normal NMRI mice and homozygous "nude" mice. *Cell Tissue Res.,* 188:409–426.
79. Städtler, F. (1973): Die normale und gestörte praepuberale Hodenentwicklung des Menschen. In: *Veröffentlichungen aus der Morphologischen Pathologie,* Vol. 92, edited by W. Giese, W. Büngeler, G. Seifert, and G. Peters. Gustav Fischer Verlag, Stuttgart.
80. Stein, L. E., and Anderson, C. H. (1979): A qualitative and quantitative study of rete ovarii development in the fetal rat: Correlation with the onset of meiosis and follicle cell appearance. *Anat. Rec.,* 193:197–212.
81. Steinberger, E., and Steinberger, A. (1972): Testis: basic and clinical aspects. In: *Reproductive Biology,* Chapt. 4, edited by H. Balin and S. Glasser. Excerpta Medica, Amsterdam.
82. Stieve, H. (1930): Harn- und Geschlechtsapparat. In: *Handbuch der Mikroskopischen Anatomie des Menschen,* Vol. 7, Part 2: *Männliche Genitalorgane,* edited by W. v. Möllendorff. Springer-Verlag, Berlin.
83. Straaten, H. W. M. van, and Wensing, C. J. G. (1978): Leydig cell development in the testis of the pig. *Biol. Reprod.,* 18:86–93.
84. Straaten, H. W. M. van, Ribbers-de Ridder, R., and Wensing, C. J. G. (1978): Early deviations of testicular Leydig cells in the naturally unilateral cryptorchid pig. *Biol. Reprod.,* 19:171–176.
85. Tsafriri, A., and Channing, C. P. (1975): An inhibitory influence of granulosa cells and follicular fluid upon porcine oocyte meiosis in vitro. *Endocrinology,* 96:922–927.
86. Vilar, O. (1970): Histology of the human testis from neonatal period to adolescence. In: *The*

Human Testis. Advances in Experimental Medicine and Biology, Vol. 10, edited by E. Rosemberg and C. A. Paulsen. Plenum Press, New York.

87. Vilar, O., Paulsen, C. A., and Moore, D. J. (1970): Electron microscopy of the human seminiferous tubules. In: *The Human Testis. Advances in Experimental Medicine and Biology,* Vol. 10, edited by E. Rosemberg and C. A. Paulsen. Plenum Press, New York.

88. Vitale, R., Fawcett, D. W., and Dym, M. (1973): The normal development of the blood-testis barrier and the effects of clomiphene and estrogen treatment. *Anat. Rec.,* 176:333–344.

89. Vossmeyer, J. (1971): Zur Cytologie der pränatalen Gonaden-Entwicklung beim Menschen. I. Die Histogenese des Hoden, an Eponschnitten untersucht. *Z. Anat. Entwicklungsgesch.,* 134:146–164.

90. Wachtel, S. S., Koo, G. C., and Ohno, S. (1977): H-Y antigen and male development. In: *The Testis in Normal and Infertile Men,* edited by P. Troen and H. R. Nankin. Raven Press, New York.

91. Wachtel, S. S., Ohno, S., Koo, G. C. and Boyse, E. A. (1975): Possible role for H-Y antigen in the primary determination of sex. *Nature,* 257:235–236.

92. Wagenen, G. van, and Simpson, M. E. (1965): *Embryology of the Ovary and Testis. Homo sapiens and Macaca mulatta.* Yale University Press, New Haven.

93. Wartenberg, H. (1974): Spermatogenese-Oogenese: Ein cytomorphologischer Vergleich. *Verh. Anat. Ges.,* 68:63–92.

94. Wartenberg, H. (1976): Comparative cytomorphologic aspects of the male germ cells, especially of the "gonia". *Andrologia,* 8:117–130.

95. Wartenberg, H. (1978): Human testicular development and the role of the mesonephros in the origin of a dual Sertoli cell system. *Andrologia,* 10:1–21.

96. Wartenberg, H. (1979): Der Mesonephros und die Gonadenentwicklung. *Verh. Anat. Ges. (Innsbruck),* 73:385–401.

97. Wartenberg, H., Holstein, A.-F., and Vossmeyer, J. (1971): Zur Cytologie der pränatalen Gonadenentwicklung beim Menschen. II. Elektronenmikroskopische Untersuchungen über die Cytogenese von Gonocyten and fetalen Spermatogonien im Hoden. *Z. Anat. Entwicklungsgesch.,* 134:165–185.

98. Watzka, M. (1962): Die entwicklungsgeschichtlichen Grundlagen der Gonaden und der Intersexualität. *Arch. Gynaekol.,* 198:319–328.

99. Wilson, K. M. (1926): Origin and development of the rete ovarii and the rete testis in the human embryo. *Carnegie Inst. Wash. Publ. No. 362., Contrib. Embryol.,* 17:69–88.

100. Witschi, E. (1914): Experimentelle Untersuchungen über die Entwicklungsgeschichte der Keimdrüse von Rana temporaria. *Arch. Mikro. Anat.,* 85:9–113.

101. Witschi, E. (1948): Migration of the germ cells of human embryos from the yolk sac to the primitive gonadal folds. *Carnegie Inst. Wash. Publ. No. 575, Contrib. Embryol.,* 32:67–80.

102. Witschi, E. (1951): Embryogenesis of the adrenal and the reproductive gland. *Rec. Prog. Horm. Res.,* 6:1-27.

103. Witschi, E. (1956): *Development of Vertebrates.* Saunders, Philadelphia.

104. Witschi, E. (1957): The inductor theory of sex differentiation; *J. Fac. Sci. Hokkaido Univ., (Ser. VI, Zool.),* 13:428–439.

105. Witschi, E. (1962): Embryology of the ovary. In: *The Ovary,* Chapt. 1, edited by H. G. Grady and D. E. Smith. Williams and Wilkins, Baltimore.

106. Witschi, E. (1965): Hormones and embryonic induction. *Arch. Anat. Microsc. Morphol. Exp.,* 54:601–611.

107. Witschi, E. (1967): Biochemistry of sex differentiation in vertebrate embryos. In: *The Biochemistry of Animal Development,* Vol. II, Chapt. 4, edited by R. Weber. Academic Press, New York.

108. Witschi, E. (1970): Embryology of the testis. In: *The Human Testis,* edited by E. Rosemberg and C. A. Paulsen. Plenum Press, New York.

109. Wolf, U. (1979): XY gonadal dysgenesis and the H-Y antigen. *Hum. Genet.,* 47:269–277.

110. Wolf, U., and Zenzes, M.-T. (1979): Gonadendifferenzierung und H-Y-Antigen. *Verh. Anat. Ges. (Innsbruck),* 73:379–384.

111. Zenzes, M.-T., Müller, U., Aschmoneit, I., and Wolf, U. (1978): Studies on H-Y antigen in different cell fractions of the testis during pubescence. *Hum. Genet.,* 45:297–303.

112. Zenzes, M.-T., Wolf, U., and Engel, W. (1978): Organization in vitro of ovarian cells into testicular structures. *Hum. Genet.,* 44:333–338.

113. Zenzes, M.-T., Wolf, U., Günther, E., and Engel, W. (1978): Studies on the function of H-Y antigen: dissociation and reorganization experiments on rat gonadal tissue. *Cytogenet. Cell Genet.,* 20:365–372.
114. Zuckerman, S., and Baker, T. G. (1977): The development of the ovary and the process of oogenesis. In: *The Ovary,* 2nd Ed., Vol. I, edited by S. Zuckerman and B. J. Weir. Academic Press, New York.

The Testis, edited by H. Burger and D. de Kretser.
Raven Press, New York © 1981.

4

Endocrinology of the Fetal Testis

*Charles Faiman, **Jeremy S. D. Winter, and †Francisco I. Reyes

*Departments of Physiology and Medicine; **Department of Paediatrics; †Departments
of Obstetrics and Gynaecology and Physiology; University of Manitoba, Health Sciences
Center, Winnepeg, Manitoba, Canada*

The study of human fetal testicular development and function has received
little attention until the last four decades when interest was aroused by the
recognition of a number of defects in genital development. The pioneering studies
of Jost in the rabbit (46–48) coupled with morphological observations in certain
cases of anomalous sexual development first allowed inferences to be made regarding human fetal testicular function. More recently, the advent of improved
technology in the area of hormone measurement has permitted direct study of
the endocrinology of fetal testicular development.

It is the purpose of this chapter to describe fetal testicular function and its
regulatory mechanisms in relation to prenatal sexual differentiation.

TESTICULAR DIFFERENTIATION AND DEVELOPMENT[1]

In human embryos primordial germ cells migrate from their original site in
the endoderm of the yolk sac to reach the genital ridges at 5 to 6 weeks postfertili-
zation (101). The earliest sign of sexual differentiation in males is the development
of testes from undifferentiated gonadal anlagen. At about 7 to 8 weeks of fetal
age strands of germ cells and presumptive Sertoli cell precursors form into
sex cords, the precursors of the seminiferous tubules. This stage of gonadal
differentiation is clearly gene related; the Y-chromosome normally contains the
determinant gene for testicular differentiation (92,96). This Y-linked testis-organ-
izing gene specifies a plasma membrane protein which can be identified immuno-
logically as the H-Y histocompatibility antigen. It has been postulated that
this H-Y locus, present in all male cells, causes the medullary cords of the
indifferent gonad to develop into a testis (63,92).

The first typical Leydig cells, containing large amounts of smooth endoplasmic

---

[1] See also chapter three.

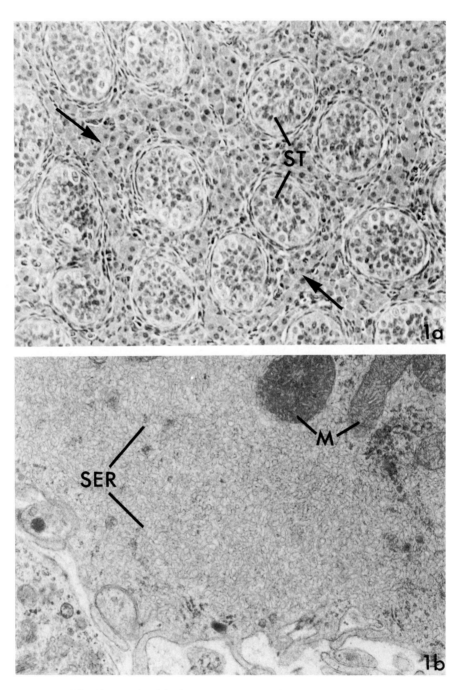

FIG. 1. a: Light micrograph of fetal testis, crown-rump length 11.4 cm (14.5 weeks). Note the numerous Leydig cells (arrows) interspersed between developing seminiferous tubules (ST). Magnification × 910. **b:** Electron micrograph of fetal testis (Fig. 1a), exhibiting numerous profiles of smooth-surfaced endoplasmic reticulum (SER). Mitochondria (M) are also seen. Magnification × 19,750.

reticulum that suggest a steroidogenic potential, appear at around 8 weeks. By 14 to 18 weeks these cells fill the space between the sex cords and make up more than half the volume of the testis (66) (see Fig. 1). At about this same time some of the medullary sex cords begin to canalize and gonocytes become transformed into spermatogonia (30,32). After the 18th week, the Leydig cells begin to involute and disappear entirely a few weeks after birth (57). By 27 weeks the seminiferous tubules are separated by only a narrow interstitium containing few Leydig cells. A well developed tunica albuginea now envelops the testis and projects its septae deep into the gonad. At this time, the fetal testis begins its journey through the inguinal canal, to reach the scrotum by 34 to 35 weeks (102).

During the last 4 months of fetal life, the structural features of the testis remain essentially unchanged, except for continuing growth of the seminiferous tubules. Spermatogenesis does not occur during fetal life and, in fact, does not commence until puberty. Unlike the ovary, meiotic division is not initiated in the testis of the fetus; the factor(s) responsible for this difference remains unknown (49,62).

FUNCTIONAL DEVELOPMENT OF THE TESTIS

The classic experiments of Jost (47–49) established a fetal testicular endocrine role. Early fetal castration in both sexes resulted in feminine genital duct differentiation. Androgens could replace the masculinizing influence of the testes but failed to inhibit Müllerian duct development. Thus, the fetal testis produces two types of morphogenetic substances: steroidal androgens and a nonsteroidal inhibitor of Müllerian duct development.

Müllerian Inhibitory Factor

The Müllerian inhibitory factor (anti-Müllerian hormone) (Fig. 2) (45) originates from the Sertoli cells and appears to be a large protein, estimated weight 200,000–320,000 daltons. Inhibitory activity of the fetal testis can be demonstrated as early as 7 to 8 weeks of fetal age by its effect upon fetal rat Müllerian ducts, that is, at the time when the testis begins to differentiate. This activity decreases when all the seminiferous tubules have completed their canalization (26 to 28 weeks); activity remains low until term, with eventual disappearance early in neonatal life. Müllerian duct regression is first observed at 8 weeks in male fetuses, just following the appearance of Müllerian inhibitory activity; after 10 weeks only vestigial duct remnants are found (30,31). The significance of the continued presence of Müllerian inhibitory activity following duct regression is unknown.

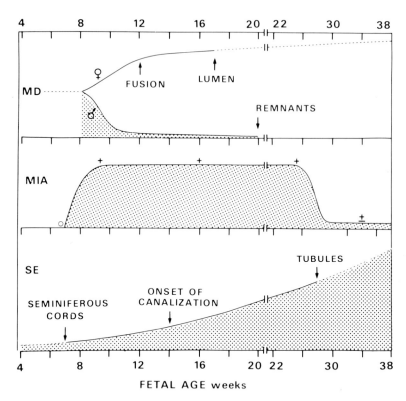

FIG. 2. Müllerian duct (MD) differentiation. Müllerian inhibitory activity (MIA), and seminiferous epithelium (SE) growth in the human, after data from different authors (see text). (From ref. 76.)

Production of Sex Steroids

The recognition of extensive Leydig cell proliferation in young fetuses (14) provided the first suggestive evidence for testicular steroid synthesis. Subsequent histochemical studies documented the presence of key enzymes for steroidogenesis (60), and ultrastructural observations (32,66) also were indicative of active steroid hormone biosynthesis.

Direct evidence that the Leydig cells of the fetal testis could produce androgens came from *in vitro* incubation and *in vivo* perfusion studies which demonstrated testosterone synthesis either from acetate or from precursor steroid sulfates (3,13,59,65,78,82,89). The temporal pattern of this synthesis coincides closely with that for differentiation of the male urogenital tract in that testosterone formation begins at about 8 weeks of fetal age and is maximal at 12 to 13 weeks (86).

Testosterone is the principal steroid found in extracts of fetal testes (41,74). The relationships of gonadal testosterone concentration, gonadal weight and

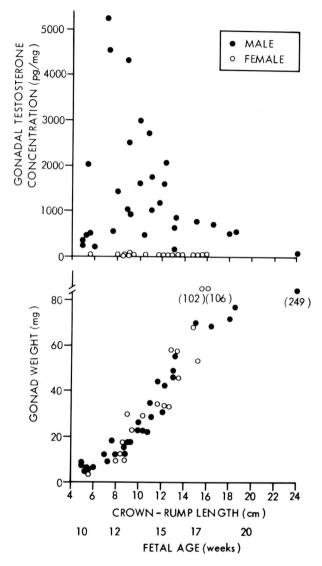

FIG. 3. Gonadal testosterone concentrations and total wet weight (organ pairs) in male and female fetuses as a function of crown-rump length and fetal age. (From ref. 74.)

fetal age in both sexes are shown in Fig. 3. Testosterone is present in the testes of the youngest fetuses studied (10 weeks). There is a brisk rise in testicular testosterone concentration to a peak at about 12 weeks, and then a decline. This pattern correlates well with the initial growth and later involution of fetal Leydig cells as well as with the timing of *in vitro* synthesis of testosterone from radiolabeled precursors (86), and thus presumably reflects testicular pro-

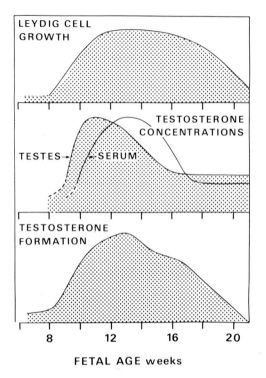

FIG. 4. Leydig cell growth and testosterone production by human fetal testes. (From refs. 30,73,74,76,86.)

duction (see Fig. 4). In contrast, testosterone concentrations are negligible in the ovaries and in the adrenals of both sexes (74). Only small amounts of estradiol are found in extracts of fetal testes which can probably be accounted for by the estradiol present in trapped serum and interstitial fluid (74).

SEX STEROIDS IN SERUM AND IN AMNIOTIC FLUID

Serum

The strong evidence, alluded to previously, implying active testosterone secretion by the fetal testis has been borne out by analysis of serum testosterone concentrations during the period of genital differentiation (2,23,73,88). As can be seen in Fig. 5, serum testosterone levels in male fetuses parallel the rise and fall of testicular testosterone concentrations (Fig. 3), whereas levels in female fetuses are substantially lower and show no change during gestation. Serum testosterone concentrations in male fetuses peak at 14 to 16 weeks, somewhat later than the peak in gonadal testosterone (Fig. 3), and can reach the adult male range (230–1,000 ng/dl). After 24 weeks of age, until term, the sex difference

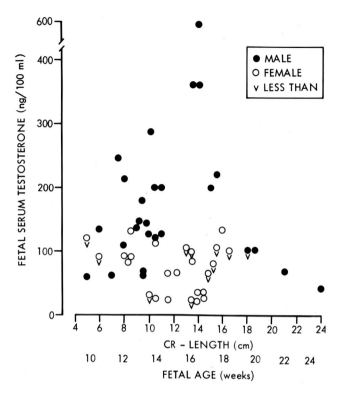

FIG. 5. Fetal serum testosterone concentrations as a function of age. (From ref. 73.)

in circulating testosterone concentrations virtually disappears (88,98) although umbilical arterial levels may be slightly higher in male than in female newborns (26). Since there is no evidence for significant testosterone synthesis by either fetal adrenals or ovaries (50,64,74,81,89), it is likely that the circulating testosterone in female fetuses, as well as a portion of that in the sera of males, reflects placental androgen production (53).

The ontogenesis of sex hormone binding globulin (SHBG) is unknown. In postnatal life the bulk of unconjugated testosterone and estradiol circulates tightly bound to SHBG; the biologically active component appears to be the small fraction of unbound or free testosterone in serum (5). The percentage of free testosterone in newborns of both sexes is approximately 3%, that is, about threefold higher than in older neonates and adults (27). Therefore, the fetus may be exposed to higher levels of biologically active testosterone than would have been predicted on the basis of total testosterone values. It is possible, however, that the large concentrations of estradiol and progesterone (see below) found in both sexes play an important protective role at the target tissue level against excessive androgenic activity (71). Unlike the situation in some other species it does not appear that α-fetoprotein binds sex steroids in the human (87).

Serum estradiol levels (Fig. 6) show no significant sex difference in human fetuses (73,84) or newborns (11,98), nor are maternal estradiol values influenced by fetal sex (73). The concentrations on both the fetal and maternal sides are similar from 10 to 18 weeks (Fig. 6). Values in the fetus show greater variability than those in the mother, and most are well above the maximum levels (approximately 30 ng/dl) seen in the nonpregnant state. The absence of a sex difference in circulating estradiol and the *in vitro* evidence indicating that the young fetal gonad is unable to aromatize (64,77) agree with the notion that the bulk of circulating estradiol in the fetus and in the mother is of placental origin (22,85). Estradiol levels increase during late gestation on both the fetal and maternal sides, but at term maternal concentrations are approximately threefold higher

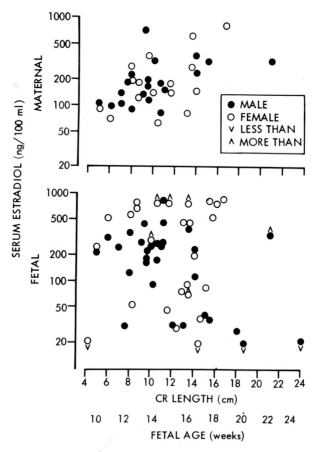

FIG. 6. Semilogarithmic plot of maternal and fetal serum estradiol-17β concentrations as a function of fetal age. (From ref. 73.)

than in the fetus. Apart from some observations in monkeys (54), and histological and histochemical findings in humans (69), there is no available evidence for fetal ovarian steroid secretion during the last weeks prior to birth.

Although the human fetal ovary is able to synthesize progesterone (64,77) most, if not all, of the circulating progesterone is of placental origin (22). No information is available on circulating progesterone levels during fetal life. Mixed umbilical cord progesterone concentrations are similar in both sexes and higher than maternal values at term (38). The finding that the umbilical venous-arterial concentration difference is greater in females, however, raises the possibilities of a sex difference in progesterone utilization and in placental progesterone production.

Amniotic Fluid

Since amniotic fluid is accessible to sampling, at least after 14 weeks gestation, a number of investigators have examined this fluid to assess whether or not it might accurately reflect the hormonal milieu in the fetal compartment.

Unconjugated testosterone concentrations in amniotic fluid show a striking parallelism to those seen in fetal serum (10,24,29,94). Concentrations in pregnancies bearing male fetuses, between 8 to 20 weeks, average approximately 20 ng/dl and are 3- to 10-fold higher than those in ones bearing females. Values in females remain low throughout gestation (<10 ng/dl). Levels decline in males from 20 weeks to term but remain slightly higher than those seen in females.

Estradiol concentrations are similar in both sexes. Levels decline slightly from 8 to 20 weeks and increase from 32 weeks to term (79,95). The pattern resembles that seen in fetal serum. Although data are limited, fetal serum concentrations also show no appreciable change until 34 weeks, following which there is a brisk rise to term (84). In contrast, maternal levels rise steadily throughout pregnancy (90).

Progesterone concentrations in amniotic fluid are highest between 10 to 19 weeks gestation, and decline late in pregnancy (94). No sex difference is apparent. This pattern cannot be compared to the situation in the fetus since no data are available on fetal serum, save for the fact that cord levels at term are high. The pattern, however, is quite different from that seen in the maternal compartment, in which levels rise throughout pregnancy and are highest at, or near, term.

Thus, amniotic fluid estimations appear to accurately reflect the fetal environment in the case of testosterone, and perhaps estradiol as well. The situation regarding progesterone requires further study.

TARGET ORGAN RESPONSES TO FETAL STEROIDS

Prior to 8 weeks of fetal age the urogenital duct system is undifferentiated. In the absence of gonadal function the internal and external anlagen differentiate

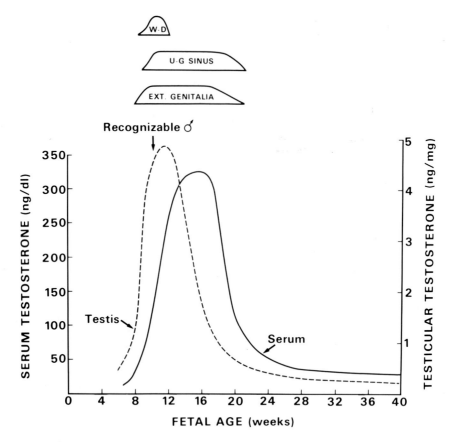

FIG. 7. The relationship of changes in mean testicular and serum testosterone concentrations to the time of development of the Wolffian ducts (W-D) and virilization of the urogenital (U-G) sinus and external genitalia in male fetuses. (From ref. 97.)

in the female pattern. Müllerian-inhibiting factor prevents development of the uterus and fallopian tubes in males (Fig. 2). The function of testosterone secretion by the testis is to stimulate the development of the epididymis, vas deferens, seminal vesicles and ejaculatory ducts from the Wolffian ducts. Moreover, testosterone promotes virilization of the urogenital sinus and the urogenital tubercle, leading to the formation of the prostate, male urethra, penis, and scrotum. The timing of these events, in relation to the patterns of testosterone concentrations in the testis and in serum, is shown in Fig. 7.

Differentiation of the male internal genitalia from the Wolffian ducts begins at about 8 weeks of fetal age. Jost has demonstrated that this early virilization represents a local rather than a systemic effect of testosterone (46), a finding that is in keeping with our observation that testosterone appears in the testes 1 to 2 weeks before serum concentrations begin to rise. This local effect of testosterone would explain why, in true hermaphrodites, male internal ducts differentiate only on the side of the testis, whereas on the opposite side one finds only Müllerian structures occasionally associated with a rudimentary vas deferens (46). Male differentiation of the urogenital sinus and external genitalia begins at 9 to 10 weeks (30,31,44) and appears to depend upon circulating testosterone. By the 10th week, male fetuses can be recognized from the appearance of the external genitalia. Coincident with the peak in serum testosterone levels (14–16 weeks), adult-like seminal vesicles become recognizable and the urethra reaches the meatus. The glans becomes covered by the prepuce and the prostate acquires its definitive form by about the 20th week.

The effective intracellular androgen for Wolffian duct development appears to be testosterone itself. Masculinization of both the urogenital sinus and external genital anlagen appears to be mediated by intracellular conversion of testosterone to its 5α-reduced metabolite, dihydrotestosterone. This is in keeping with the finding that these latter tissues have the capacity for enzymatic conversion prior to male differentiation (86) and would serve to explain the observations in recently described male pseudohermaphrodites in whom urogenital sinus and tubercle derivatives fail to masculinize (5α-reductase deficient) whereas Wolffian differentiation is entirely normal (67,93).

GONADOTROPIN CONTROL OF FETAL TESTICULAR DEVELOPMENT AND FUNCTION

Although it is possible that secretion of testosterone by the fetal testis is programmed directly by a genetic mechanism, and evidence suggests that at least Leydig cell differentiation can occur in the absence of gonadotropin stimulation (68), it seems likely that the testis in prenatal life, as in postnatal life, responds to gonadotropic stimulation. Certainly the fetal testis has receptors for luteinizing hormone (LH) and chorionic gonadotropin (CG) (15,28,42) and responds *in vitro* to CG with increased formation of cyclic AMP and synthesis of testosterone (1,4,42). Circulating gonadotropins in human and other mammalian fetuses may originate from either the fetal hypophysis or the placenta. This dual origin of gonadotropins raises the question as to whether testosterone secretion, and therefore genital differentiation, depends upon chorionic and/or pituitary gonadotropin stimulation.

Circulating Gonadotropins in Fetal Life

CG appears in the maternal circulation shortly after implantation of the blastocyst, about 9 to 13 days postovulation (16,52). Maternal serum CG levels peak at 8 to 10 weeks postconception and then decline to a nadir at 17 to 19 weeks (58,91). This pattern bears a close temporal correlation to the pattern of fetal testicular testosterone production and suggests that secretion of CG into fetal serum might be the major stimulus to fetal Leydig cell function.

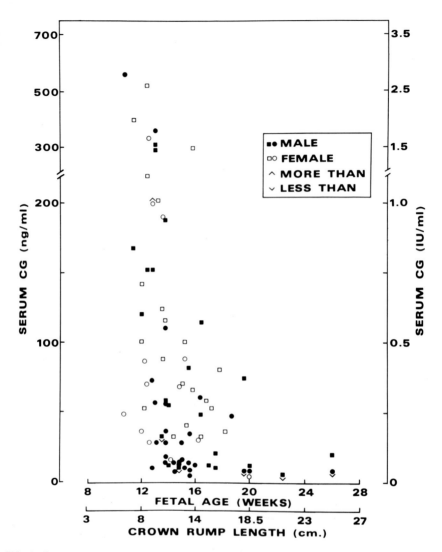

FIG. 8. Serum concentrations of CG in male and female fetuses as a function of crown-rump length and fetal age. Values shown by squares were obtained with a radioimmunoassay method utilizing an HCG antiserum and values shown by circles with an assay using an HCG β-subunit antiserum. (From ref. 18.)

Fetal serum CG concentrations are shown in Fig. 8. The pattern of fetal CG levels parallels that of maternal serum (18). However, in paired specimens the fetal concentrations are on an average $\frac{1}{31}$ of those in maternal serum (73). A close correlation is also seen with amniotic fluid concentrations (Fig. 9). The earliest amniotic fluid specimens examined (8–10 weeks) showed substantial

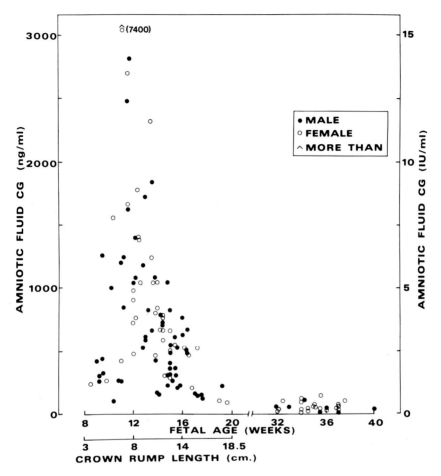

FIG. 9. Amniotic fluid CG concentrations by β-CG assay, expressed in nanograms pure CG and as IU of the 2nd International Standard of HCG/ml as a function of fetal age. (From ref. 18.)

amounts of CG. Peak levels were seen at 11 to 14 weeks followed by a decline in levels toward term. Thus, the CG patterns closely parallel the one observed for testosterone concentrations in the male fetus. Fetal sex does not influence maternal, fetal, or amniotic fluid CG concentrations during the time of sexual differentiation (18).

The fetal pituitary does not contain detectable amounts of CG (18). Synthesis and release of LH and FSH by fetal pituitaries in organ culture cannot be demonstrated until 11 weeks postconception (35); however, immunoreactive gonadotropins can be detected in pituitary extracts as early as 10 weeks fetal age (18,40,51) when LH cells first appear (7). Fetal pituitary concentrations of LH and FSH increase rapidly to peak levels at about 20 to 25 weeks and

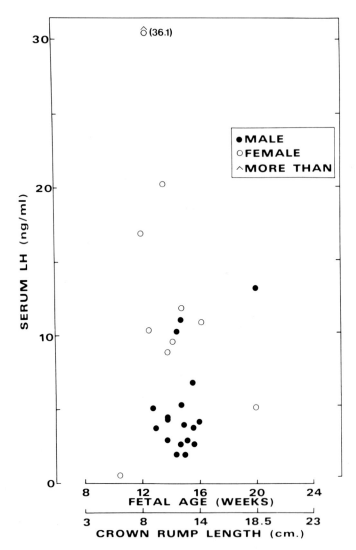

FIG. 10. Serum concentrations of LH measured by a specific LH β-subunit assay, as a function of crown-rump length and fetal age. (From ref. 18.)

then decline; in midgestation, pituitary concentrations of both gonadotropins are significantly higher in female than in male fetuses.

Concentrations of LH in fetal serum and in amniotic fluid are shown in Figs. 10 and 11; since maternal concentrations of LH (and FSH) are low or undetectable (75), amniotic fluid gonadotropins appear to be of fetal origin. In both sexes, LH appears in the fetal serum and amniotic fluid at about 11 to 12 weeks, later than the appearance of CG, and following by some 3 to 4

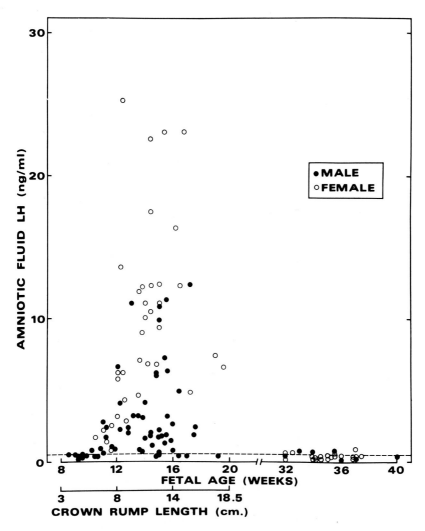

FIG. 11. Amniotic fluid concentrations of LH (determined by β-subunit assay) as a function of crown-rump length and fetal age. The horizontal dashed line indicates the limit of sensitivity of the assay. (From ref. 18.)

weeks the onset of testosterone production by the testis. LH concentrations rise to peak levels at 12 to 16 weeks and then decline in the latter half of pregnancy (39,51). From 12 to 20 weeks, serum and amniotic fluid LH levels are significantly higher in female fetuses (18,56).

Concentrations of FSH in fetal serum are shown in Fig. 12. The pattern for amniotic fluid is similar (18). As is the case for LH, FSH is low, or undetectable, prior to 12 weeks; values peak between 13 to 30 weeks and decline to

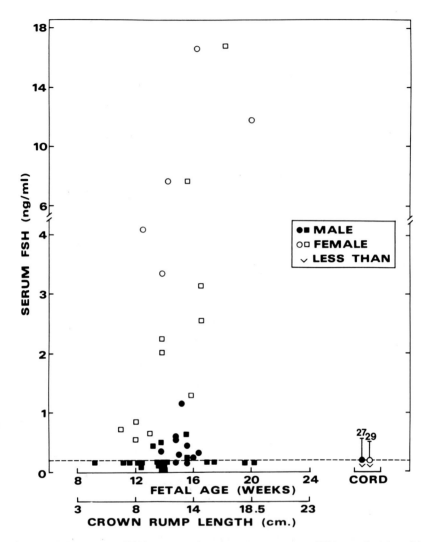

FIG. 12. Individual serum FSH concentrations in nanograms pure FSH as a function of fetal age. Cord values are shown as median and range with numeral above indicating number of samples. The dotted line indicates the detection limit of the assay (0.2 ng/ml). (From ref. 18.)

low values thereafter to term (18,39,51,56,88). The sex difference in FSH levels is striking: female fetal serum levels attain the adult castrate range, whereas male serum levels only occasionally reach the low normal adult range. By term, the major detectable gonadotropic components in fetal serum are CG and go-nadotropin α-subunit (39).

The Fetal Pituitary-Testicular Axis

The relationships in the male fetus of circulating concentrations of CG, LH and FSH, testicular development, and serum testosterone levels are summarized in Fig. 13. There is a close temporal relationship between patterns of CG and of testosterone; levels of both are clearly elevated during the critical period of Leydig cell and genital differentiation (8 to 12 weeks). Since LH is not detectable at this time, it seems reasonable to conclude that CG initiates these processes. During the later stages of genital differentiation (12–16 weeks), pituitary LH secretion begins and may influence Leydig cell function; but throughout gestation CG concentrations (in gravimetric terms) remain higher than those of LH.

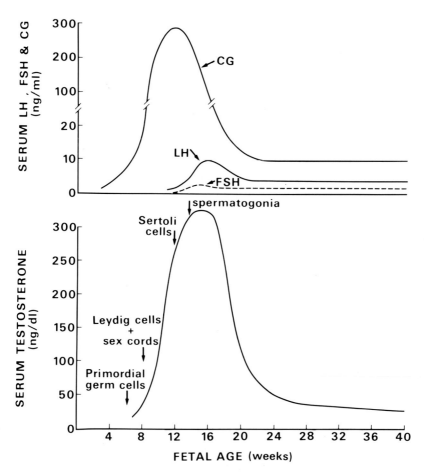

FIG. 13. A schematic summary of the temporal relationships between mean serum concentrations of CG, LH, and FSH, mean serum testosterone concentrations and morphologic development of the fetal testis. (From ref. 97.)

The various descriptions of normal male genital differentiation in apituitary and anencephalic fetuses (9,12,17,103) provide further indication that testicular testosterone secretion during the first trimester is mediated primarily by CG rather than LH. The occurrence of hypotrophic external genitalia and reduced numbers of testicular Leydig cells in these fetuses, however, indicates that LH may be instrumental in promoting androgen secretion after genital differentiation is complete.

It is of interest that both Sertoli cell differentiation and the transformation of primordial germ cells into spermatogonia occur when FSH appears in the fetal circulation. This coincidence does not confirm FSH's role in the differentiation of spermatogonia and Sertoli cells. But, taken together with the finding of retarded seminiferous tubule maturation in anencephalic or hypogonadotropic individuals (9,12,17,103) it does imply that such a role may exist. Further support for this contention comes from the recent studies by Gulyas et al. (36), who found a striking reduction in testicular weight and in the numbers of spermatogonia following fetal hypophysectomy in rhesus monkeys at 16 weeks gestation (average length of gestation 24 weeks).

Testicular Descent

Hypogonadotropic patients (8,80), like anencephalic fetuses (103), are frequently cryptorchid. The mechanism for testicular descent is unknown. Although there is negative evidence regarding an hormonal influence upon testicular descent (25), which occurs at a time (27–35 weeks) when gonadotropin levels and testicular androgen production have declined, recent findings in the rodent suggest a role for pituitary LH and testicular androgen in this process (37,70).

FETAL HYPOTHALAMIC AND PITUITARY REGULATION

In postnatal life, secretion of gonadotropins is regulated by the hypothalamic LH-releasing hormone (LH-RH) which reaches the pituitary gland via the hypothalamo-hypophyseal portal system. In turn, secretion of LH-RH is influenced by circulating sex steroids, which may also modulate the pituitary response to LH-RH.

Hypothalamic Regulation of Gonadotropin Secretion

There is a close temporal relationship between the anatomical and functional development of the fetal hypothalamus and pituitary. The median eminence of the tuber cinereum and the primordial pituitary are recognizable by 8 weeks of age (6,43). LH-RH immunoreactivity has been detected in the fetal hypothalamus at this time (100), while pituitary gonadotropins become identifiable 1 to 2 weeks later (18,51). Preliminary observations of fetal hypothalamic LH-RH content are shown in Fig. 14. In an unpublished study of 43 hypothalami from

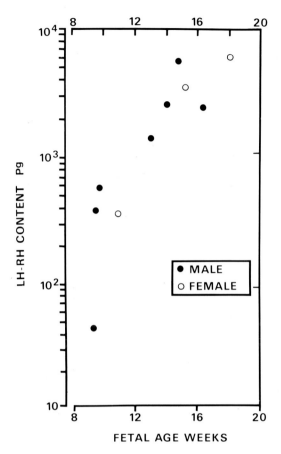

FIG. 14. Semilogarithmic plot of hypothalamic LH-RH content (by radioimmunoassay) from human fetuses in relation to age. (From ref. 76.)

8 to 18 week fetuses, an approximate 250-fold increment from 20 to 5,000 pg/hypothalamus was observed over this age span (19); no sex difference in values was seen. After 29 weeks, biologically assayed hypothalamic gonadotropin-releasing activity declines (55). The temporal relationship in patterns between hypothalamic LH-RH activity and circulating pituitary gonadotropins in the fetus, coupled with the findings that as early as 10 to 20 weeks the fetal pituitary is capable of enhanced synthesis and release of FSH and LH in response to LH-RH administration both *in vitro* (33,34) and *in vivo* (88), strongly suggest that the fetal pituitary is under the influence of hypothalamic regulation.

The establishment of a direct connection between the primary and the secondary plexuses of the hypothalamo-hypophyseal portal vasculature may not occur until 18 to 20 weeks of age (21,61). Thus, prior to this time if the hypothalamus is to influence pituitary secretion it may only act by local diffusion of regulatory factors. Gonadotropin-releasing hormone could diffuse either directly [the pars tuberalis and the tuber cinereum are distinctly vascularized from early stages (6)] or indirectly via the cerebrospinal fluid of the infundibular recess into the pars distalis. The possibility remains, however, that secretion of FSH and LH in younger fetuses, at least, is independent of hypothalamic regulation.

Development of Feedback Mechanisms

The striking sex difference in circulating FSH and LH levels in midgestation (Figs. 10 and 12) suggests that testosterone in the male fetus (Fig. 5) suppresses gonadotropin release. Preliminary observations *(unpublished)* in rhesus monkey fetuses support this contention: orchidectomy, which is known to result in a diminution in circulating testosterone levels (72), results in increased FSH and LH levels, whereas ovariectomy has no apparent effect. Since, as previously mentioned, hypothalamic LH-RH content is the same in both sexes, the implication is that the sexual dimorphism in regulation of pituitary gonadotropin secretion at this time involves feedback recognition at the level of the pituitary.

The absence of gonadotropin suppression in the midgestation human female fetus, despite generous levels of circulating levels of estradiol (Fig. 6), indicates the absence of hypothalamic or pituitary receptors for estrogen-mediated feedback. The subsequent decline in gonadotropin concentrations to low levels by term in both sexes, as well as the apparently concomitant fall in hypothalamic LH-RH activity (55), presumably reflect maturation of this feedback mechanism. The recent finding of specific estrogen-binding cytosol receptors in the pituitary, hypothalamus, and other neural structures from midgestation fetuses of both sexes (20) is in accord with this hypothesis.

SUMMARY AND CONCLUSIONS

Normal male genital differentiation requires fetal testicular secretion of both testosterone and the nonsteroidal Müllerian-inhibitory factor. It appears that secretion of testosterone, at least during the critical period of differentiation, occurs in response to stimulation by CG, although pituitary LH may influence Leydig cell function in later fetal life. Fetal pituitary gonadotropin secretion appears to be required for germ cell proliferation and possibly for testicular descent into the scrotal position as well.

The pattern of FSH and LH secretion in the fetus reflects gradual maturation of a functional hypothalamo-pituitary unit responsive to feedback inhibition by sex steroids. The higher levels of gonadotropins in female fetuses from 12 to 30 weeks suggest either that maturation occurs earlier in males than in females, or, more probably, that feedback recognition of androgens is established before that of estrogens. The decline in FSH and LH production in both sexes later in gestation seems to indicate the acquisition of an estrogen-mediated feedback mechanism at this time, as does the appearance of estrogen receptors in the pituitary and hypothalamus.

The decline in testosterone secretion later in gestation in male fetuses is probably a reflection of decreased chorionic and pituitary gonadotropin stimulation, although additional influences, such as prolactin or estradiol, may directly inhibit Leydig cell function at this time (83,99).

Thus, the interrelationships among testicular, pituitary, and hypothalamic development and function during fetal life are complex. Although much information has recently become available, it is obvious that further exploration is needed to clarify the intricacies of this endocrine axis. Furthermore, to what extent exposure of the mother and developing fetus to environmental or pharmacological agents may perturb the system and lead to possible problems postnatally, such as in the onset and course of puberty, future fertility, and adult sex-related behavior, remains unknown and subjects worthy of future investigation.

ACKNOWLEDGMENTS

The studies from the author's laboratory were supported by the Medical Research Council of Canada (Grant PG-5) and the Children's Hospital Research Foundation. We are grateful to Dr. Jim Thliveris for providing us with Fig. 1. We thank Cheryl Hunter for typing this manuscript.

REFERENCES

1. Abramovich, D. R., Baker, T. G., and Neal, P. (1974): Effect of human chorionic gonadotrophin on testosterone secretion by the foetal human testis in organ culture. *J. Endocrinol.,* 60:179–185.
2. Abramovich, D. R., and Rowe, P. (1973): Foetal plasma testosterone levels at midpregnancy and at term: relationship to foetal sex. *J. Endocrinol.,* 56:621–622.
3. Acevedo, H. F., Axelrod, L. R., Ishikawa, E., and Takaki, F. (1963): Studies in fetal metabolism. II. Metabolism of progesterone-4-C^{14} and pregnenolone-7α-H$_3$ in human fetal testes. *J. Clin. Endocrinol. Metab.,* 23:885–890.
4. Ahluwalia, B., Williams, J., and Verma, P. (1974): In vitro testosterone biosynthesis in the human fetal testis. II. Stimulation by cyclic AMP and human chorionic gonadotropin (hCG). *Endocrinology,* 95:1411–1415.
5. Anderson, D. C. (1974): Sex-hormone-binding globulin. *Clin. Endocrinol.,* 3:69–96.
6. Atwell, W. J. (1926): The development of the hypophysis cerebri in man, with special reference to the pars tuberalis. *Am. J. Anat.,* 37:159–179.
7. Baker, B. L., and Jaffe, R. B. (1975): The genesis of cell types in the adenohypophysis of the human fetus as observed with immunocytochemistry. *Am. J. Anat.,* 143:137–162.
8. Bardin, C. W., Ross, G. R., Rifkind, A. B., Cargille, C. M., and Lipsett, M. B. (1969): Studies of the pituitary-Leydig cell axis in young men with hypogonadotropic hypogonadism and hyposmia. *J. Clin. Invest.,* 48:2046–2056.
9. Bearn, J. G. (1968): Anencephaly and the development of the male genital tract. *Acta Paediatr. Acad. Sci. (Hung.),* 9:159–180.
10. Belisle, S., Fencl, M. deM., and Tulchinsky, D. (1977): Amniotic fluid testosterone and follicle-stimulating hormone in the determination of fetal sex. *Am. J. Obstet. Gynecol.,* 128:514–519.
11. Bidlingmaier, F., Versmold, H., and Knorr, D. (1974): Plasma estrogens in newborns and

infants. In: *Sexual Endocrinology of the Perinatal Period,* edited by M. G. Forest and J. Bertrand, pp. 299–314. Editions INSERM, Paris.

12. Blizzard, R. M., and Alberts, M. (1956): Hypopituitarism, hypoadrenalism and hypogonadism in the newborn infant. *J. Pediatr.,* 48:782–783.
13. Bloch, E. (1964): Metabolism of 4-^{14}C-progesterone by human fetal testes and ovaries. *Endocrinology,* 74:833–845.
14. Bouin, P., and Ancel, P. (1903): Sur la signification de la glande interstitielle du testicule embryonnaire. *C.R. Soc. Biol.,* 55:1682–1684.
15. Catt, K. J., Dufau, M. L., Neaves, W. B., Walsh, P. C., and Wilson, J. D. (1975): LH-hCG receptors and testosterone content during differentiation of the testis in the rabbit embryo. *Endocrinology,* 97:1157–1165.
16. Catt, K. J., Dufau, M. L., and Vaitukaitis, J. L. (1975): Appearance of hCG in pregnancy plasma following the initiation of implantation of the blastocyst. *J. Clin. Endocrinol. Metab.,* 40:537–540.
17. Ch'in, K. Y. (1938): The endocrine glands of anencephalic foetuses. *Chin. Med. J.,* (Suppl. 2): 63–90.
18. Clements, J. A., Reyes, F. I., Winter, J. S. D., and Faiman, C. (1976): Studies on human sexual development: III. Fetal pituitary, serum and amniotic fluid concentrations of LH, CG and FSH. *J. Clin. Endocrinol. Metab.,* 42:9–19.
19. Clements, J. A., Reyes, F. I., Winter, J. S. D., and Faiman, C. (1980): Ontogenesis of gonadotropin releasing hormone in the human fetal hypothalamus. *Proc. Soc. Exp. Biol. Med. (in press).*
20. Davies, I. J., Naftolin, F., Ryan, K. J., and Siu, V. (1975): A specific, high affinity, limited-capacity estrogen binding component in the cytosol of human fetal pituitary and brain tissues. *J. Clin. Endocrinol. Metab.,* 40:909–912.
21. D'Espinasse, P. G. (1933): The development of the hypophyseal portal system in man. *J. Anat.,* 68:11–18.
22. Diczfalusy, E., and Troen, P. (1961): Endocrine functions of human placenta. *Vitam. Horm.,* 19:229–311.
23. Diez D'Aux, R. C., and Murphy, B. E. P. (1974): Androgens in the human fetus. *J. Steroid Biochem.,* 5:207–210.
24. Dörner, G., Stahl, F., and Baumgarten, G. (1972): Signifikante Unterschiede im Testosteronund 11-OHCS-Gehalt des Fruchtwassers zwischen männlichen und weiblichen Föten. *Endokrinologie,* 60:285–288.
25. Elger, W. (1966): Die Rolle der fetalen Androgene in der Sexual-differenzierung des Kaninchens und ihre Abgrenzung gegen andere hormonale und somatische Faktoren durch Anwendung eines starken Antiandrogens. *Arch. Anat. Microsc. Morphol. Exp.,* 55:657–743.
26. Forest, M. G., and Cathiard, A. M. (1975): Pattern of plasma testosterone and Δ^4-androstenedione in normal newborns: evidence for testicular activity at birth. *J. Clin. Endocrinol. Metab.,* 41:977–980.
27. Forest, M. G., Cathiard, A. M., and Bertrand, J. A. (1973): Total and unbound testosterone levels in the newborn and in normal and hypogonadal children. *J. Clin. Endocrinol. Metab.,* 36:1132–1142.
28. Frawein, J., and Engel, W. (1974): Constitutivity of the HCG-receptor protein in the testis of rat and man. *Nature,* 249:377–379.
29. Giles, H. R., Lox, C. D., Heine, M. W., and Christian, C. D. (1974): Intrauterine fetal sex determination by radioimmunoassay of amniotic fluid testosterone. *Gynecol. Invest.,* 5:317–323.
30. Gillman, J. (1948): The development of the gonads in man with a consideration of the role of the fetal endocrines and the histogenesis of ovarian tumors. *Contrib. Embryol. Carnegie Inst.,* 32:81–131.
31. Glenister, T. W. (1962): The development of the utricle and of the so-called middle or median lobe of the human prostate. *J. Anat.,* 96:443–455.
32. Gondos, B., and Hobel, C. J. (1971): Ultrastructure of germ cell development in the human fetal testis. *Z. Zellforsch.,* 119:1–20.
33. Goodyer, C. G., St. George Hall, C., Guyda, H., Robert, F., and Giroud, C. J.-P. (1977): Human fetal pituitary in culture: hormone secretion and response to somatostatin, luteinizing hormone releasing factor, thyrotropin releasing factor and dibutyryl cyclic AMP. *J. Clin. Endocrinol. Metab.,* 45:73–85.

34. Groom, G. V., and Boyns, A. R. (1973): Effect of hypothalamic releasing factors and steroids on release of gonadotrophins by organ cultures of human foetal pituitaries. *J. Endocrinol.,* 59:511–522.
35. Groom, G. V., Groom, M. A., Cooke, I. D., and Boyns, A. R. (1971): The secretion of immuno-reactive luteinizing hormone and follicle-stimulating hormone by the human foetal pituitary in organ culture. *J. Endocrinol.,* 49:335–344.
36. Gulyas, B. J., Tullner, W. W., and Hodgen, G. D. (1977): Fetal or maternal hypophysectomy in rhesus monkeys (Macaca mulatta): effects on the development of testes and other endocrine organs. *Biol. Reprod.,* 17:650–660.
37. Hadziselimovic, F., and Girard, J. (1977): Pathogenesis of cryptorchidism. *Hormone Res.,* 8:76–83.
38. Hagemenas, F. C., and Kittinger, G. W. (1973): The influence of fetal sex on the levels of plasma progesterone in the human fetus. *J. Clin. Endocrinol. Metab.,* 36:389–391.
39. Hagen, C., and McNeilly, A. S. (1975): The gonadotropic hormones and their subunits in human maternal and fetal circulation at delivery. *Amer. J. Obstet. Gynecol.,* 121:926–930.
40. Hagen, C., and McNeilly, A. S. (1975): Identification of human luteinizing hormone, follicle-stimulating hormone, luteinizing hormone β-subunit and gonadotropin α-subunit in foetal and adult pituitary glands. *J. Endocrinol.,* 67:49–57.
41. Huhtaniemi, I., Ikonen, M., and Vihko, R. (1970): Presence of testosterone and other neutral steroids in human fetal testes. *Biochem. Biophys. Res. Commun.,* 38:715–720.
42. Huhtaniemi, I. T., Korenbrot, C. C., and Jaffe, R. B. (1977): hCG binding and stimulation of testosterone biosynthesis in the human fetal testis. *J. Clin. Endocrinol. Metab.,* 44:963–967.
43. Hyyppä, M. (1972): Hypothalamic monoamines in human fetuses. *Neuroendocrinology,* 9:257–266.
44. Jirasek, J. E. (1977): Morphogenesis of the genital system in the human. In: *Birth Defects,* Original Article Series, Vol. 13, No. 2: Morphogenesis and Malformation of the Genital System, edited by R. J. Blandau and D. Bergsma, pp. 13–39. Alan R. Liss, New York.
45. Josso, N., Picard, J. Y., and Tran, D. (1977): The anti-Müllerian hormone. In: *Birth Defects,* Original Article Series, Vol. 13, No. 2: Morphogenesis and Malformation of the Genital System, edited by R. J. Blandau and D. Bergsma, pp. 59–84. Alan R. Liss, New York.
46. Jost, A. (1947): Sur le rôle des gonades foetales dans la différenciation sexuelle somatique de l'embryon de lapin. *C.R. Assoc. Anat.,* 34:255–262.
47. Jost, A. (1947): Recherches sur la différenciation sexuelle de l'embryon de lapin: II. Action des androgens de synthese sur l'histogenèse génitale. *Arch. Anat. Microsc. Morphol. Exp.,* 36:242–270.
48. Jost, A. (1947): Recherches sur la différenciation sexuelle de l'embryon de lapin. III. Rôle des gonades foetales dans la différenciation sexuelle somatique. *Arch. Anat. Microsc. Morphol. Exp.,* 36:271–315.
49. Jost, A., Vigier, B., Prépin, J., and Perchelet, J. P. (1973): Studies on sex differentiation in mammals. *Recent Prog. Horm. Res.,* 29:1–35.
50. Jungmann, R. A., and Schweppe, J. S. (1968): Biosynthesis of sterols and steroids from acetate-^{14}C by human fetal ovaries. *J. Clin. Endocrinol. Metab.,* 28:1599–1604.
51. Kaplan, S. L., Grumbach, M. M., and Aubert, M. L. (1976): The ontogenesis of pituitary hormones and hypothalamic factors in the human fetus: maturation of central nervous system regulation of anterior pituitary function. *Recent Prog. Horm. Res.,* 32:161–243.
52. Kosasa, T. S., Levesque, L. A., Taymor, M. L., and Goldstein, D. P. (1974): Measurement of early chorionic activity with a radioimmunoassay specific for human chorionic gonadotropin following spontaneous and induced ovulation. *Fertil. Steril.,* 25:211–216.
53. Lamb, E., Mancuso, S., Dell' Acqua, S., Wiqvist, H., and Diczfalusy, E. (1967): Studies on the metabolism of C-19 steroids in the human foetoplantal unit. *Acta. Endocrinol.,* 55:263–277.
54. Lemons, J. A., Foster, D. L., and Jaffe, R. B. (1974): Aromatization by the immature rhesus ovary. *Endocrinology,* 94:1181–1184.
55. Levina, S. E. (1971): Sexual differentiation in epiphyseal and hypothalamic regulation of the secretion of follicle-stimulating hormone and luteinizing hormone by fetal hypophyses cultured in vitro. In: *Hormones in Development,* edited by M. Hamburgh and E. J. W. Barrington, pp. 547–552. Appleton-Century-Crofts, New York.

56. Levina, S. E. (1972): Times of appearance of LH and FSH activities in human fetal circulation. *Gen. Comp. Endocrinol.,* 19:242–246.
57. Mancini, R. E., Vilar, O., Lavieri, J. C., Andrada, J. A., and Heinrich, J. J. (1963): Development of Leydig cells in the normal human testis. *Am. J. Anat.,* 112:203–210.
58. Marshall, J. R., Hammond, C. B., Ross, G. T., Jacobson, A., Rayford, P., and Odell, W. D. (1968): Plasma and urinary chorionic gonadotropin during early human pregnancy. *Obstet. Gynecol.,* 32:760–764.
59. Mathur, R. S., Wiqvist, N., and Diczfalusy, E. (1972): De novo synthesis of steroids and steroid sulphates by the testicles of the human foetus at midgestation. *Acta Endocrinol.,* 71:792–800.
60. Niemi, M., Ikonen, M., and Hervonen, A. (1967): Histochemistry and fine structure of interstitial tissue in human foetal testis. In: *Endocrinology of the Testes, Ciba Found. Colloq. Endocrinol.,* 16:31–55.
61. Niminieva, K. (1949): Observations on the development of the hypophyseal portal system. *Acta Paediatr. Scand.,* 39:366–377.
62. O, W-S., and Short, R. V. (1977): Sex determination and differentiation in mammalian germ cells. In : *Birth Defects,* Original Article Series, Vol. 13, No. 2: Morphogenesis and Malformation of the Genital System, edited by R. J. Blandau and D. Bergsma, pp. 1–12. Alan R. Liss, New York.
63. Ohno, S. (1977): Testosterone and cellular response. In: *Birth Defects,* Original Article Series, Vol. 13, No. 2: Morphogenesis and Malformation of the Genital System, edited by R. J. Blandau and D. Bergsma, pp. 99–106. Alan R. Liss, New York.
64. Payne, A. H., and Jaffe, R. B. (1974): Androgen formation from pregnenolone sulfate by the human fetal ovary. *J. Clin. Endocrinol. Metab.,* 39:300–304.
65. Payne, A. H., and Jaffe, R. B. (1975): Androgen formation from pregnenolone sulfate by fetal, neonatal, prepubertal and adult human testes. *J. Clin. Endocrinol. Metab.,* 40:102–107.
66. Pelliniemi, L. J., and Niemi, M. (1969): Fine structure of the human foetal testis. *Z. Zellforsch.,* 99:507–522.
67. Peterson, R. E., Imperato-McGinley, J., Gautier, T., and Sturla, E. (1977): Male pseudohermaphroditism due to steroid 5α-reductase deficiency. *Am. J. Med.,* 62:170–191.
68. Picon, R. (1976): Testosterone secretion by foetal rat testes in vitro. *J. Endocrinol.,* 71:231–238.
69. Pinkerton, J. H. M., McKay, D. G., Adams, E. C., and Hertig, A. G. (1961): Development of the human ovary—a study using histochemical techniques. *Obstet. Gynecol.,* 18:152–181.
70. Raifer, J., and Walsh, P. C. (1977): Testicular descent. In: *Birth Defects,* Original Article Series, Vol. 13, No. 2: Morphogenesis and Malformation of the Genital System, edited by R. J. Blandau and D. Bergsma, pp. 107–122. Alan R. Liss, New York.
71. Resko, J. A. (1975): Fetal hormones and their effect on the differentiation of the central nervous system in primates. *Fed. Proc.,* 34:1650–1655.
72. Resko, J. A., Malley, A., Begley, D., and Hess, D. L. (1973): Radioimmunoassay of testosterone during fetal development of the rhesus monkey. *Endocrinology,* 93:156–161.
73. Reyes, F. I., Boroditsky, R. S., Winter, J. S. D., and Faiman, C. (1974): Studies on human sexual development. II. Fetal and maternal serum gonadotropin and sex steroid concentrations. *J. Clin. Endocrinol. Metab.,* 38:612–617.
74. Reyes, F. I., Winter, J. S. D., and Faiman, C. (1973): Studies on human sexual development. I. Fetal gonadal and adrenal sex steroids. *J. Clin. Endocrinol. Metab.,* 37:74–78.
75. Reyes, F. I., Winter, J. S. D., and Faiman, C. (1976): Pituitary gonadotropin function during human pregnancy: Serum FSH and LH levels before and after LH-RH administration. *J. Clin. Endocrinol. Metab.,* 42:590–592.
76. Reyes, F. I., Winter, J. S. D., and Faiman, C. (1976): Gonadotropin-gonadal interrelationships in the fetus. In: *Diabetes and other Endocrine Disorders During Pregnancy and in the Newborn,* edited by M. I. New and R. H. Fiser, Jr., pp. 83–106. Alan R. Liss, New York.
77. Rice, B. F., Jacks, K., Smith, B., and Sternberg, W. H. (1971): Steroid hormone synthesis by human fetal adrenal and gonadal tissues. *Prog. Endocr. Soc.,* 53rd Meeting, Abstract, p. 249.
78. Rice, B. F., Johanson, C. A., and Sternberg, W. H. (1966): Formation of steroid hormones from acetate-1-^{14}C by a human fetal testis preparation grown in organ culture. *Steroids,* 7:79–89.

79. Robinson, J. D., Judd, H. L., Young, P. E., Jones, O. W., and Yen, S. S. C. (1977): Amniotic fluid androgens and estrogens in midgestation. *J. Clin. Endocrinol. Metab.,* 45:755–761.
80. Santen, R. J., and Paulsen, C. A. (1973): Hypogonadotropic eunuchoidism. II. Gonadal responsiveness to exogenous gonadotropins. *J. Clin. Endocrinol. Metab.,* 36:47–54.
81. Schindler, A. F., and Friedrich, E. (1975): Steroid metabolism of foetal tissues. I. Metabolism of pregnenolone-4-¹⁴C by human foetal ovaries. *Endokrinologie,* 65:72–79.
82. Serra, G. V., Pérez-Palacios, and Jaffe, R. B. (1970): De novo testosterone biosynthesis in the human fetal testis. *J. Clin. Endocrinol. Metab.,* 30:128–130.
83. Sholiton, L. J., Srivastava, L., and Taylor, B. B. (1975): The in-vitro and in-vivo effects of diethylstilbestrol on testicular synthesis of testosterone. *Steroids,* 26:797–806.
84. Shutt, D. A., Smith, I. D., and Shearman, R. P. (1974): Oestrone, oestradiol-17β and oestriol levels in human foetal plasma during gestation and at term. *J. Endocrinol.,* 60:333–341.
85. Siiteri, P. K., and MacDonald, P. C. (1966): Placental estrogen biosynthesis during human pregnancy. *J. Clin. Endocrinol. Metab.,* 26:751–761.
86. Siiteri, P. K., and Wilson, J. D. (1974): Testosterone formation and metabolism during male sexual differentiation in the human embryo. *J. Clin. Endocrinol. Metab.,* 38:113–125.
87. Swartz, S. K., and Soloff, M. S. (1974): The lack of estrogen binding by human α-fetoprotein. *J. Clin. Endocrinol. Metab.,* 39:589–591.
88. Takagi, S., Yoshida, T., Tsubata, K., Ozaki, H., Fujii, T. K., Nomura, Y., and Sawada, M. (1977): Sex differences in fetal gonadotropins and androgens. *J. Steroid Biochem.,* 8:609–620.
89. Taylor, T., Coutts, J. R. T., and Macnaughton, M. C. (1974): Human foetal synthesis of testosterone from perfused progesterone. *J. Endocrinol.,* 60:321–326.
90. Tulchinsky, D. (1973): Placental secretion of unconjugated estrone, estradiol, and estriol into the maternal and fetal circulation. *J. Clin. Endocrinol. Metab.,* 36:1079–1087.
91. Varma, K., Larraga, L., and Selenkow, H. A. (1971): Radioimmunoassay of serum human chorionic gonadotropin during normal pregnancy. *Obstet. Gynecol.,* 37:10–18.
92. Wachtel, S. S., Ohno, S., Koo, G. C., and Boyce, E. A. (1975): Possible role of H-Y antigen in the primary determination of sex. *Nature,* 257:235–236.
93. Walsh, P. C., Madden, J. D., Harrod, M. J., Goldstein, J. L., MacDonald, P. C., and Wilson, J. D. (1974): Familial incomplete male pseudohermaphroditism, Type 2; decreased dihydrotestosterone formation in pseudovaginal perineoscrotal hypospadias. *N. Engl. J. Med.,* 291:1097–1103.
94. Warne, G. L., Faiman, C., Reyes, F. I., and Winter, J. S. D. (1977): Studies on human sexual development. V. Concentrations of testosterone, 17-hydroxyprogesterone and progesterone in human amniotic fluid throughout gestation. *J. Clin. Endocrinol. Metab.,* 44:934–938.
95. Warne, G. L., Reyes, F. I., Faiman, C., and Winter, J. S. D. (1978): Studies on human sexual development. VI. Concentrations of unconjugated dehydroepiandrosterone, estradiol and estriol in amniotic fluid throughout gestation. *J. Clin. Endocrinol. Metab.,* 47:1363–1367.
96. Welshons, W. J., and Russell, L. B. (1959): The Y-chromosome as the bearer of male determining factors in the mouse. *Proc. Natl. Acad. Sci. USA,* 45:560–566.
97. Winter, J. S. D., Faiman, C., and Reyes, F. I. (1977): Sex steroid production by the human fetus: its role in morphogenesis and control by gonadotropins. In: *Birth Defects,* Original Article Series, Vol. 13, No. 2: Morphogenesis and Malformation of the Genital System, edited by R. J. Blandau and D. Bergsma, pp. 41–58. Alan R. Liss, New York.
98. Winter, J. S. D., Hughes, I. A., Reyes, F. I., and Faiman, C. (1976): Pituitary-gonadal relations in infancy: 2. Patterns of serum gonadal steroid concentrations in man from birth to two years of age. *J. Clin. Endocrinol. Metab.,* 42:679–686.
99. Winters, A. J., Colston, C., MacDonald, P. C., and Porter, J. C. (1975): Fetal plasma prolactin levels. *J. Clin. Endocrinol. Metab.,* 41:626–629.
100. Winters, A. J., Eskay, R. L., and Porter, J. C. (1974): Concentration and distribution of TRH and LRH in the human fetal brain. *J. Clin. Endocrinol. Metab.,* 39:960–963.
101. Witschi, E. (1951): Gonad development and function. *Recent Prog. Horm. Res.,* 6:1–23.
102. Wyndham, N. R. (1943): A morphological study of testicular descent. *J. Anat.,* 88:179–188.
103. Zondek, L. H., and Zondek, T. (1965): Observations on the testis in anencephaly with special reference to the Leydig cells. *Biol. Neonat.,* 8:329–347.

The Testis, edited by H. Burger and D. de Kretser.
Raven Press, New York © 1981.

5

Endocrine Control of Testicular Function From Birth to Puberty

Ronald S. Swerdloff and David Heber

Department of Medicine, Harbor General Hospital Campus, UCLA School of Medicine, Los Angeles, California 90509

ENDOCRINE CONTROL OF TESTICULAR FUNCTION FROM BIRTH TO PUBERTY

Testicular function is controlled throughout life by a complex interacting system involving the extrahypothalamic central nervous system (CNS), the hypothalamus, the pituitary gland, and the gonads (see Fig. 1). Current evidence indicates that during the process of sexual maturation, physiological changes important to the control of testicular function occur at each of these anatomical levels. This chapter will review these phenomena and attempt to integrate them with our overall understanding of reproductive function. Before considering the specific mechanisms of sexual maturation, an overview of the male reproductive control system will be provided. While most of the information reviewed will deal with data obtained in human subjects, important information gleaned from experimental animal models will be included where the physiological insights gained seem relevant to human physiology.

Overall Endocrine Control of Testicular Function: Extrahypothalamic Central Nervous System

It has long been known that factors such as light, emotion, and olfaction, representing inputs originating in the extrahypothalamic CNS, affect the control of reproductive function. It is likely that CNS neurons influence the hypothalamic secretion of gonadotropin-releasing hormone (GnRH), which mediates the secretion of luteinizing hormone (LH) and follicle stimulating hormone (FSH) from the pituitary. Dopamine (DA), norepinephrine (NE) and serotonin (5-HT) are three CNS monoamine neurotransmitters involved in the control of hypothalamic GnRH secretion. Since only a small fraction of all CNS neurons

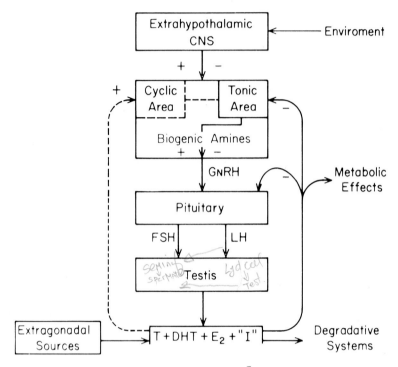

FIG. 1. Hypothalamic-pituitary gonadal feedback system of the male. The extragonadal sources of androgen referred to include androgens and androgen precursors produced by the adrenal glands. The testis directly secretes testosterone, dihydrotestosterone, and estradiol. Other substances have been postulated to be secreted by the testes which are believed to have an influence on FSH secretion. Such substances referred to as "I" in the diagram have been various names, including inhibin. (From ref. 69a.)

(17) contain these neurotransmitters it remains possible that other neurotransmitters may be involved in the control of reproductive function.

The effects of light on reproductive function have been observed in humans and studied extensively in lower species. During periods of darkness, the pineal gland in rodents increases its production of melatonin, a biogenic amine which has been shown to regulate gonadal function under special experimental circumstances. For example, blind hamsters undergo gonadal atrophy unless they are also pinealectomized (80). The activity of pineal enzymes producing melatonin is regulated by a light-dependent biological clock resulting in increased melatonin production during periods of darkness (81). When pharmacologic amounts of melatonin are administered to experimental animals both pituitary gonadotropin secretion and gonadal function are inhibited (81). The implications of these findings for human physiology must await further studies since the differences in qualitative response to pinealectomy may vary even between closely related species. Despite this reservation there are indications that visual stimuli may affect reproductive function in humans. For instance, menarche is known to occur earlier in blind girls (83). Similar studies on the effects of light have not been performed in boys, but blind men have been reported to have abnormal night-day patterns in circulating levels of LH, FSH, and gonadal steroids (5).

The effects of emotion on the reproductive axis have long been observed in females, where emotional stress has been known to cause abnormalities of the menstrual cycle. Anorexia nervosa represents an extreme example of the effect of emotional stress on reproductive function. In females with this disorder, a reversible regression of hypothalamic-pituitary function to a prepubertal state has been shown to occur (32). The pathophysiologic mechanisms responsible for these changes remain unclear. In men, serum testosterone levels have been shown to be depressed during periods of psychological stress (28). Whether this effect is mediated by the CNS directly or via increased adrenal glucocorticoid secretion remains controversial.

Olfactory stimuli may also influence reproductive function in mature and immature animals. For example, female rats placed in a room with male rat urine will undergo accelerated sexual maturation (9). Olfactory stimuli originating from female genital secretions have been shown to affect sexual behavior in male primates (37). The role, if any, of olfaction in human reproductive function is unknown.

Prostaglandin E_2 when injected into the cerebral ventricles of rats has been shown to stimulate pituitary LH and FSH secretion (14). Inhibitors of prostaglandin synthetase do not appear to affect menstrual cycles in females (70), and the physiologic importance of brain prostaglandins in reproductive function is not established.

The Hypothalamus

The hypothalamus acts as an integrating center for inputs from the extrahypothalamic CNS, the pituitary, and the gonads. Both the preoptic area and the medial basal hypothalamus are involved in the control of reproduction. GnRH is found in highest concentration in the median eminence, arcuate nucleus, suprachiasmatic nucleus, and preoptic nucleus (49). Norepinephrine-containing neurons distinct from those containing GnRH originate in the midbrain and end in the median eminence. Dopamine-containing neurons and GnRH-containing neurons travel from the arcuate nucleus to the median eminence (3). Present evidence indicates that norepinephrine stimulates GnRH release and dopaminergic neurons exert a tonic inhibitory effect on GnRH release (59). Receptors for testosterone and estradiol have been identified in the hypothalamus and represent a potential site of steroid modulation of GnRH secretion (22).

The Pituitary Gland

The hypothalamic hypophyseal portal vessels connect the median eminence with the pituitary gland and carry GnRH to the pituitary gonadotrophs. Immunocytochemical evidence indicates that GnRH binds to the gonadotrophs (68) and that both LH and FSH are secreted by a single cell type. GnRH stimulates the release of both LH and FSH *in vivo* and *in vitro,* and there is no convincing evidence for the existence of separate releasing factors for LH and FSH (60,82). These gonadotropins mediate both testicular androgen biosynthesis and spermatogenesis.

The Gonads

The testis consists of two major functional compartments. The Leydig cells which are the primary source of intratesticular and circulating testosterone, and the spermatogenic tubules which constitute 80 to 90% of testicular mass and mediate the process of spermatogenesis.

LH secreted by the pituitary binds to a specific Leydig cell membrane receptor in the testis (24), stimulating adenyl cyclase-dependent protein kinase (13), and resulting in the production of enzymes involved in testosterone biosynthesis. In addition to testosterone, the testis secretes lesser amounts of dehydroepian-drosterone, Δ^4-androstenedione, estrogen, and dihydrotestosterone (DHT). Ninety-five percent of circulating testosterone results from direct testicular secretion and testosterone is the major steroidal product secreted by the testis (50). In many target tissues such as the sex accessory glands, testosterone is converted to DHT by the enzyme 5 α-reductase. Direct testicular secretion of DHT accounts for only 10% of daily DHT production. DHT or testosterone can then combine with a specific nuclear receptor to induce masculine end-organ effects. In some tissues such as vas deferens, epididymis, muscle, and bone, there is no 5 α-reductase and testosterone is thought to exert its effects directly. The syndrome of testicular feminization results from the absence of testosterone receptors, and these patients are phenotypic females with female habitus, breasts, female external genitalia, and intraabdominal testes (10). Thus, normal male sexual maturation depends both on testicular production of testosterone and end-organ sensitivity to its effects.

The process of spermatogenesis is dependent on FSH, LH, and testosterone (67). The effects of LH on spermatogenesis seem to be mediated through the stimulation of testosterone synthesis. The administration of either LH or testosterone to immature or chronically hypophysectomized adult animals results in partial induction of spermatogenesis (spermatid stage 14–15). Further maturation requires the addition of FSH (for review see Steinberger and Steinberger ref. 66). In sexually mature animals where spermatogenesis has already been initiated, the administration or implantation of large amounts of testosterone alone immediately after acute hypophysectomy will maintain the normal process of sperm maturation. In either case, high concentrations of intratesticular testosterone must be produced to effect these changes.

Feedback Control of the Gonad on the Hypothalamic-Pituitary Axis

In the female both stimulatory and inhibitory feedback effects of gonadal hormones on gonadotropin secretion exist. The male differs from the female in that the gonads exert only inhibitory effects on the hypothalamic-pituitary unit. Removal of the testes results in marked elevations of LH and FSH, and subsequent administration of gonadal products returns gonadotropin levels toward normal (21,72). By this negative feedback mechanism, gonadal secretions maintain the basal or tonic serum concentration of gonadotropins. The nature of the inhibitory testicular substances and whether the inhibition occurs at the hypothalamic, pituitary, or at both levels remain controversial. In addition, there is some evidence that LH may inhibit its own secretion via short-loop negative feedback (38).

Most investigations have considered the effects of gonadal products on pituitary gonadotropin secretion. Döcke and Dörner (12) proposed that gonadal steroids inhibited LH and FSH secretion by decreasing the sensitivity of the pituitary gonadotrophs to GnRH. This concept would allow for changing levels of LH and FSH despite constant levels of GnRH secretion from the hypothalamus. An alternative view is that gonadal steroids inhibit LH and FSH secretion by decreasing hypothalamic GnRH secretion. Difficulty in measuring GnRH in hypophyseal portal blood under the required experimental conditions has hampered the resolution of this controversy. It is our opinion that the data support the concept of inhibitory effects of gonadal steroids at both a hypothalamic and pituitary level.

Two steroids produced by the testes, testosterone and estradiol, have been implicated in the control of gonadotropin secretion. Both of these steroids when administered in pharmacologic amounts will inhibit the postgonadectomy rise in gonadotropins (21,72), but the primacy of one of these steroids as the physiological inhibitor of gonadotropin secretion remains controversial. While serum testosterone levels in men are much higher than estradiol levels, estradiol is more potent than testosterone in inhibiting LH secretion in both men and experimental animals (21,71,72,76). Naftolin et al. (41) had actually proposed that all the effects of testosterone on the central nervous system might be due to brain aromatization of testosterone to estrogens. A number of studies showed that certain androgens which could not be converted to estrogens (because of their chemical structure) could nonetheless inhibit gonadotropin secretion in man and laboratory animals (40,74). When testosterone and estradiol were infused into normal men in physiologic amounts (58), similar suppression of mean LH levels occurred, but divergent effects on pulsatile LH secretion were observed. Testosterone increased LH pulse amplitude and frequency, while estradiol decreased pulse amplitude with no effect on pulse frequency. In addition, estradiol infusion decreased pituitary LH release in response to a single dose of GnRH, while testosterone had no effect on pituitary GnRH responsiveness. Based on current knowledge, it appears that physiologic concentrations of testosterone and estradiol have independent inhibitory effects on LH and FSH secretion, although the precise anatomical level and physiological mechanisms by which they act remain controversial.

While there is general agreement that gonadal steroids are the effective inhibitors of LH secretion, it has been proposed that an additional factor may specifically influence FSH secretion. There is a great deal of evidence suggesting that FSH and LH secretion may, in part, be separately controlled and that a seminiferous tubule factor may selectively inhibit FSH secretion. McCullagh and Walsh in 1935 (34) suggested that a substance which they called inhibin, originating in germinal epithelium, inhibited FSH production. They based this hypothesis on the observation that in conditions where germinal epithelium was selectively injured, serum FSH was elevated in the face of normal serum LH and testosterone. This phenomenon has been observed following testes irradiation (51), use of antispermatogenic agents (75), experimentally induced cryptorchidism in rats (62,73), and in patients with "Sertoli cell only" syndrome (56). Patients with severe oligospermia or azoospermia have also been observed to have elevated serum levels of FSH and normal LH levels (11,30,54). Several groups have isolated a peptide substance with selective FSH-inhibiting activity from the semen and testes of experimental animals (2,8,19). The control of inhibin secretion and its detailed actions on the reproductive axis must await its futher purification and structural characterization.

THE REPRODUCTIVE AXIS DURING SEXUAL MATURATION

The Process of Puberty

Through the process of sexual maturation, a boy acquires both the physical appearance of a man and the capacity to produce offspring. The many physical changes associated with puberty in the male occur in androgen-sensitive tissues such as the larynx, the apocrine sweat glands, skeletal muscles, bone epiphyses, external genitalia, and facial, axillary, and pubic hair follicles. The androgens, primarily secreted by the testes, thus mediate the familiar changes associated with male sexual maturation including increased phallic size, increased muscle mass, body fat redistribution, the pubertal growth spurt, epiphyseal closure, and the appearance of pubic, axillary, and facial hair. These changes occur gradually over several years and the age at which they each occur may vary considerably between individuals. Marshall and Tanner (33) carefully documented these changes in boys and girls. The sequence and approximate timing of the physical changes associated with puberty in boys is shown in Fig. 2. In order to improve the clinical evaluation of patients and to enable clinicians and researchers to correlate maturational appearances with hormonal events, a standardized classification of the composite stages of sexual maturation was developed (see Table 1). In addition to variation between individuals in the same society, the age at which these changes occur varies on a geographical basis. Nutrition and climate have been proposed as important environmental influences on the timing of sexual maturation.

On first observing the changes occurring in puberty without the benefit of modern techniques of measurement, researchers in the 1940s (25) advanced the theory that increases in end-organ responsiveness to constant levels of andro-

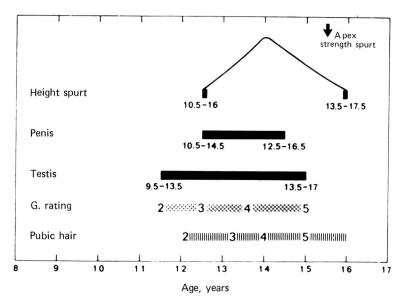

FIG. 2. Sequence of development of physical changes associated with puberty in boys. The large numbers refer to the Tanner stages of pubic hair and genital development. (From ref. 33.)

gens caused puberty. While some studies in animals supported this concept (48), studies by Odell and Swerdloff (44) in the rat revealed no significant differences between mature and immature animals in sex accessory gland responses to testosterone. While careful studies relating stage of sexual maturation to responsiveness of androgen target tissues have not been performed in boys during puberty, the data from animals coupled with measured increases in testosterone

TABLE 1. *Composite stages of sexual development in males*

Stage	Description
P–1	Preadolescent; largest testis diameter $\leq$ 2.4 cm; no pubic hair or penile enlargement
P–2	Sparse pubic hair, mainly at base of penis; testis diameter 2.4 to 3.2 cm; scrotal skin reddened; little penile enlargement
P–3	Pubic hair darker, coarser, but limited in distribution; early penis enlargement; sparse axillary hair; testis diameter 3.3 to 4.0 cm; scrotal skin darker
P–4	Adult pubic hair; moderate axillary hair; testis diameter 4.1 to 4.5 cm
P–5	Adult secondary characteristics; testis diameter greater than 4.5 cm

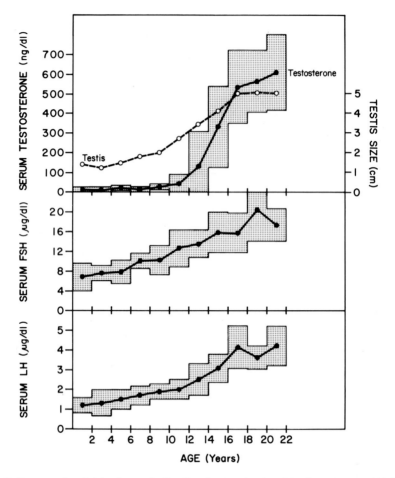

FIG. 3. Cross-sectional data demonstrating the changes in size of testis and serum LH, FSH, and testosterone during sexual maturation in boys. The absolute levels of serum LH and FSH differ among laboratories but the relative changes with age are representative of most studies. (From ref. 69a.)

during maturation (see below) suggest that changes in end-organ sensitivity are unimportant in puberty in humans.

Since the testes are the primary source for the androgens mediating the changes of sexual maturation, the activation of testicular function is central to the process of puberty. The testes, under the influence of pituitary gonadotropins, increase their production of testosterone as shown in Fig. 3. In the human, LH and FSH also increase through puberty, but the rate of increase in gonadotropins is gradual compared to the steep rise in testosterone levels between the ages of 10 and 16 (see Fig. 3). Thus, the change in gonadotropin levels is amplified at the gonadal level. The pattern of changes in gonadotropin secretion during sexual maturation varies between species. For example, gonadotropin levels in bulls do not rise at all during sexual maturation while testosterone secretion is markedly increased (43). In such species, the amplification process may be of even greater importance than it is in the human. Thus, both the pattern of gonadotropin secretion during sexual maturation and the changes occurring in gonadal sensitivity to gonadotropin stimulation are important aspects of the pubertal process.

Gonadotropin Secretion During Sexual Maturation

Gonadotropin levels at birth are low in the human (23). They rise transiently during the first few months of life, but from 6 months of age until approximately 10 years of age, remain low in the face of low testosterone levels (15). The concept of a gonadostat governing the feedback sensitivity of the hypothalamic-pituitary unit to gonadal hormonal inhibition of pituitary gonadotropin secretion has been proposed to explain the changing pattern of serum LH and FSH concentrations from birth to puberty. The transient rise in gonadotropins early in life has been ascribed to immaturity of the gonadostat (26). However, once established, the gonadostat maintains a high level of sensitivity during childhood to the negative feedback effects of low circulating prepubertal testosterone concentrations. The increases in gonadotropins and testosterone levels during puberty can be explained by a resetting of the sensitivity of the gonadostat. Thus, as the gonadostat becomes less sensitive to feedback inhibition, pituitary gonadotropin secretion and testosterone secretion both increase until they again come to equilibrium at the higher adult levels. The work of many groups measuring LH and FSH levels in children during various stages of sexual maturation was reviewed by Faiman and Winter (16), and supports the concept that gonadotropins increase coincident with biologic evidence of androgen effects during sexual maturation. In these studies, statistically significant increases in LH and FSH were found to correlate with advancing stages of sexual maturation, but there was great overlap among individuals classified in the different pubertal stages.

The greater sensitivity of the prepubertal reproductive hypothalamic-pituitary unit was first demonstrated in animal studies. Ramirez and McCann (52) demonstrated that immature rats were more sensitive than adult animals to androgenic suppression of gonadotropin secretion. The greater sensitivity of the gonadostat in children is suggested by a study utilizing clomiphene, an estrogen antagonist with weak estrogen effects in adults. In this study (29) a very small dose of clomiphene (1% of the dose used to routinely elevate gonadotropins in adults as part of the widely used clomiphene test) suppressed gonadotropins when administered to children. From these observations it was inferred that the weak estrogen effects of this antiestrogen drug were perceived by the highly sensitive prepubertal gonadostat, resulting in suppression of gonadotropin levels. This concept was also supported by studies in girls (27) showing that prepubertal females were more sensitive to suppressive effects of estrogen on gonadotropin secretion. However, gonadal inhibition does not explain all the known features of the prepubertal pattern of gonadotropin secretion, and modulation by the extrahypothalamic and hypothalamic CNS may be important in puberty.

CNS Modulation of Gonadotropin Secretion

There is evidence that extrahypothalamic CNS modulation of gonadotropin secretion is important both during the prepubertal years and during the process of sexual maturation. During the prepubertal years, castration results in a limited rise in gonadotropins to well below adult castrate levels (78). Furthermore, in individuals with gonadal dysgenesis and other agonadal conditions, where steroidal inhibition is absent, there is a further rise in their already elevated gonadotropins at the time when puberty would be expected to occur in normal individuals (78). These observations have been interpreted as providing evidence for extrahypothalamic CNS suppression of gonadotropins during the prepubertal years and for a maturation of the extrahypothalamic CNS at the time of puberty (45). Hypothalamic neurotransmitter secretion (norepinephrine turnover) increases during sexual maturation in the rat, thereby providing a possible neuroendocrine mechanism for increasing gonadotropins during puberty (52a). Further evidence for CNS modulation of gonadotropin secretion is provided by the observation of nocturnal pulses in gonadotropins which occur in humans at the onset of puberty (6). As shown in Fig. 4, these pulses occur during sleep. Early in puberty these nocturnal pulses occur only during sleep, but as puberty progresses, they increase in magnitude and occur throughout the day and night (7). Although pulsatile LH secretion may be mediated by changes at several levels in the reproductive axis, the initial correlation with sleep suggests that there is progressive maturation of extrahypothalamic CNS pathways during sexual maturation.

Hypothalamic-Pituitary Changes with Puberty

The rise in gonadotropins which is observed in humans during sexual maturation may be mediated by changes at a hypothalamic and pituitary level as well. Recently, an immunoreactive GnRH-like peptide has been measured in human urine, and its production has been found to be greater in postpubertal than in prepubertal children (53). If this peptide reflects hypothalamic GnRH secretion, this observation would suggest that increased hypothalamic releasing factor secretion may mediate the observed increases in pituitary gonadotropin secretion. Alternatively, changes in the physiological state of the gonadotroph have been observed to occur through puberty. Roth et al. (55) demonstrated increased LH secretion in response to GnRH with progressive stages of sexual maturation in boys. In addition, more FSH than LH is secreted in response to GnRH prepubertally, whereas more LH than FSH is secreted postpubertally in response to GnRH. Since a single cell type secretes both LH and FSH in

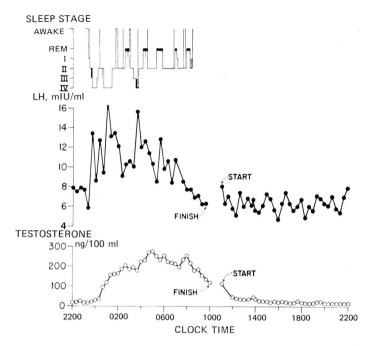

FIG. 4. Plasma LH and testosterone sampled every 20 min for 24 hr in a normal 14-year-old pubertal boy. A sleep histogram is shown above the period of nocturnal sleep. Sleep stages are awake and REM (rapid eye movement) stages 1 to 4 is indicated by the depth of the line graph. (From ref. 6a.)

response to GnRH, some modulation is occurring at the pituitary gonadotroph level to cause this change. In rats, Aiyer et al. (1) have demonstrated that GnRH induces greater sensitivity to itself with a lag time of about 60 min. This phenomenon, called the "self-priming" action of GnRH, has also been observed in human females (77). Thus, increasing GnRH secretion during puberty may in itself amplify the response of the pituitary glands to releasing hormone stimulation. Unfortunately, difficulty in measuring portal blood concentrations of GnRH make it impossible to critically test this hypothesis in humans.

Gonadal Changes During Puberty

An amplification process also occurs at the gonadal level such that the gradual rise observed in gonadotropin levels results in a steep rise in testosterone biosynthesis and secretion during puberty. This process involves both changes in testicular sensitivity to gonadotropin stimulation and changes in androgen biosynthetic pathways leading to increased testosterone production.

Considerable information about the processes mediating the increased gonadal sensitivity to gonadotropins during sexual maturation has been derived from

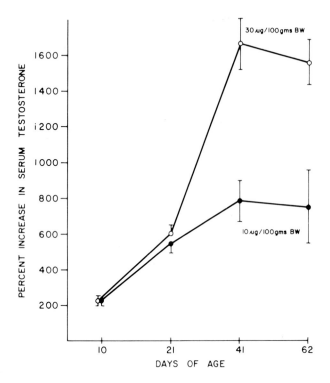

FIG. 5. Percent increase in serum testosterone plotted against age of male intact rats for two doses of NIH-LH-β7. Note that for both doses, with increasing age, a greater change in serum testosterone occurred in response to a constant dose of LH. (From ref. 46.)

studies on laboratory animals. In the male rat, LH falls between 10 and 20 days of age, and then rises slowly through the stages of sexual maturation. FSH reaches a peak at 30 to 40 days of age and then actually falls during sexual maturation (73). The rat testis becomes more responsive to these gonadotropins during puberty. For example, the immature rat testis does not respond to LH administered 5 days after hypophysectomy (47) while the adult male rat testis does. Furthermore, immature rats secrete much less testosterone in response to LH than do mature rats (Fig. 5). The LH responsiveness of the immature rat testis increases gradually with age to adult levels (46), and the number of LH receptors per testis increases with age (45) as shown in Fig. 6. Several observations suggested that the pituitary gonadotropins mediated the increasing gonadal sensitivity to LH observed with age in the immature male rat. FSH administration normalized the response to LH in hypophysectomized immature male rats suggesting that FSH somehow induced LH sensitivity in the immature testis (47). These findings were confirmed in immature intact male rats (46).

A potential mechanism for this FSH-induced effect, is the observed increase

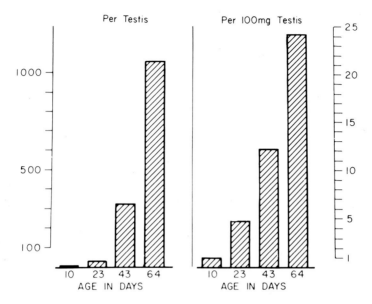

FIG. 6. LH receptors determined by Scatchard analyses of binding data in intact male rats at different ages. The results indicate that the relative receptor populations, expressed either per testis (left) or per testis weight (right), increase progressively with sexual maturation. (From ref. 45.)

in testicular LH receptors in immature hypophysectomized male rats treated with FSH as shown in Fig. 7. In this experiment, 21-day-old rats were hypophysectomized and treated 5 days later with either FSH or saline for 5 consecutive days. The testes were then removed, and a greater than 100% increase in testicular LH receptors per testis was observed in the FSH-treated group. Thus, FSH could affect testicular sensitivity to another hormone by inducing synthesis of

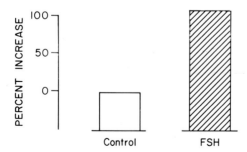

FIG. 7. FSH induction of LH receptors in the 5-day hypophysectomized rat. Male animals were hypophysectomized at 21 days of age and, 5 days later, treated for 5 days with either saline or FSH (16.2 µg/day). The testes were removed and LH receptors quantified. There was greater than 100% increase in LH receptors in the FSH-treated group as shown. (From ref. 45.)

the LH receptor. It is not known how FSH mediates this effect, since Leydig cell binding of FSH has not been demonstrated.

Data in humans support the generalization of this concept of the gonad as an active participant in the process of sexual maturation. Several groups (20, 57,79) have demonstrated decreased responsiveness of the prepubertal testis compared to the adult testis. The magnitude of the testosterone response to human chorionic gonadotropin (hCG), which has largely LH-like activity, increases with age and correlates with both basal LH and FSH levels (79). Sizonenko et al. (61) reported that basal serum FSH concentration correlated best with testicular hCG responsiveness in boys.

Another potential site for the mediation of the sharp increase in gonadal function observed with puberty, is at the level of testicular androgen biosynthesis. Studies to date have concentrated on the description of changes in androgen biosynthetic pathways in human and animal testes studies *in vitro*. The mechanisms by which the observed changes occur have not yet been studied, but represent important areas for future investigation.

The detailed description of androgen biosynthetic pathways is outside the scope of this chapter. However, it is important to realize that the nature of precursor androgens produced by the testis depends on which enzymatic pathways are most active. Thus, any clinical or animal study attempting to document gonadal changes in androgen biosynthesis during puberty must include measurement of key intermediate precursor androgens as well as testosterone.

A number of investigators have suggested that the immature testis metabolizes precursor steroids in a different manner than the mature testis. For example, the ratio of production of androstenedione to testosterone is much greater in the immature rat, bull, and guinea pig testes than in their adult counterpart (4,31,42,69). In addition, *in vitro* studies of rat testicular tissue have demonstrated changes in 5α-reductase activity during development. During the perinatal period rat testicular tissue is capable of converting precursors to testosterone at rates similar to or higher than that found for mature rat testes (63). At 20 to 25 days of age, a decreased ability to synthesize testosterone occurs in conjunction with an increase in 5α-reductase activity with formation of 5α-androstenediol and androsterone. As development progresses there is a gradual return to predominant testosterone production with decreased synthesis of 5α-reduced androgens (64,78). The seminiferous tubules are capable of converting testosterone to 5α-androstenediol (65), and may play a role in the observed changes in androgen biosynthesis with development.

Studies of androgen metabolism in human testes *in vitro* have been carried out using testicular biopsy specimens incubated with ^{3}H-progesterone (65). In studies of two prepubertal patients with hypogonadotropic hypogonadism, ^{3}H-progesterone was adequately metabolized (76% and 61%) but only small amounts (1.0% and 0.26%) were converted to testosterone. Compared to normal adults there was increased conversion of precursor steroids to 5α-reduced metabolites. In addition, one patient with oligospermia was studied and found to have evidence of increased 5α-reductase activity, which decreased as testosterone production increased with gonadotropin therapy of this individual. This suggestive evidence awaits further studies on the key steps in the differentiation of androgen biosynthetic pathways with sexual maturation.

The Development of the Ability to Reproduce

Puberty consists of both the secondary sexual development described earlier and the development of reproductive (spermatogenic) capacity. The control of spermatogenesis by LH, FSH and testosterone has already been considered in the section on overall control of the reproductive system. Maturation of the germinal epithelium appears to occur early during the pubertal process. Increases in serum LH and FSH have been described above. As the serum level of gonadotropins increase and the Leydig cells became more responsive to LH intratesticular testosterone increases providing the milieu for sperm maturation. It is of interest that mature sperm have been described in the urine of children before secondary sexual development is obvious. This suggests that the critical level of gonadotropins and testosterone are present in the testis before there is evidence of increased circulating testosterone.

As described earlier, FSH has a critical role in the production of mature sperm. Evidence from animal studies indicates that FSH induces these effects at a Sertoli cell level (35,36,39). It has been suggested (67) that FSH, by its induction of increased androgen binding protein synthesis by the Sertoli cell, increases the availability of testosterone to the spermatogenic tubule, and that these increased levels of androgen-protein complexes are essential to the completion of spermatogenesis. This exciting area of research will doubtless reveal other steps in the maturation of spermatogenic function by the testis.

Adrenarche

The development of pubic and axillary hair in the female is believed to result from increased secretion of androgens or androgen precursors from the adrenal glands (adrenarche). Since the testis is the primary source of androgens in the male and the adrenal is only a minor contributor to overall androgen production, the importance of adrenarche in male sexual maturation remains speculative.

Integration of the Process of Puberty with Hormonal Events

Sexual maturation or puberty is a complex physiologic process that results in the maturation of the gonads. The mature gonad provides for both adult reproductive capacity and the production of circulating male hormones which stimulate the development of secondary sexual characteristics.

TABLE 2. *The hormonal events of puberty*

Anatomical level	Changes	Results
Central nervous system	Decreasing sensitivity of the gonadostat Increased stimulatory neurotransmitter production Pulsatile release of LH	Increased LRH
Pituitary gland	Increased pituitary sensitivity to GnRH Increased LH to FSH ratio in response to GnRH	Increased gonadotropins
Gonads	Increased gonadal sensitivity to gonadotropins Alterations in androgen biosynthetic pathways Sertoli cell activation	Increased testosterone levels Production of mature sperm
Adrenal	Increased adrenal androgen production	Early axillary and pubic hair

These gonadal changes are the result of maturational events occurring at multiple levels of the reproductive hormonal axis (see Table 2).

Testosterone secretion increases during puberty both as a result of increasing gonadotropin secretion and increased gonadal sensitivity to gonadotropins. The rise in FSH levels precedes that of LH and appears to sensitize the Leydig cell to LH stimulation. This process may occur as a result of the induction of LH receptors by FSH and may be associated with changes in androgen biosynthetic pathways. The coupled effects of LH, FSH, and testosterone are also responsible for sperm maturation.

The mechanisms which result in increased gonadotropin secretion during puberty are less well understood. It appears that changes in extrahypothalamic CNS maturation during puberty may decrease the sensitivity of the reproductive hypothalamic-pituitary unit (gonadostat) to inhibition by gonadal steroids. This resetting of the gonadostat results in increases of both testosterone and gonadotropins to a new equilibrium state at higher adult levels. Changes in both hypothalamic GnRH secretion and the physiologic state of the pituitary gonadotrophs may be responsible for the observed increased sensitivity of the pituitary gland to exogenous GnRH stimulation as puberty progresses. The inability to measure GnRH in human portal blood under appropriate conditions hampers efforts to understand puberty at this anatomical level.

Much further work will be necessary in many of the exciting areas of research discussed in this chapter, before the multiple hormonal events outlined can be interrelated to form an integrated picture of the fascinating process that converts boys to men.

REFERENCES

1. Aiyer, M. S., Chiappa, A., Fink, G., and Greig, F. (1973): A priming effect of luteinizing hormone releasing factor on the anterior pituitary gland in the female rat. *J. Physiol. (Lond),* 234:81.
2. Baker, H. W. G., Burger, H. G., deKretser, D. M., Dulmanis, A., Eddie, L. W., Hudson, B., Keogh, E. J., Lee, V. W. K., and Rennie, G. C. (1976): Testicular control of follicle-stimulating hormone secretion. *Recent Prog. Horm. Res.,* 32:429.
3. Barry, J., Dubois, M. P., and Poulain, F. (1973): LRF-producing cells of the mammalian hypothalamus. *Z. Zellforsch. Mikrosk. Anat.,* 146:351.
4. Becker, W. G., and Snipes, C. A. (1968): Shift with age in steady-state concentrations of androstenedione and testosterone in incubations of guinea-pig testis. *Biochem. J.,* 107:35.
5. Bodenheimer, S., Winter, J. S. D., and Faiman, C. (1973): Diurnal rhythms of serum gonadotropins, testosterone, estradiol, and cortisol in blind men. *J. Clin. Endocrinol. Metab.,* 37:472.
6. Boyar, R., Finkelstein, J., Roffway, H., Kapen, S., Weitzman, E., and Hellman, L. (1972): Synchronization of LH secretion with sleep during puberty. *N. Engl. J. Med.,* 287:582.
6a. Boyar, R. M., Rosenfeld, R. S., Kapen, S., Finkelstein, J. W., Roffwarg, H. P., Weitzman, E. D., and Hellman, L. (1974): Simultaneous augmented secretion of luteinizing hormone and testosterone during sleep. *J. Clin. Invest.,* 54:609.
7. Boyar, R., Perlow, M., Hellman, L., Kapen, S., and Weitzman, E. (1972): Twenty-four hour pattern of luteinizing hormone secretion in normal men with sleep stage recording. *J. Clin. Endocrinol. Metab.,* 35:73.
8. Braunstein, G. D., and Swerdloff, R. S. (1977): Effect of aqueous extracts of bull and rat testicles on serum FSH and LH in the acutely castrate male rat. *J. Clin. Endocrinol. Metab.,* 35:281.
9. Bronson, F. H. (1968): Pheromonal influences on mammalian reproduction. In: *Perspectives in Reproduction and Sexual Behavior,* edited by M. Diamond, p. 341. Indiana University Press, Bloomington.
10. Bullock, L. P., and Bardin, C. W. (1972): Androgen receptors in testicular feminization. *J. Clin. Endocrinol. Metab.,* 35:935.
11. de Kretser, D. M., Burger, H. G., Fortune, D., Hudson, B., Long, A. R., Paulsen, C. A., and Taft, H. P. (1972): Hormonal, histological and chromosomal studies in adult males with testicular disorders. *J. Clin. Endocrinol. Metab.,* 35:392.
12. Döcke, F., and Dörner, G. (1965): The mechanism of the induction of ovulation by estrogens. *J. Endocrinol.,* 33:491.
13. Dorrington, J. H., and Fritz, I. B. (1974): Effects of gonadotropins on cyclic AMP production by isolated seminiferous tubule and interstitial cell preparations. *Endocrinology,* 94:395.
14. Eskay, R. L., Waberg, J., Mical, R. S., and Porter, J. C. (1975): Prostaglandin E_2-induced release of LHRH into hypophyseal portal blood. *Endocrinology,* 97:816.
15. Faiman, C., and Winter, J. S. D. (1971): Sex differences in gonadotrophin concentrations in infancy. *Nature,* 232:130.
16. Faiman, C., and Winter, J. S. D. (1974): Gonadotropins and sex hormone patterns in puberty: Clinical data. In: *The Control of the Onset of Puberty,* edited by M. M. Grumbach, G. D. Grave, and F. E. Mayer, P. 32. Wiley, New York.
17. Fernstrom, J. D., and Wurtman, R. J. (1977): Brain monoamines and reproductive function. In: *International Review of Physiology II,* Vol. 13, edited by R. O. Greep, p. 23. University Park Press, Baltimore.
18. Ficher, M., and Steinberger, E. (1968): Conversion of progesterone to androsterone by testicular tissue at different stages of maturation. *Steroids,* 12:491.
19. Franchimont, P., Chari, S., Hazee-Hagelstein, M. T., Debruche, M. L., and Duraiswami, S. (1977): Evidence for the existence of inhibin. In: *The Testis in Normal and Infertile Men,* edited by P. Troen and H. R. Nankin, p. 253. Raven Press, New York.
20. Frasier, S. D., Gafford, F., and Horton, R. (1969): Plasma androgens in childhood and adolescence. *J. Clin. Endocrinol. Metab.,* 29:1404.
21. Gay, V. L., and Dever, N. W. (1971): Effects of testosterone propionate and estradiol benzoate—alone or in combination—on serum LH and FSH in orchidectomized rats. *Endocrinology,* 89:161.
22. Greeley, G. H., Muldoon, T. G., and Mahesh, V. B. (1975): Correlative aspects of LHRH sensitivity and cytoplasmic estrogen receptor concentration in the anterior pituitary and hypothalamus of the cycling rat. *Biol. Reprod.,* 13:505.

23. Grumbach, M. M., and Kaplan, S. L. (1973): Ontogenesis of growth hormone, insulin, prolactin, and gonadotropin secretion in the human fetus. In: *Fetal and Neonatal Physiology,* Proc. Sir Joseph Barcroft Centenary Symposium, p. 462. Cambridge University Press, Cambridge.
24. Hall, P. F., and Eik-Nes, K. B. (1962): The action of gonadotropic hormones upon rabbit testis in vitro. *Biochim. Biophys. Acta,* 63:411.
25. Hooker, C. W. (1942): Pubertal increase in responsiveness to androgen in the male rat. *Endocrinology,* 30:77.
26. Kaplan, S. L., Grumbach, M. M., and Aubert, M. L. (1976): Fetal pituitary and hypothalamic hormones. *Recent Prog. Horm. Res.,* 32:161.
27. Kelch, R. P., Kaplan, S. L., and Grumbach, M. M. (1973): Suppression of urinary and plasma follicle-stimulating hormone by exogenous estrogens in prepubertal and pubertal children. *J. Clin. Invest.,* 52:1122.
28. Kreutz, L. E., Rose, R. M., and Jennings, R. (1972): Suppression of plasma testosterone levels and psychological stress. *Arch. Gen. Psychiatry,* 26:479.
29. Kulin, H. E., Grumbach, M. M., and Kaplan, S. L. (1972): Gonadal-hypothalamic interaction in prepubertal and pubertal man: Effect of clomiphene citrate on urinary follicle-stimulating hormone, luteinizing hormone and plasma testosterone. *Pediatr. Res.,* 6:162.
30. Leonard, J. M., Leach, R. B., Couture, M., and Paulsen, C. A. (1972): Plasma and urine follicle-stimulating hormone levels in oligospermia. *J. Clin. Endocrinol. Metab.,* 34:209.
31. Lindner, H. R., and Mann, T. (1960): Relationship between the content of androgenic steroids in the testes and the secretory activity of the seminal vesicles in the bull. *J. Clin. Endocrinol. Metab.,* 21:341.
32. Marshall, J. C. and Fraser, T. R. (1971): Amenorrhea in anorexia nervosa: Assessment and treatment with clomiphene citrate. *Br. Med. J.,* 4:590.
33. Marshall, W. A., and Tanner, J. M. (1970): Variations in pattern of pubertal changes in boys. *Arch. Dis. Child.,* 45:13.
34. McCullagh, D. R., and Walsh, E. L. (1935): Experimental hypertrophy and atrophy of the prostate gland. *Endocrinology,* 19:466.
35. Means, A. R. (1971): Concerning the mechanism of FSH action: Rapid stimulation of testicular synthesis of nuclear RNA. *Endocrinology,* 89:981.
36. Means, A. R., and Hall, P. F. (1968): Protein biosynthesis in the testis: I. Comparison between stimulation by FSH and glucose. *Endocrinology,* 82:597.
37. Michael, R. P., and Kaverne, E. B. (1968): Pheromones in the communication of sexual status in primates. *Nature,* 218:746.
38. Molitch, M., Edmonds, M., Jones, E. E., and Odell, W. D. (1976): Short-loop feedback control of luteinizing hormone in the rabbit. *Am. J. Physiol.,* 230:907.
39. Murad, F., Strauch, S., and Vaughn, M. (1969): The effect of gonadotropins on testicular adenyl cyclase. *Biochim. Biophys. Acta,* 177:591.
40. Naftolin, F., Feder, H. H. (1973): Suppression of LH secretion in male rats by 5α-androstan-17β-ol-3-one propionate. *J. Endocrinol.,* 56:155.
41. Naftolin, F., Ryan, K. J., and Petro, Z. (1972): Aromatization of androstenedione by the anterior hypothalamus of adult male and female rats. *Endocrinology,* 90:295.
42. Nayfeh, S. H., and Baggett, B. (1966): Metabolism of progesterone by rat testicular homogenates. I. Isolation and identification of metabolites. *Endocrinology,* 78:460.
43. Odell, W. D., Hescox, M. A., and Kiddy, C. A. (1970): Studies of hypothalamic-pituitary-gonadal interrelations in prepubertal cattle. In: *Gonadotrophins and Ovarian Development,* edited by W. R. Butt, A. C. Crooke, and M. Ryle, p. 371. Livingstone, Edinburgh.
44. Odell, W. D., and Swerdloff, R. S. (1974): The role of the gonads in sexual maturation. In: *The Control of the Onset of Puberty,* edited by M. M. Grumbach, G. D. Grave, and F. E. Mayer, p. 313. Wiley, New York.
45. Odell, W. D., and Swerdloff, R. S. (1976): Etiologies of sexual maturation: A model system based on the sexually maturing rat. *Recent Prog. Horm. Res.,* 32:245.
46. Odell, W. D., Swerdloff, R. S., Bain, J., Wollesen, F., and Grover, P. K. (1974): The effect of sexual maturation on testicular response to LH stimulation of testosterone secretion in the intact rat. *Endocrinology,* 95:1380.
47. Odell, W. D., Swerdloff, R. S., Jacobs, H. S., and Hescox, M.A. (1973): FSH induction of sensitivity to LH: One cause of sexual maturation in the male rat. *Endocrinology,* 92:160.
48. Ojeda, S. R., and Ramirez, V. D. (1972): Plasma LH and FSH in maturing rats: response to hemigonadectomy. *Endocrinology,* 90:466.

49. Palkovits, M., Arimura, A., Brownstein, M., Schally, A. V., and Saavedra, J. M. (1974): LHRH content of the hypothalamic nuclei in the rat. *Endocrinology,* 96:554.
50. Paulsen, C. A. (1974): The testis. In: *Textbook of Endocrinology,* edited by R. H. Williams, p. 323. Saunders, Philadelphia.
51. Paulsen, C. A. (1968): Effect of human chorionic gonadotrophin therapy on testicular function. In: *Gonadotropins,* edited by E. Rosemberg, p. 491. Geron-X, Los Altos, California.
52. Ramirez, V. D., McCann, S. M. (1965): Inhibitory effect of testosterone on luteinizing hormone secretion in immature and adult rats. *Endocrinology,* 76:412.
52a. Raum, W. J., Glass, A. R., and Swerdloff, R. S. (1978): The role of hypothalamic catecholamines in the process of sexual maturation in the female Wistar rat. *Clin. Res.,* 26:171A.
53. Root, A. W., Reiter, E. O., and Duckett, G. E. (1977): Urinary excretion of immunoreactive GnRH-like material in prepubertal and pubertal children. *J. Clin. Endocrinol. Metab.,* 44:909.
54. Rosen, S. W., and Weintraub, B. D. (1971): Monotropic increase of serum FSH correlated with low sperm count in young men with idiopathic oligospermia and aspermia. *J. Clin. Endocrinol. Metab.,* 32:410.
55. Roth, J. C., Grumbach, M. M., and Kaplan, S. L. (1973): Effect of synthetic luteinizing hormone-releasing factor on serum testosterone and gonadotropins in prepubertal, pubertal, and adult males. *J. Clin. Endocrinol. Metab.,* 37:680.
56. Ryan, R. J., Cloutier, M. D., Hayles, A. B., Paris, J., and Randall, R. V. (1970): The clinical utility of radio-immunoassays for serum follicle-stimulating hormone (FSH) and luteinizing hormone (LH). *Med. Clin. North Am.,* 54:1049.
57. Saez, J. M., and Bertrand, J. (1968): Studies on testicular function in children: Plasma concentrations of testosterone dehydroepiandrosterone, and its sulfate before and after stimulation with hCG. *Steroids,* 12:749.
58. Santen, R. J. (1977): Independent effects of testosterone and estradiol on the secretion of gonadotropins in men. In: *The Testis in Normal and Infertile Men,* edited by P. Troen and H. R. Nankin, p. 197. Raven Press, New York.
59. Sawyer, C. H. (1975): Some recent developments in brain pituitary ovarian physiology. *Neuroendocrinology,* 17:97.
60. Schally, A. V., Arimura, A., Kastin, A. J., Matsuo, H., Baba, Y., Redding, T. W., Nair, R. M. G., and Debeljuk, L., (1971): Gonadotropin-releasing hormone: One polypeptide regulates secretion of luteinizing and follicle-stimulating hormones. *Science,* 173:1036.
61. Sizonenko, P. C., Cuendet, A., and Paunier, L. (1973): FSH I. Evidence for its mediating role on testosterone secretion in cryptorchidism. *J. Clin. Endocrinol. Metab.,* 37:68.
62. Steinberger, E., and Duckett, G. E. (1968): Effect of testosterone on the release of FSH from the pituitary gland. *Acta Endocrinol. (Kbh),* 57:289.
63. Steinberger, E., and Ficher, M. (1968): Conversion of progesterone to testosterone by testicular tissue at different stages of maturation. *Steroids,* 11:351, 1968.
64. Steinberger, E., and Ficher, M. (1969): Differentiation of steroid biosynthetic pathways in developing testes. *Biol. Reprod.,* (Suppl. 1):119.
65. Steinberger, E., Smith, K. D., Tcholakian, R. K., Chowdhury, M., Steinberger, A., Ficher, M., and Paulsen, C. A. (1974): Steroidogenesis in human testes. In: *Male Fertility and Sterility,* edited by R. E. Mancini, and L. Martini, p. 149. Academic Press, London.
66. Steinberger, E., and Steinberger, A. (1969): The spermatogenic function of the testes. In: *The Gonads,* edited by K. W. McKerns, p. 715. Appleton-Century-Crofts, New York.
67. Steinberger, E., Steinberger, A., and Sanborn, B. (1974): Endocrine control of spermatogenesis. In: *Physiology and Genetics of Reproduction,* edited by E. M. Coutinho and F. Fuchs, part A, p. 163. Plenum Press, New York.
68. Steinberger, L. A., Petrali, J. P., Joseph, S. A., Meyer, H. G., and Mills, K. R. (1978): Specificity of the immunocytochemical luteinizing hormone-releasing hormone receptor reaction. *Endocrinology,* 102:63.
69. Stylianou, M., Forchielli, E., and Dorfman, R. I. (1961): The metabolism of 4-C14-testosterone in rat testis homogenate. *J. Biol. Chem.,* 236:1318.
69a. Swerdloff, R. S. (1978): Physiological control of puberty. *Med. Clin. N. Am.,* 62:351.
70. Swerdloff, R. S., and Greenway, F. (1978): Effect of aspirin (prostaglandin synthetase inhibitor) on the menstrual cycle. *Fertil. Steril.,* 30:364.
71. Swerdloff, R. S., and Odell, W. D. (1968): Feedback control of LH and FSH secretion. *Lancet,* 2:683.
72. Swerdloff, R. S., and Walsh, P. C. (1973): Testosterone and estradiol suppression of LH and

FSH in adult male rats: Duration of castration, duration of treatment and combined treatment. *Acta Endocrinol. (Kbh),* 73:11.

73. Swerdloff, R. S., Walsh, P. C., Jacobs, H. S., and Odell W. D. (1971): Serum LH and FSH during sexual maturation in the male rat: Effect of castration and cryptorchidism: *Endocrinology,* 88:120.

74. Swerdloff, R. S., Walsh, P. C., and Odell, W. D. (1972): Control of LH and FSH secretion in the male: Evidence that aromatization of androgens to estradiol is not required for inhibition of gonadotropin secretion. *Steroids,* 20:13.

75. Van Thiel, D. H., Sherins, R. J., Myers, G. H., and DeVita, V. T., (1972): Evidence for a specific seminiferous tubule factor affecting follicle-stimulating hormone secretion in man. *J. Clin. Invest.,* 51:1009.

76. Walsh, P. C., Swerdloff, R. S., and Odell, W. D. (1973): Feedback control of FSH in the male: Role of estrogen. *Acta Endocrinol. (Kbh),* 74:449.

77. Wang, C. F., Lasley, B. L., Lein, A., and Yen, S. S. C (1976): The functional changes of the pituitary gonadotrophs during the menstrual cycle. *J. Clin. Endocrinol. Metab.,* 42:718.

78. Winter, J. S. D., and Faiman, C. (1972): Serum gonadotropin concentrations in agonadal children and adults. *J. Clin. Endocrinol. Metab.,* 35:561.

79. Winter, J. S. D., and Faiman, C. (1972): Pituitary-gonadal relations in male children and adolescents. *Pediatr. Res.,* 6:126.

80. Wurtman, R. J. (1967): Effect of light and visual stimuli on endocrine function. In: *Neuroendocrinology,* Vol. 2, edited by W. F. Gruong and L. Martini, pp. 19–59. Academic Press, New York.

81. Wurtman, R. J., and Cardinali, D. P. (1974): The pineal organ. In: *Textbook of Endocrinology,* edited by R. H. Williams, p. 832. Saunders, Philadelphia.

82. Yen, S. S. C., Rebar, G., Vandenberg, G., Naftolin, F., Eheara, Y., Engblom, S., Ryan, K. J., Benirschke, K., Rivier, J., Amoss, M., and Guillemin, R. (1972): Synthetic luteinizing hormone-releasing factor: A potent stimulator of gonadotropin release in man. *J. Clin. Endocrinol. Metab.,* 34:1108.

83. Zacharias, L., and Wurtman, R. J. (1964): Blindness: Its relation to age of menarche. *Science,* 144:1154.

The Testis, edited by H. Burger and D. de Kretser.
Raven Press, New York © 1981.

6

Endocrine Control of Adult Testicular Function

Gere S. diZerega and Richard J. Sherins

*Developmental Endocrinology Branch, Pregnancy Research Branch, National Institute
of Child Health and Human Development, Bethesda, Maryland 20014*

Endocrine control of testicular function in the adult is composed of intra-
and extratesticular elements (Fig. 1). Luteinizing hormone (LH) and follicle
stimulating hormone (FSH) of anterior pituitary origin regulate both Leydig
cell and seminiferous tubule function. In turn, Leydig cell sex steroids and
seminiferous tubule non-sex steroid factor(s) modulate peripheral concentrations
of the gonadotropins by their interaction at the hypothalamus and pituitary.
Recent studies also suggest an important interaction between Leydig cells and
adjacent tubule cells (2,34).

This chapter will discuss recent advances in reproductive physiology. Most
of the data presented have been obtained from human investigation, however,
studies in other species will be included when applicable. This chapter is not
intended to be an exhaustive literature review, rather to highlight some of the
important endocrine factors which regulate adult testicular function.

REGULATION OF LEYDIG CELL FUNCTION

Luteinizing Hormone

LH binds and acts primarily on the Leydig cell (Fig. 1). The major effect
is to stimulate steroidogenesis. LH action is mediated through surface membrane
proteins which are specific and of high affinity (13). LH receptor binding leads
to increased adenylate cyclase activity followed by a rise in intracellular cyclic
AMP (73). Newly formed cyclic AMP binds to the regulatory portion of protein
kinase located in the cytoplasm. Following cyclic AMP binding this holoenzyme
dissociates, releasing its regulatory subunit which then activates protein substrates (23).

LH increases the conversion of 20- and 22α-hydroxycholesterol to pregnenolone, a testosterone precursor, through action of cholesterol-esterase and choles-
terol-side chain cleavage enzymes (29,30). LH also accelerates cholesterol entry

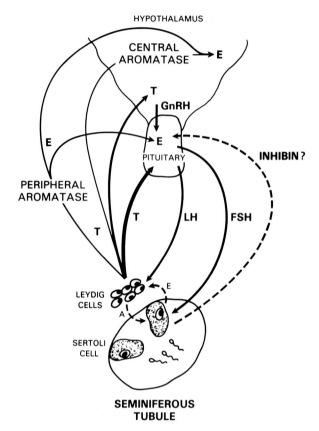

FIG. 1. Schematic representation of the complex interactions between hypothalamus, pituitary, and testis in adult men.

into mitochondria wherein the above-mentioned reactions are thought to take place. Thus, the major effect of LH upon steroidogenesis is to increase the availability of steroid substrate by accelerating the metabolism of cholesterol (31).

A variety of steroids are secreted by the Leydig cell which include testosterone, 17α-hydroxyprogesterone and estradiol. In normal men 7 mg of testosterone is produced per day, predominantly from direct Leydig cell secretion (5). By contrast, half of the testosterone produced in women (0.35 mg/day) is derived from peripheral conversion of adrenal precursors, principally androstenedione. In man, the majority of circulating testosterone is bound to a high affinity β-globulin, testosterone-estradiol binding globulin (TeBG). Most current studies suggest that only the free or unbound level of testosterone is available for cellular entry and androgen action (32).

While the total testosterone level is usually an adequate reflection of Leydig cell function, in some cases measurement of total serum testosterone concentration may give a misleading impression of biologic availability. In patients with primary testicular failure, i.e., Klinefelter's syndrome, hepatic cirrhosis, senescent male, total testosterone levels are within the normal range yet serum gonadotropin concentrations are elevated (51). In these circumstances, the TeBG levels are markedly elevated accounting for increased plasma testosterone binding (75). Since testosterone secretion is reduced in those patients the decrease in free testosterone level more accurately reflects the disease state. The hepatic production of TeBG is sensitive to sex steroid modulation (15). Estrogen increases the TeBG level while testosterone decreases its concentration. It has been proposed that the ratio of estrogen to androgen determines the hepatic TeBG production (15). This seems a plausible mechanism to explain the elevated TeBG levels in patients with primary testicular failure because estrogen levels are maintained despite the fall in androgen production.

Only one-third of the total daily production of estradiol is from direct testicular secretion, the rest derives from conversion (aromatization) of testosterone in peripheral tissues (5). Considerable controversy exists as to the role of the Sertoli cell in the production of estradiol. While the Sertoli cell has been shown to contain an aromatase capable of converting testosterone to estradiol (20), there is considerable doubt that this mechanism provides a quantitatively important source of estradiol. This is best illustrated in men with severely damaged tubules (51) (Klinefelter's syndrome) where estradiol production rates are normal despite absence of seminiferous tubules. Until more data are available, localization of cellular estradiol production in the testis will remain unclear.

Follicle Stimulating Hormone

While FSH has been shown to bind and act upon the seminiferous tubule (Fig. 1), recent evidence indicates that FSH also influences Leydig cell function. In the rabbit (35), hypophysectomized immature rat (49), and hypogonadotropic men (60) FSH enhances LH stimulation of testosterone secretion. This effect is probably the result of an FSH mediated increase in Leydig cell LH receptors. Although a permissive role for FSH in augmenting LH induced steroid secretion is clear, direct FSH binding to Leydig cells has not been demonstrated.

Prolactin

There is considerable controversy regarding the role of prolactin in the regulation of testicular function (7,10). Most of the evidence that prolactin may interact with testicular tissue comes from investigation in the rodent (8). Prolactin enhances LH induced testosterone secretion by increasing the conversion of cholesterol to pregnenolone (29,30). In the sexually immature rat prolactin augments human chorionic gonadotropin (HGG) stimulated peripheral testosterone levels and the growth of androgen target tissues. This effect is thought to be mediated through prolactin binding to Leydig cells (22). Prolactin receptors have also been located in the testis of man. Increases of testosterone concentration have been shown to follow experimentally induced elevations of plasma prolactin levels (52). However, under normal physiologic conditions it remains unclear as to whether prolactin has an important role in modulating human testicular function.

REGULATION OF SEMINIFEROUS TUBULE FUNCTION

Follicle Stimulating Hormone

Of the multiple cellular elements comprising the seminiferous tubule only the Sertoli cell has been shown to contain FSH receptors (46). There is no evidence to date that LH directly effects any of the seminiferous tubule components. FSH stimulates adenylate cyclase to produce cyclic AMP which activates the regulatory subunit of protein kinase (16,21,46).

One of the major actions of FSH is to stimulate protein synthesis (46). Increased amino acid incorporation into protein following FSH exposure has been demonstrated both *in vivo* and in isolated Sertoli cell cultures from immature rats. In addition to general protein synthesis, FSH stimulates the production of at least four specific proteins (45). These include androgen binding protein (ABP) (32,46) and plasminogen activator (38), both of which are secreted into the rete testis fluid, and two proteins which remain in the Sertoli cell, a protein kinase inhibitor and gamma glutamyl transpeptidase (37).

Production of ABP has been best characterized in the immature rat (71). Evidence for this protein in man is controversial since distinguishing between ABP and TeBG has been difficult technically (78). Recent evidence suggests that human ABP has a higher affinity and lower binding capacity for androgen than TeBG circulating in the plasma (33). However, the physical properties of human and rat ABP are thus far indistinguishable.

To date studies have demonstrated an FSH action only in testes of immature rats and little if any stimulation of protein synthesis, cyclic AMP, or ABP have been found in the mature rat. Although the Sertoli cell becomes refractory to FSH by 25 days of age, recent data indicate that hypophysectomy can restore Sertoli cell FSH sensitivity in the sexually mature animal (45,53). The loss of cellular response to FSH in the adult rat is owing to a defect in the production of cyclic AMP secondary to increased phosphodiesterase activity and not from a decrease in FSH receptors, as the receptor number increases with age.

In addition to stimulation of protein synthesis, FSH also appears to influence the Sertoli cell cytoskeleton (45) and the distribution of intracellular calcium by stimulation of a calcium dependent regulatory protein. This protein modulates the adenyl cyclase system through phosphodiesterase suppression and alters cellular secretion and motility by microfilament realignment.

Considerable controversy exists over the steroidogenic potential of the seminiferous tubule. While Sertoli cells of 10-day-old rats can convert androstenedione to testosterone (17β-oxidoreductase activity) when stimulated by FSH (4,20), no conversion to testosterone can be demonstrated when cholesterol is added to seminiferous tubule preparations. Since Sertoli cells from older rats do not exhibit increased steroid synthesis in response to FSH, an important role for Sertoli cell steroidogenesis appears limited to the immature developing testis.

Spermatogenesis

Endocrine control of spermatogenesis is a complex process requiring the presence of FSH and high intratesticular levels of testosterone. Although there have been numerous studies in rodents and man (11,24,66), controversy remains over the relative contribution of FSH and testosterone to the spermatogenic process. Steinberger presented convincing evidence in the hypophysectomized, immature rat that testosterone alone could account for the initiation of spermatogenesis and that FSH was required only for its completion (spermatid to spermatozoa) (66,68). Several studies in boys with precocious puberty because of interstitial cell testicular tumors also support the concept that high intratesticular levels of testosterone are necessary for initiation of spermatogenesis. The tubules adjacent to the androgen producing tumor undergo germinal maturation while the contralateral testis remains unstimulated despite virilizing peripheral serum concentrations of testosterone.

Unlike the rat, exogenous administration of testosterone to hypogonadotropic men does not induce spermatogenesis (42). This failure in the human is most likely owing to the practical limits of the dose which can be administered. By contrast HCG administration stimulates an increase in intratesticular testosterone and promptly initiates spermatogenesis (60). In the absence of exogenous FSH maturation of the seminiferous epithelium does not progress beyond the spermatid stage in men with complete hypogonadotropism. Although FSH alone does not initiate spermatogenesis, the addition of FSH to HCG primed hypogonadotropic men results in completion of spermatogenesis and production of adequate numbers of sperm for impregnation. In this regard, an important role for FSH in spermiogenesis (completion of spermatid to mature spermatozoa) is similar in both rat and man.

An important role for FSH in the maintenance of spermatogenesis, however, is more controversial. Two lines of evidence in the human suggest that spermatogenesis may be maintained by high intratesticular levels of androgen (1,17) in the absence of normal levels of FSH. Studies in sexually mature men have demonstrated that sperm output can be maintained after suppression of FSH when high levels of intratesticular androgen are achieved by HCG administration (58). More recently, studies in hypogonadotropic men show that spermatogenesis can be maintained by HCG alone once adequate sperm production has been achieved utilizing both HCG and FSH (60). Additional information will be required to define a precise role of FSH in the maintenance of spermatogenesis.

REGULATION OF GONADOTROPIN SECRETION

Leydig cell

There is abundant evidence that a variety of sex steroids are capable of modifying both LH and FSH concentrations in the peripheral circulation (59,62,63). The Leydig cell normally secretes testosterone, estradiol, and 17-OH progesterone. Early studies suggested that testosterone was the principal regulator of LH secretion while estradiol was an important modifier of FSH release (26). More recently studies of sex steroid secretion demonstrated that testosterone serves as an important prohormone for estradiol production (5). In normal men two-thirds to three-fourths of the total daily production of estradiol (30–40 µg/day) is derived from conversion of testosterone in peripheral tissues while only 30% is secreted directly from the testis (Fig. 2) (41). Similarly, testosterone serves as the prohormone for dihydrotestosterone (DHT) production. Virtually all of the daily DHT production (300 µg/day) is derived from conversion of testosterone in peripheral tissues. Since both androgens and estrogens alter LH and FSH levels, the relative contribution of testosterone and estradiol upon gonadotropin concentrations must take into account these peripheral conversions.

Recent studies have shown that androgens and estrogens have differential effects on gonadotropin regulation (54,69,79). When testosterone is administered to normal men in physiologic dosage the mean concentrations of LH and FSH are equally suppressed (59,79). Administration of estradiol at levels which are achieved by peripheral conversion of physiologic concentrations of testosterone, produces the same degree of FSH suppression as that produced by testosterone

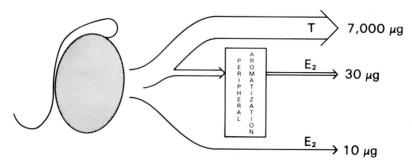

FIG. 2. Schematic representation of direct testicular secretion of testosterone (7,000 µg/day) and estradiol (10 µg/day) and production of estradiol (30 µg/day) by peripheral aromatization of the secreted testosterone.

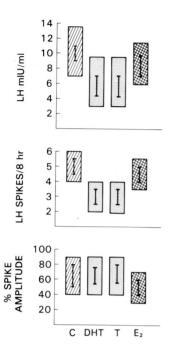

FIG. 3. The effect in normal men of dihydro-testosterone (DHT), testosterone (T) and es-tradiol (E₂) on mean LH concentration *(top)*, the number of LH spikes per 8 hr *(middle)*, and LH spike amplitude *(bottom)*. The range of values for each group is shown by the closed rectangle. Standard deviation is indicated within the rectangle. Pretreatment basal values are indicated as group C.

itself and 60% of the decrease seen in the LH level by testosterone. To determine whether aromatization explains all of the testosterone effect on LH and FSH concentrations, nonaromatizable androgens have been administered in similar kinetic studies. These "pure androgens" decrease mean LH levels but fail to alter FSH concentration. Thus, testosterone modulates gonadotropin concentrations both as an androgen and as a prohormone for estradiol (79).

The androgenic and estrogenic components of testosterone action alter pulsatile LH release by different mechanisms (Fig. 3) (55,79). The pulse frequency of episodic LH bursts in plasma is decreased following administration of testosterone and pure androgens, while no change in pulse frequency occurs following estradiol administration. On the other hand, the decrease in mean LH level following estradiol administration is associated with a proportional reduction in pulse amplitude while no such effect is seen following pure androgen administration (55,79). The importance of aromatization in testosterone's modulation of gonadotropin concentrations is further emphasized by the failure of testosterone to suppress LH and FSH levels in men pretreated with the antiestrogen clomiphene (79). In recent studies it has also been possible to selectively inhibit the aromatization of testosterone to estradiol in normal men without diminishing testosterone secretion (43). In this setting both LH and FSH concentrations rise in response to the selective lowering of estradiol levels.

Some studies of men with primary gonadal failure have suggested a relative insensitivity of gonadotropin levels to suppression by androgen. However, recent analysis of the regulation of LH concentrations in both castrate men and men with primary gonadal failure has shown that there is a loss only of the pure androgenic component of testosterone action (80). Unlike normal men, testosterone administration produces a decrease in LH pulse amplitude in these patients, but no change in pulse frequency. In addition, administration of pure androgen fails to produce any change in mean LH level or pulse frequency. These data support the concept that testosterone acts both as an androgen and as an estrogen.

In men, where seminiferous tubule injury results in selective germ cell depletion, a monotropic increase in FSH level occurs (19,28,40,61,75), while there is maintenance of essentially normal Leydig cell function (Fig. 4). These data suggest a difference in gonadal regulation of FSH and LH. Since testosterone administration produces equimolar LH and FSH suppression when infused into normal men at physiologic doses (59,79), the apparent difference in FSH regulation may not be related to testosterone action. At present, no selective deficit in any sex steriod examined has been found which accounts for the monotropic increase in FSH level among men with germ cell depletion (70). These data suggest that there may be another testicular factor, independent of sex steroids, which regulates FSH concentration.

Seminiferous tubule

To explain the elevation in FSH but not LH concentration following germ cell depletion, McCullagh (44) in 1932 hypothesized that the seminiferous tubule produced a factor capable of selective FSH suppression which he termed inhibin. During the last decade, numerous laboratories have corroborated these results. More recently, a series of studies utilizing seminal plasma, rete testis fluid, and aqueous testis extracts have provided direct evidence for a factor which appears capable of selectively lowering FSH levels (6,27,74). Inhibin is thought to be a protein with a molecular weight between 5,000 to 20,000 daltons. A similar factor has now been isolated from ovarian follicular fluid which suggests that there may be an analogous non-sex steroid FSH inhibitor in the female (57). Thus, it appears that regulation of FSH secretion, unlike that of LH, may involve two testicular products: testosterone and a seminiferous tubule protein.

Recent investigations have identified the Sertoli cell as the most likely site of inhibin production. Germ cell depletion states can be achieved in the rat during which FSH levels remain within normal limits. However, the most direct evidence for Sertoli cell production of inhibin comes from studies where Sertoli cells are co-cultured with pituitary cells; and FSH levels are decreased in the media (64,65). Sertoli cell preparations have also been found to suppress FSH response to GnRH and to decrease synthesis of FSH in rat pituitary cultures (67). Together, these data provide provocative evidence that an inhibin exists and is probably produced by the Sertoli cell.

Although clinical observations and direct studies employing other species

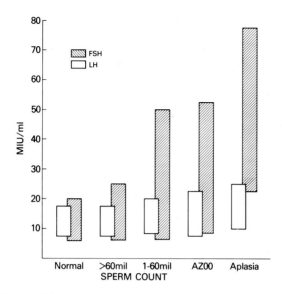

FIG. 4. Levels of serum FSH and LH concentration in normal and infertile men with varying sperm counts and germ cell deficiencies: High sperm output (<60 ml), low sperm output (1–60 ml), azoospermia with maturation arrest (azoo), and germinal aplasia (aplasia). The range of values for each group is indicated in the enclosed rectangle.

support the existence of a testicular protein capable of specific FSH inhibition, sufficient evidence also exists from primate studies to seriously question the physiologic role of inhibin in man. When physiologic amounts of testosterone are given to Rhesus monkeys immediately following castration, FSH and LH levels remain at precastration values indicating that in the Rhesus no other testicular product is required for suppressive control of FSH (50). Until further investigation of human castrates following testosterone replacement or purification and synthesis of the putative testicular protein capable of selective FSH suppression occurs, the physiologic role of inhibin in the human will remain in question.

LEYDIG-SERTOLI CELL INTERACTION

Whereas the pituitary-testicular axis is the principal pathway for endocrine control, recent studies provide provocative evidence for the existence of an intratesticular Leydig-Sertoli cell interaction (Fig. 5) (2,22,34). *In vitro* studies demonstrate that Sertoli cells are capable of converting androgen precursors into estrogen in the absence of Leydig cells (20). In rats (9) estrogens reduce testosterone synthesis independently of LH suppression. This effect is mediated through a decrease in Leydig cell LH receptors as well as inhibition of $17\text{-}\alpha$ hydroxylase and 17-desmolase enzymes (22). Similar effects have been reported in men with prostatic carcinoma treated with synthetic estrogens (7), where testosterone con-

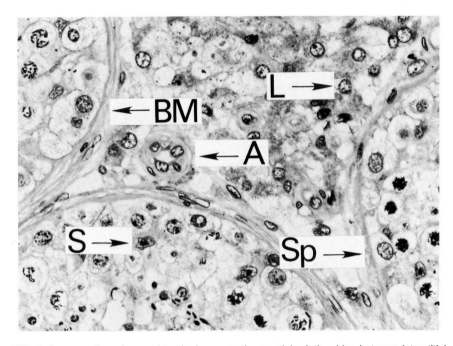

FIG. 5. Cross section of normal testis demonstrating spatial relationships between interstitial Leydig cells (L) and seminiferous tubule sertoli cells (S). Spermatocytes, basement membrane (Bm) and arterioles (A) are shown for further orientation (HE. ×500).

centration is suppressed to about 20% of pretreatment levels without significant LH suppression. A possible candidate for this local Leydig cell regulator is estradiol (34,36) since rat Leydig cells have been shown to contain estradiol but not androgen receptors (47). These data suggest the presence of a closed loop feedback system where Leydig cell androgens are aromatized by the Sertoli cell to estrogens which diffuse back into the interstitial tissue to regulate Leydig cell function.

REFERENCES

1. Ahmad, N., Haltmeyer, G. V., and Eik-Nes, K. B. (1975): Maintenance of spermatogenesis with testosterone or dihydrotestosterone in hypophysectomized rats. *J. Reprod. Fert.,* 44:103–107.
2. Aoki, A., and Fawcett, D. W. (1978): Is there a local feedback from the seminiferous tubules affecting activity of the Leydig cell. *Biol. Reprod.,* 19:144–158.
3. Aragma, C., and Frieson, H. C. (1975): Specific prolactin binding sites in the prostate and testis of rats. *Endocrinology,* 97:677–684.
4. Armstrong, D. T., Moon, Y. S., Fritz, I. B., and Dorrington, J. H. (1975): Synthesis of estradiol-17 by Sertoli cells in culture: Stimulation of FSH and dibutyryl cyclic AMP. In: *Hormonal Regulation of Spermatogenesis,* edited by F. S. French, pp. 85–96. Plenum Press, New York.
5. Baird, D., Horton, R., Longcope, C., and Tait, J. F. (1968): Steroid pre-hormones, *Perspect. Biol. Med.,* 1:384–421.

6. Baker, H. W. G., Bremner, W. J., Burger, H. G., de Kretser, D. M., Dulmanis, A., Eddie, L. W., Hudson, P., Keogh, E. J., Lee, V. W., and Rennie, G. C. (1976): Testicular control of follicle stimulating hormone secretion. *Recent Prog. Horm. Res.,* 32:429–476.

7. Baker, H. W. G., Burger, H. C., de Kretser, D. M., Hudson, B., and Straffon, W. G. (1973): Effects of synthetic oral estrogen in normal men and patients with prostatic carcinoma. Lack of gonadotropin suppression by chlorotrianesine. *Clin. Endocrinol.,* 2:297–306.

8. Bartke, A. (1976): Pituitary-testis relationships; Role of prolactin in the regulation of testicular function. In: *Progress in Reproductive Biology-Sperm Action,* Vol. 1, edited by P. O. Hubinot and M. L. Hermite, p. 136. Karger, Basel.

9. Bartke, A. K., Williams, I. H., and Dalterio, S. (1977): Effects of estrogens on testicular testosterone production in vitro. *Biol. Reprod.,* 171:645–649.

10. Besser, G. M., and Thorner, M. O. (1975): Prolactin and gonadal function. *Pathol. Biol. (Paris),* 23:779–782.

11. Burger, H. G., Franchimont, P., de Kretser, D. M., and Hudson, B. (1975): Gonadotropins in spermatogenesis control. In: *Recent Progress in Reproductive Endocrinology,* edited by P. G. Crosignani and V. H. T. James, p. 605. Academic Press, New York.

12. Boccabella, A. V. (1963): Reinitiation and restoration of spermatogenesis with testosterone propionate and other hormones after a long-term post hypophysectomy regression period. *Endocrinology,* 72:787–798.

13. Catt, K. J., Tsuruhara, T., Mendelson, C., Ketelslegers, J. M., and Dufau, M. L. (1974): Gonadotrophin binding and activation of the interstitial cell of the testis. In: *Hormone Binding and Target Cell Activation in the Testis,* edited by M. L. Dufaw and A. R. Means, p. 237. Plenum Press, New York.

14. Charreau, E. H., Attramadal, A., Lorjesen, P. A., Purvis, K., Calandra, R., and Hansson, V. (1977): Prolactin binding in rat testis: specific receptors in interstitial cells. *Mol. Cell. Endocrinol.,* 6:303–308.

15. Chopra, I. J., Tulchinsky, D., and Greenway, F. L. (1973): Estrogen androgen imbalance in hepatic cirrhosis. *Ann. Intern. Med.,* 79:198–203.

16. Chowdhury, M., Steinberger, A., and Steinberger, E. (1978): Inhibition of de novo synthesis of FSH by the Sertoli cell factor (SCF). *Endocrinology,* 103:644–647.

17. Davies, A. G., Courot, M., and Gresham, P. (1974): Effect of testosterone on spermatogenesis in adult mice during treatment with estradiol. *J. Endocrinol.,* 60:37–45.

18. de Jong, F. H., Hey, A. H., and Van der Molen, H. J. (1973): Effect of gonadotrophins on the secretion of estradiol 17β and testosterone by the rat testis. *J. Endocrinol.,* 57:277–284.

19. de Kretser, D. M., Burger, H. G., and Hudson, B. (1974): Relationship between serum FSH levels and germinal cells in males with infertility. *J. Clin. Endocrinol. Metab.,* 38:787–793.

20. Dorrington, J. H., and Armstrong, D. T. (1975): Follicle stimulating hormone stimulates estradiol-17β synthesis in cultured Sertoli cells. *Proc. Natl. Acad. Sci.,* 72:2677–2681.

21. Dorrington, J. H., and Fritz, I. B. (1974): Effects of gonadotropins on cyclic AMP production by isolated seminiferous tubule and insterstitial cell preparations. *Endocrinology,* 94:395–403.

22. Dufau, M., Hsueh, A. J., Cigorraga, S., Backal, A. J., and Catt, K. J. (1978): Inhibition of Leydig cell function through hormonal regulatory mechanism. *Int. J. Androl.* Suppl. 2:193–239.

23. Dufau, M., Tsuruhara, T., Horner, K. A., Podesta, E. J., and Catt, K. J. (1977): Intermediate role of adenosine cyclic monophosphate and protein kinase during gonadotrophin induced steroidogenesis in testicular interstitial cells. *Proc. Natl. Acad. Sci. USA,* 74:3419–3423.

24. Elkington, J. S. H., and Blackshaw, A. W. (1974): Studies on testicular function. I. Quantitative effects of FSH, LH, testosterone, and dihydrotestosterone on restoration and maintenance of spermatogenesis in the hypophysectomized rat. *Aust. J. Biol. Sci.,* 27:47–57.

25. Elkington, J. S. H., Sanborn, B. M., Martin, M. W., Chowdhury, A. K., and Steinberger, E. (1977): Effect of testosterone proprionate on ABP levels in rats hypophysectomized at different ages using individual sampling. *Mol. Cell. Endocrinol.,* 6:203–210.

26. Franchimont, P., Chari, S., and Demoulin, A. (1975): Hypothalamus- pituitary-testis interaction. *J. Reprod. Fert.,* 44:335–350.

27. Franchimont, P. S., Chari, S., Hagelstein, M. I., and Duraiswami, S. (1975): Existence of a follicle-stimulaing hormone inhibiting factor inhibin in bull seminal plasma. *Nature,* 257:402–404.

28. Franchimont, P., Millet, D., Vendrely, E., Letarve, J. Legros, J. J., and Netter, A. (1972):

Relationship between spermatogenesis and serum gonadotropin levels in azoospermia and oligospermia. *J. Clin. Endocrinol. Metab.,* 34:1003–1008.

29. Hafiez, A., Bartke, A., and Lloyd, C. W. (1972): The role of prolactin in the regulation of testis function: the synergistic effects of prolactin and LH on the incorporation of C^{14}-acetate into testosterone and cholesterol by testis from hypophysectomized rats in vitro. *J. Endrocrinol.,* 53:223–230.

30. Hafiez, A. A., Philpott, J. E., and Bartke, A. (1971): The role of prolactin in the regulation of testicular function: the effect of prolactin and luteinizing hormone on 3β hydroxysteroid dehydrogenase activity in the testis of mice and rats. *J. Endocrinol.,* 50:619–623.

31. Hall, P. F., Irby, D. C., and de Kretser, D. M. (1967): Conversion of cholesterol to androgens by rat testis. Comparison of interstitial cells and seminiferous tubules. *Endocrinology,* 84:488–496.

32. Hansson, V. M., Ritzen, M., French, F. S., and Nayfeh, S. N. (1975): Androgen transport and receptor mechanisms in testis and epididymis. In: *Handbook of Physiology,* Vol. V, edited by R. Greep and D. W. Hamilton, pp. 173–202. American Physiological Society, Washington, D.C.

33. Hsu, Aiv-Fel, and Troen, P. (1978): An androgen binding protein in the testicular cytosol of human testis. *J. Clin. Invest.,* 61:1611–1619.

34. Hsueh, A. J., Dufau, M., and Catt, K. J. (1978): Inhibitory effects of estrogen on Leydig cell function: studies of FSH treated hypophysectomized rat. *Endocrinology,* 103:1069–1102.

35. Johnson, B. H., and Ewing, L. L. (1971): Follicle-stimulating hormone and the regulation of testosterone secretion in rabbit testis. *Science,* 73:635–637.

36. Jones, T. M., Fang, V. S., Landau, R. L., and Rosenfield, R. (1975): Direct inhibition of Leydig cell function by estradiol. *Proceedings: American Endocrine Society,* 57th Annual Meeting, Abstract 196.

37. Krueger, P. M., Hodgen, G. D., Sherins, R. J. (1974): New evidence for the role of the Sertoli cell and spermatogonia in feedback control of FSH secretion in male rats. *Endocrinology,* 95:955–962.

38. Lacroix, M., Smith, F. E., and Fritz, I. B. (1977): Secretion of plasminogen activation by Sertoli cell-enriched cultures. *Mol. Cell. Endocrinol.,* 9:227–236.

39. Lee, P. A., Hoffman, W. H., White, J. J., Engle, R. M. E., and Blizzard, E. M. (1974): Serum gonadotropins in cryptorchidism. *Am. J. Dis. Child.,* 127:530–532.

40. Leonard, J. M., Leach, R. B., Couture, M., and Paulsen, C. A. (1972): Plasma and urinary follicle stimulating hormone levels in oligospermia. *J. Clin. Endocrinol. Metab.,* 34:209–214.

41. Longcope C., Kato, T., and Horton, R. (1969): Conversion of blood androgens to estrogens in normal men and women. *J. Clin. Invest.,* 48:2191–2201.

42. MacLeod, J. (1970): The effects of urinary gonadotropin following hypophysectomy and in hypogonadotropic eunuchoidism. In: *The Human Testis,* edited by E. Rosenberg and C. A. Paulsen, pp. 577–590. Plenum Press, New York.

43. Marynick, S. P., Loriaux, D. L., Sherins, R. J., Pita, J. C., and Lipsett, M. B. (1979): Evidence that testosterone acts on both an androgen and an estrogen in suppressing pituitary gonadotropin secretion in men. *J. Clin. Endocrinol. Metab.,* 49:396–398.

44. McCullagh, D. R. (1932): Dual endocrine activity of the testis. *Science,* 76:19–21.

45. Means, A. R., Dedman, J. R., Tindall, D. J., and Welsh, M. J. (1978): Hormonal regulation of Sertoli cell. *Int. J. Androl.* [Suppl 2], 2:403–421.

46. Means, A. R., Fakunding, J. L., Huckins, C., Tindall, D. J., and Vitale, R. (1976): Follicle-stimulating hormone, the Sertoli cell and spermatogenesis. *Recent Prog. Horm. Res.,* 32:477.

47. Mulder, E., Van Beurden-Lamers, W. M. O., De Boer, W., Brinkman, A. O., and Van der Molen, H. J. (1974): Testicular estradiol receptors in the rat. In: *Hormone Binding and Target Cell Activation in the Testis,* edited by M. L. Dufau and A. R. Means, pp. 343–356. Plenum Press, New York.

48. Naftolin, F., Ryan, K. J., Davies, I. J., Reddy, V. V., Flores, F., Petro, Z., and Kuhn, M. (1975): The formation of estrogens by central neuroendocrine tissue. *Recent Prog. Horm. Res.,* 31:249–314.

49. Odell, W. D., Swerdloff, R. S., Jacobs, H. S., and Hescox, M. A. (1973): FSH induction of sensitivity to LH: one cause of sexual maturation in the male rat. *Endocrinology,* 92:160–165.

50. Plant, T. M., Hess, D. L., Hotchkiss, J., and Knobil, E. (1978): Testosterone and the control of gonadotropin secretion in the male rhesus monkey. *Endocrinology,* 103:535–541.

51. Ruder, H. J., Loriaux, D. L., Sherins, R. J., and Lipsett, M. B. (1974): Leydig cell function in men with disorders of spermatogenesis. *J. Clin. Endocrinol. Metab.,* 38:244–247.
52. Rubin, R. T., Poland, R., Sobel, I., Towin, B., and Odell, W. (1978): Effects of prolactin and prolactin plus luteinizing hormone on plasma testosterone levels in normal adult men. *J. Clin. Endocrinol. Metab.,* 47:447–452.
53. Sanborn, B. M., Elklington, J. S. H., Chowdhury, M., Tcholakian, R. K., and Steinberger, E. (1975): Hormonal influences on the level of testicular androgen binding activity: effect of FSH following hypophysectomy. *Endocrinology,* 96:304–312.
54. Santen, R. J. (1975): Is aromatization of testosterone to estradiol required for inhibition of LH secretion in men. *J. Clin. Invest.,* 56:1555–1563.
55. Santen, R. J., and Bardin, C. W. (1973): Episodic luteinizing hormone secretion in man. Pulse analysis, clinical interpretation, physiologic mechanisms. *J. Clin. Invest.,* 52:2617–2628.
56. Santen, R. J., Leonard, J. M., Sherins, R. J., Gandy, H. M., and Paulsen, C. A. (1971): Short and long-term effects of clomiphene citrate on the pituitary-testicular axis. *J. Clin. Endocrinol. Metab.,* 33:970–976.
57. Schwartz, N. B., Channing, C. P. (1977): Evidence for ovarian "inhibin": suppression of the secondary rise in serum follicle stimulating hormone levels in proestrus rats by injection of porcine follicular fluid. *Proc. Natl. Acad. Sci. USA,* 74:5721–5723.
58. Sherins, R. J. (1974): Clinical aspects of treatment of male infertility with gonadotropins: Testicular response of some men given hCG with and without pergonal. In: *Male Infertility and Sterility. Proceedings of the Serono Symposia,* Vol. 5, edited by R. E. Mancini and L. Martini, pp. 545–565. Academic Press, New York.
59. Sherins, R. J., and Loriaux, D. L. (1973): Studies on the role of sex steroids in the feedback control of FHS concentrations in men. *J. Clin. Endocrinol. Metab.,* 36:886–893.
60. Sherins, R. J., Winters, S. J., and Wachslicht, H. (1977): Studies of the role of HCG and low dose FSH in initiating spermatogenesis in hypogonadotropic men. *Proceedings: American Endocrine Society,* 59th Annual Meeting, Abstract No. 312.
61. Sina, D. R., Schumann, R., Abraham, R., Taubert, H. D., and Dericks-Tan, J. S. E. (1973): Increased serum FSH levels correlated with low and high sperm counts in male infertile patients. *Andrologia,* 7:31–37.
62. Sizonenko, P. C., Cuendet, A., Paunier, L. (1973): FSH. I. Evidence for its mediating role on testosterone secretion in cryptorchidism. *J. Clin. Endocrinol. Metab.,* 37:68–73.
63. Stewart-Bently, M., Odell, W., and Horton, R. (1974): The feedback control of luteinizing hormone in normal adult men. *J. Clin. Endocrinol. Metab.,* 38:545–553.
64. Steinberger, A., Heindel, J. J., Lindsey, J. N., Elkington, J. S. H., Sanborn, B. M., and Steinberger, E. (1975): Isolation and culture of FSH responsive cells. *Endocr. Res. Commun.,* 2:261–270.
65. Steinberger, A., and Steinberger, E. (1976): Secretion of an FSH inhibiting factor by cultured Sertoli cells. *Endocrinology,* 99:918–921.
66. Steinberger, E. (1971): Hormonal control of mammalian spermatogenesis. *Physiol. Rev.,* 51:1–22.
67. Steinberger, E., and Chowdhury, M. (1974): Control of pituitary FSH in male rats. *Acta Endocrinol. (Kbh),* 76:235–241.
68. Steinberger, E. A., Root, A., Ficher, M., and Smith, K. D. (1973): The role of androgens in the initiation of spermatogenesis in the rat. *J. Clin. Endocrinol. Metab.,* 37:746–751.
69. Swerdloff, R. S., Walsh, P. C. (1973): Testosterone and estradiol suppression of LH and FSH in adult male rats: Duration of castration, duration of treatment and combined treatment. *Acta Endocrinol. (Kbh),* 73:11–21.
70. Swerdloff, R. S., Grover, P. K., Jacobs, H. S., and Bain, J. (1973): Search for a substance which selectively inhibits FSH-Effects of steroids and prostaglandins on serum FSH and LH levels. *Steroids,* 21:703–722.
71. Thanki, K. N., and Steinberger, A. (1977): Effect of age and hypophysectomy on FSH binding by rat testis. *Andrologia,* 9:307.
72. Tindall, D. J., Mena, C. R., and Means, A. R. (1978): Hormonal regulation of androgen-binding protein in the hypophysectomized rat. *Endocrinology,* 103:589–594.
73. Tsuruhara, T., Dufau, M., Cigurraga, S., and Catt, K. J. (1977): Hormonal regulation of testicular luteinizing hormone receptors. Effects on cyclic AMP and testosterone responses in isolated Leydig cells. *J. Biol. Chem.,* 252:9002–9009.
74. Van Beurden, W. M. O., Roodnat, B., and Van der Molen, H. J. (1978): Effects of estrogens

and FSH on LH stimulation of steroid production by testis Leydig cells from immature rats. *Int. J. Androl.,* Suppl. 2:374–384.

75. Van Thiel, D. H., Lester, R., and Sherins, R. J. (1974): Hypogonadism in alcoholic liver disease: Evidence for a double defect. *Gastroenterology,* 67:1188–1199.

76. Van Thiel, D. H., Sherins, R. J., Myers, G. H., and DeVita, V. T. (1972): Evidence for a specific seminiferous tubular factor affecting FSH secretion in man. *J. Clin. Invest.,* 51:1009–1019.

77. Vigersky, R. A., Easley, R. B., and Loriaux, D. L. (1976): Effect of fluoxymesterone on the pituitary-gonadal axis: The role of testosterone-estradiol-binding globulin. *J. Clin. Endocrinol. Metab.,* 43:1–9.

78. Vigersky, R. A., Loriaux, D. L., Howards, S. S., Hodgen, G. D., Lipsett, M. B., and Chrambach, A. (1976): Androgen binding proteins of testis, epididymis and plasma in man and monkey. *J. Clin. Invest.,* 58:1061–1068.

79. Winters, S. J., Janick, J., Loriaux, D. L., and Sherins, R. J. (1979): Studies on the role of sex steroids in the feedback control of gonadotropin concentrations in men. II: Use of the estrogen antagonist clomiphene citrate. *J. Clin. Endocrinol. Metab.,* 48:222–227.

80. Winters, S. J., Sherins, R. J., and Loriaux, D. L. (1979): Studies on the role of sex steroids in the feedback control of gonadotrophin concentrations in men. III: Androgen resistance in primary gonadal failure. *J. Clin. Endocrinol. Metab.,* 48:553–558.

81. Wollesen, F., Swerdloff, R. S., Peterson, M., and Odell, W. D. (1974): Testosterone modulation of pituitary response to LRH: Differential effects on luteinizing hormone and follicle-stimulating hormone. *J. Clin. Invest.,* 53:85–90.

The Testis, edited by H. Burger and D. de Kretser.
Raven Press, New York © 1981.

7

The Cytology of the Human Testis

J. B. Kerr and D. M. de Kretser

Department of Anatomy, Monash University, Clayton, Victoria, Australia

The past twenty years have seen a marked expansion in our knowledge of the cytology of the testis, especially by the use of improved techniques for fixation and the availability of electron microscopy. Many of these studies have used tissue from species other than man but their findings have subsequently been shown to be relevant to human testicular tissue. Owing to the limitation of space, this chapter will be confined to an outline of the cytology of the human testes which has been subdivided into three areas: (a) The seminiferous tubule; (b) the lamina propria of the tubule or peritubular tissue; (c) the interstitial or Leydig cells (Fig. 1).

SPERMATOGENESIS AND THE SEMINIFEROUS TUBULE

The detailed studies by Clermont (19) on the light microscopy and kinetics of spermatogenesis on many mammalian species have demonstrated an orderly sequence of development which is characterized for each species including the time taken for the entire process. In a comprehensive light microscopic account of human spermatogenesis, Clermont (21) identified six cellular associations which constituted the human seminiferous cycle (Figs. 2 and 3) and, by the intratesticular injection of tritiated thymidine, showed that the development of a sperm from spermatogonia took 70 ± 4 days (58). The process can be subdivided into three phases: (a) The replication of stem cells or spermatogonia; (b) Meiosis involving the primary and secondary spermatocytes; (c) Spermiogenesis, the complex metamorphosis resulting in the transformation of a "conventional" cell, the spermatid, to the spermatozoon.

Replication of Stem Cells

Spermatogonia are situated adjacent to the basement membrane of the tubule (Figs. 4–6) and Clermont (21) described three distinct types based mainly on differences in their nuclear structure, features only identifiable in appropriately

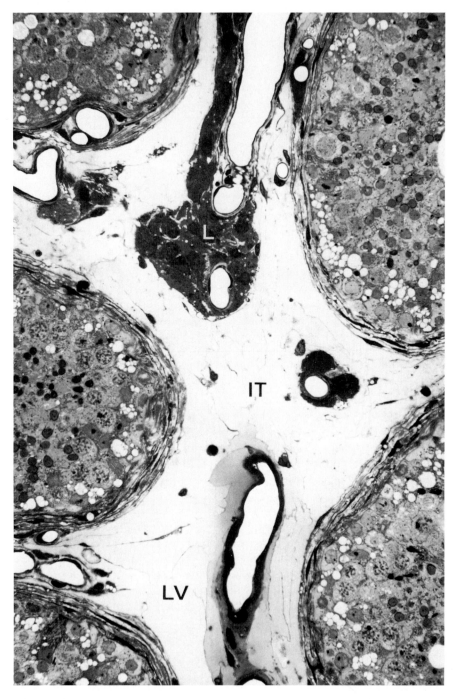

FIG. 1. Light micrograph of human testis fixed by perfusion, illustrating the intertubular tissue (IT) between five seminiferous tubules which contains islands of Leydig cells (L) and a lymphatic vessel (LV). ×400.

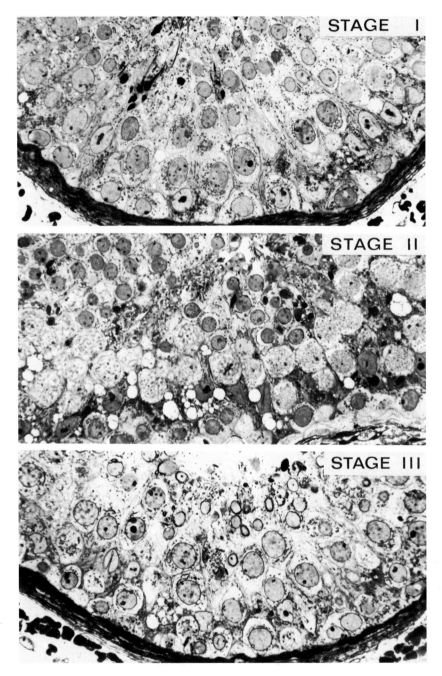

FIG. 2. Stages of the human spermatogenic cycle illustrated with 1 μm Epon-araldite sections stained with Toluidine blue. Stage I, II, and III of the human seminiferous epithelium. ×640.

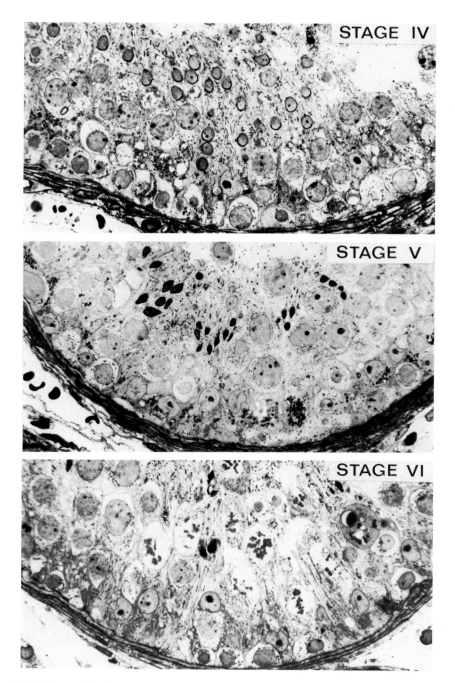

FIG. 3. Stages of the human spermatogenic cycle illustrated with 1 μm Epon-araldite sections stained with Toluidine blue. Stage IV, V, and VI of the human seminiferous epithelium. ×640.

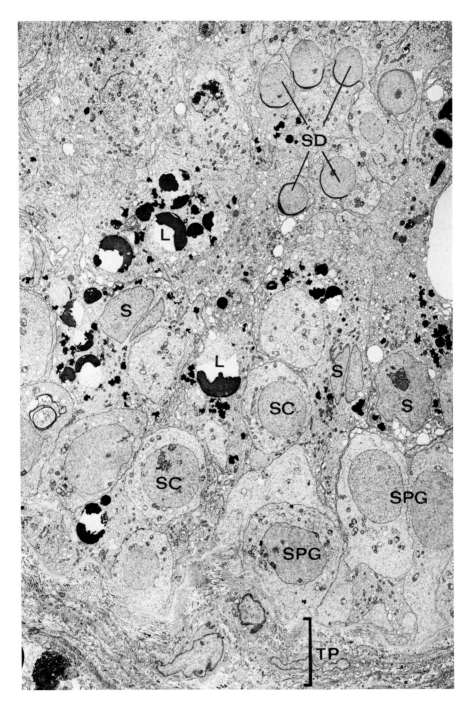

FIG. 4. Electron micrograph of the human seminiferous epithelium at stage IV, showing basally situated spermatogonia (SPG) supported by the tunica propria (TP), primary spermatocytes (SC), and round spermatids (SD). Sertoli cell nuclei (S) and many Sertoli cell lipid inclusions (L) also are illustrated. ×1,800.

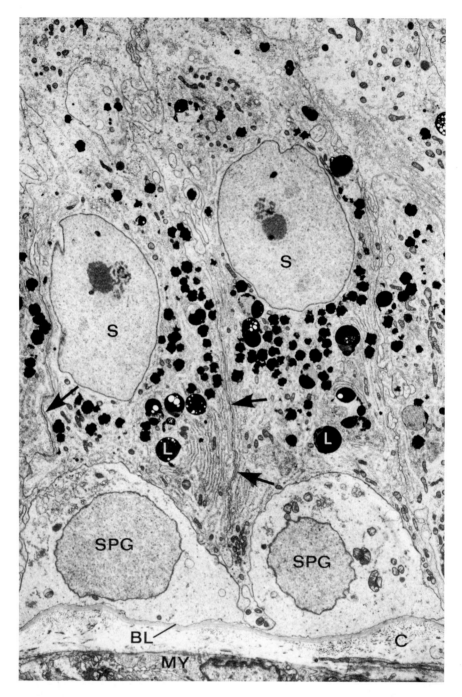

FIG. 5. Electronmicrograph of adjacent Sertoli cells with irregular nuclei (S) each containing a prominent nucleolus. Junctional specializations are observed at the apposed surfaces of the Sertoli cells (arrows), and many lipid inclusions (L) are present within the basal Sertoli cell cytoplasm. Basally positioned spermatogonia (SPG) rest upon the peritubular tissue, consisting of a basal lamina (BL), collagen fibres (C), and myoid cells (MY). ×4,000.

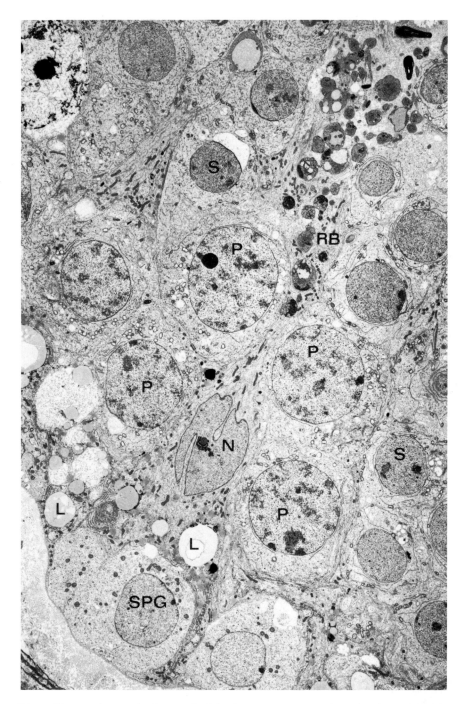

FIG. 6. Electronmicrograph of stage II of the human spermatogenic cycle, characterized by the appearance of many residual bodies (RB) within a columnar cytoplasmic trunk of a Sertoli cell, also exhibiting a basally positioned nucleus (N), and Sertoli cell lipid inclusions (L). Spermatogonia (SPG), pachytene primary spermatocytes (P), and round spermatids (S) are illustrated. ×2,000.

fixed tissue. The three types consisted of (a) the dark type A (Ad); (b) pale
type A (Ap); and (c) type B. In a later study (20), he suggested the type Ad
spermatogonia divide to produce type Ap which in turn produce type B cells.
The latter divide subsequently to produce the preleptotene primary spermatocytes which enter meiosis. Many aspects of stem cell renewal, as they pertain
to spermatogonia, have been investigated extensively in the rat with the identification of a number of subclasses, the demonstration of clusters of spermatogonia
linked by intercellular bridges, and the suggestion that "reserve stem cells"
exist which do not enter the seminiferous cycle (22,61–63).

The type Ad spermatogonia are characterized by a spherical nucleus containing fine granular deeply staining chromatin frequently showing a paler nuclear
vacuole which often contained a nucleolus. The type Ap are identified by an
ovoid nucleus containing palely staining granular chromatin with one or two
nucleoli attached to the nuclear membrane (Figs. 4–6). The type B are distinguished by a nucleus containing fine chromatin granulation in which several
heavily stained chromatin masses are dispersed, some of which are usually associated with the nuclear membrane. The cytoplasm of all spermatogonia stain
palely, and electron microscopy clearly demonstrates intercellular cytoplasmic
bridges (Fig. 4). A number of ultrastructural studies have assessed the nuclear
features of human spermatogonia and though the above characteristics have
been identified, many intermediate forms appeared to exist (27,91,105). The
type Ad have electron-lucent cytoplasm with dispersed glycogen granules and
mitochondria which form perinuclear collections. Between the mitochondria
are aggregations of electron-dense material identified in other species as germ
plasm (3,68). Occasionally small crystals—the crystals of Lubarsch (75) are
seen and consist of fibrils separated by electron-dense granules. The Golgi complex is poorly developed in Ad spermatogonia but increases in size in the type
B. In the sequence of cell divisions which result in type B spermatogonia, the
cytological characteristics change involving a decrease in glycogen content, a
dilatation of the intracristal spaces of mitochondria, and an increase in the
number of vesicles of smooth endoplasmic reticulum. Each type is separated
from adjacent Sertoli cells by a well-defined intercellular space of 200 to 250Å.

Meiosis—Primary and Secondary Spermatocytes

The spermatocyte is the male germ cell in the process of meiosis, the term
primary referring to the diploid germ cell during the first meiotic division and
the term secondary referring to the haploid germ cells during the second meiotic
division. Hence primary spermatocytes result from the division of type B spermatogonia, lose their contact with the basement membrane of the tubule and begin
the long prophase of meiosis which can be subdivided into the classical stages
of leptotene, zygotene, pachytene, diplotene, and diakinesis (Figs. 2 and 3).
This classification is based on the changes in chromatin configuration summarized by Clermont (21) commencing with the appearance of filamentous thread-

like chromosomes (leptotene). The filaments become coarser during zygotene, shortening, thickening, and pairing to form bivalents during the pachytene stage. Further thickening and repulsion between bivalents characterize the relatively short diplotene and diakinetic stages. This sequence of changes constituting the prophase of the first meiotic division took approximately 24 days to complete (58).

Sachs (95) noticed a densely staining rounded body in the nucleus of pachytene primary spermatocytes which resulted from the segregation of the sex chromosomes, the structure being termed the sex vesicle. Ultrastructurally, the sex vesicle consisted of electron-dense "cores" and chromatin fibrils and no true synaptinemal complexes indicating the possibility of crossing-over between the sex chromosomes could be seen (103). Ultrastructurally, the synaptinemal complexes consist of two lateral electron-dense elements together with a central element composed of interlacing microfibrillar elements extending from the inner aspect of both lateral elements. Considerable evidence now exists indicating that the synaptinemal complex is the ultrastructural counterpart of the paired chromosomes or bivalent which appears at the pachytene stage of meiosis, the number of bivalents for any one species being equal to the number of synaptinemal complexes (110,111). The appearance of single electron-dense threads representing the lateral element of the synaptinemal complex enables the identification of the leptotene stage of meiosis.

The cytoplasm of the primary spermatocyte is more electron-dense than the spermatogonia and adjacent cells are joined by intercellular bridges (Figs. 4–6). The Golgi complex is large and consists of a perinuclear aggregation of vesicles and crescentic arrays of membranous lamellae. The mitochondria are frequently aggregated together with intermitochondrial material identical to that seen in spermatogonia. The dilatation of the intracristal spaces in the mitochondria is even more marked than in type B spermatogonia and is similar to that seen in other species though not as marked as in the rat (3). Structures termed annulate lamellae, consisting of parallel interconnected lamellae, are often seen but their function is unknown.

The secondary spermatocytes are seen infrequently in a section of the testis since their life span is relatively short (58) as they rapidly divide to form spermatids. They are smaller than the primary spermatocytes and larger than their daughter cells, the spermatids. As with the other germ cells, they remain interconnected by cytoplasmic intercellular bridges.

Spermiogenesis

The sequence of changes which result in the transformation of the spermatid into a spermatozoon are collectively termed spermiogenesis. No cell division occurs in the process which consists of a highly coordinated reorganization of nucleus and cytoplasm together with the development of the flagellum. The light microscopic descriptions by earlier workers were incorporated by Clermont

(21) into a classification of human spermiogenesis (Fig. 7). Many of the cytological details (Fig. 7) of this process have now been observed by the use of electron microscopy (28) and can be subdivided into the following areas:

Changes in the nucleus; development of the acrosome; formation of the tail; redistribution and loss of the cytoplasm; spermiation.

Changes in the Nucleus

Early in spermiogenesis the nucleus is centrally placed but as the process continues the nucleus becomes eccentric lying adjacent to the cell membrane of the cranial pole of the spermatid but separated from it by the acrosomal cap (Fig. 8). Associated with the change in nuclear position, the chromatin becomes progressively more granular and electron dense (Figs. 9 and 10). In the later phases, the size of the chromatin complexes increases and owing to a reduction in the size of the nuclear volume; the space between the chromatin condensations decreases producing an extremely electron-dense nucleus. The nuclear membrane, made extremely redundant by the decrease in nuclear volume, forms complex folds at the abacrosomal pole, adjacent to the indentation wherein the tail of the sperm articulates with the head.

Development of the Acrosome

One of the earliest features of spermiogenesis is the appearance of a large, irregular vacuole, termed the acrosomal vesicle, in the Golgi region of the spermatid cytoplasm (Fig. 8). The vesicle contains a flocculent material which appears to increase in quantity and electron density as spermiogenesis progresses, the increase occurring by fusion of smaller vesicles from the Golgi complex. The acrosomal vesicle becomes lodged in a shallow indentation of the nucleus at the pole which lies adjacent to the cell membrane. This vesicle spreads to form a cap-like structure, the acrosome, which covers the cranial half of the nucleus (Figs. 9 and 10) and is known to contain substances necessary for the successful penetration of zona pellucida of the ovum (see ref. 14 for review). Having formed the acrosome, the Golgi complex migrates to the caudal pole of the spermatid and is eventually shed.

Formation of the Tail

The cilial-type structure forming the core of the spermatid tail develops early in spermiogenesis from one of the pair of centrioles located near the Golgi complex. A considerable length of the core, or axial filament, which consists of nine peripheral doublet microtubules surrounding a central pair, develops before the tail establishes an articulation with the abacrosomal pole of the nucleus. The centriole giving rise to the axial filament is termed the longitudinal centriole and the other, which lies at right angles, is termed the proximal centriole. Both centrioles are located in a complex structure forming the neck of

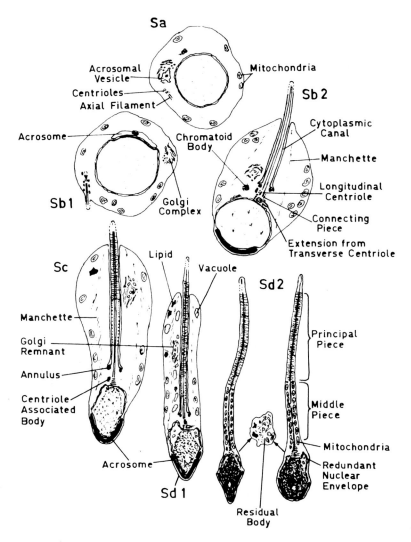

FIG. 7. The ultrastructural features of human spermiogenesis are illustrated diagramatically and arranged to correspond to the light microscopic staging utilized by Clermont (21). (From ref. 28.)

the spermatid close to the point of articulation with the nucleus (Fig. 10). From this electron-dense structure, an outer set of nine electron-dense coarse fibers extend caudally to surround the axial filament over those regions giving rise to the middle-piece and principal-piece of the tail (Fig. 10). The system of nine outer fibers becomes attenuated in the region of the principal-piece though two persist and link with the transversely disposed ribs of the principal-piece (Fig. 9).

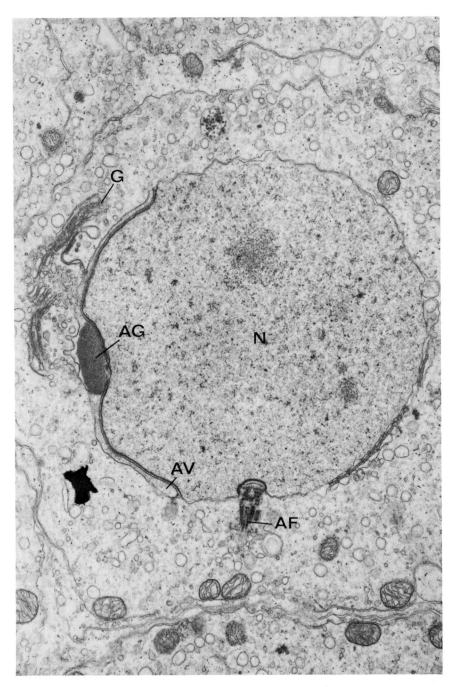

FIG. 8. A spermatid at the Sb$_1$ stage illustrates the formation of the acrosome by aggregation of material from the Golgi complex (G) to the acrosomal vesicle (AV) and granule (G). Note the early development of the axial filament (AF). ×15,200.

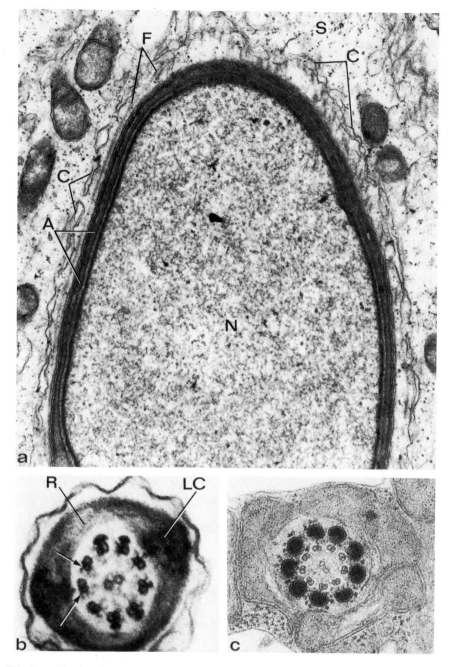

FIG. 9. a. The head of the spermatid at the S_c stage of spermatogenesis shows nucleus (N), acrosome (A), and specialized spermatid-Sertoli cell junction: S = Sertoli cell cytoplasm, C = cisternae of smooth endoplasmic reticulum, F — microfilaments close to the Sertoli cell membrane. ×58,300. **b.** Cross-section of sperm tail in region of principal-piece illustrating microtubules of axial filament with dynein arms (arrows), and ribs (R), and longitudinal columns (LC) of the coarse fiber system. ×101,500. **c.** Cross-section of sperm tail in region of middle-piece, illustrating the mitochondrial sheath (M), outer coarse fibers (CF) and doublets of axial filament (arrows). Note the absence of dynein arms since these sperm were obtained from a patient with the immotile cilia syndrome. ×60,900.

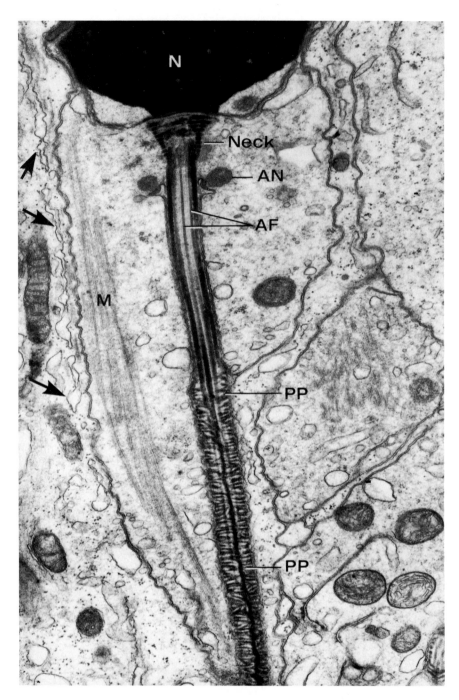

FIG. 10. A spermatid at the Sd₁ demonstrates condensed nucleus (N), the complicated structure of the neck, the annulus (N) which will migrate to the commencement of the principal-piece (PP) thereby delineating the region forming the middle-piece. Note axial filament microtubules (AF), microtubules of manchette (M) and extreme distribution of specialized Sertoli-spermatid cell junctions (arrows). ×11,350.

The mitochondria which early in spermiogenesis are located peripherally in the cell form a helical arrangement extending from the neck to the annulus, an electron-dense ring surrounding the axial filament and nine outer fibers. The mitochondrial helix delineates the region of the sperm termed the middle-piece and is formed late in spermiogenesis just preceding the release of sperm from the epithelium (Fig. 9).

The terminal region of the tail consists of the axial filament surrounded by the cell membrane (Fig. 9). The two centrally-placed single microtubules appear to be connected to the nine peripheral doublets by tenuous radial spokes termed nexin linkages. One of the microtubules forming each pair of doublets is smaller than the other which has a more electron-dense core. The smaller tubule, termed subfiber A, extends a pair of arms toward the adjacent doublet. The arms, consisting of a protein termed dynein are absent in some men with immotile sperm (Fig. 9) (1).

Redistribution and Loss of Cytoplasm

Associated with the movement of the nucleus to an eccentric position adjacent to the cell membrane of the spermatid, there is a relative change in the disposition of the cytoplasmic contents and particularly a migration of the Golgi complex to the caudal region. It is thought that these alterations are associated with the appearance of a palisade of microtubules, termed the manchette, which extend as a cylindrical sheath from the region situated just caudal to the termination of the acrosomal cap (Fig. 10).

Spermiation

Much of this cytoplasm is lost when spermatids are released from the epithelium in the process termed spermiation. At this stage, vacuoles in the spermatid cytoplasm appear to be invaginated by processes of Sertoli cell cytoplasm thereby suggesting that the Sertoli cell may actively participate in release of sperm from the epithelium and retention of the residual cytoplasm (28). The latter, termed residual bodies (Fig. 6), are phagocytosed by the Sertoli cell being progressively degraded by lysosomal action (34).

The definition of the ultrastructural features of spermiogenesis have enabled their correlation with the staging proposed by Clermont (21). It is thus possible to identify ultrastructurally an equivalent to the Sa, Sb_1, Sb_2, S_c, S_{d_1} and S_{d_2} staging of spermatid development and this in turn permits staging of the seminiferous epithelium at an electron microscopic level (Fig. 7).

The Sertoli Cell

A number of studies (6,10,15,36,38,44,46,79,82,96,97) have shown that the cytological characteristics of the human Sertoli cell are similar to those of other mammalian species. The Sertoli cell extends radially from the basement membrane of the seminiferous epithelium to the lumen of the tubule. The basal aspects of adjacent Sertoli cells are separated by spermatogonia which also lie in contact with the basement membrane of the tubule (Fig. 5). More centrally adjacent Sertoli cells meet and exhibit specialized cell junctions. The luminal extensions of the Sertoli cell are not visible by light microscopy since they consist of thin cytoplasmic processes which extend between spermatocytes and spermatids forming an arborizing network (41). This complex three-dimensional array of Sertoli cell cytoplasm is brought about by the necessity of the cell to surround a constantly dividing and mobile germ cell population which move from the basal to the luminal aspects of the epithelium (21,39).

The nuclei of the human Sertoli cells frequently form a single row lying central to the spermatogonia, though some changes in nuclear position occur in relation to the spermatogenic cycle (Figs. 2–4). In the region of the nucleus, the Sertoli cell cytoplasm is abundant and contains the major proportion of the cytoplasmic organelles. It has been shown that in the monkey, the relative volume of the Sertoli cell fluctuates between 25 to 33% of the total volume of the seminiferous epithelium (13). Similar changes have not been noted in the human though the studies have not been extensive and utilized immersion-fixed biopsy material (96). Where possible, studies designed to evaluate changes in the form and structure of the Sertoli cell during the spermatogenic cycle should utilize perfusion-fixed material. Physical disruption accompanies the use of small pieces of tissue obtained by biopsy and immersion fixation may result in unequal penetration of the fixative thereby permitting structural modification to occur. Thus the use of perfusion-fixed material can demonstrate that at Stage II of the cycle columnar cytoplasmic channels extend from the nuclear region to the lumen of the tubule (Fig. 6).

Nucleus

The nucleus of the human Sertoli cell has a pleomorphic shape owing to the complex infolding of the nuclear membrane. The nucleus is usually aligned perpendicular to the basal lamina and exhibits a uniformly homogeneous nucleoplasm, occasionally interrupted by small patches of loosely condensed euchromatin (Fig. 5). Peripheral concentrations of heterochromatin associated with the nuclear membrane are not observed in human Sertoli cells. The well-developed nucleolus forms a tripartite structure (44) consisting of a central dense core and peripheral reticular ramifications of the nucleolonema. Occasionally several associate satellite bodies of heterochromatin are observed. Although the functional significance of this complex nucleolar structure is unknown, the nucleolus is poorly developed and peripherally located before puberty becoming conspicuous during pubertal maturation and the attendant rise in FSH and LH levels. The observation that nucleolar development can be stimulated by gonadotrophic hormone treatment (29) suggests that the attainment of the adult morphology within the Sertoli cell nucleus is related to the action of FSH on the seminiferous tubule (55,78).

Cytoplasm

The basal and intermediate regions of the human Sertoli cell contain a rich supply of cytoplasmic organelles and various inclusion bodies. Mitochondria are commonly ovoid or slender structures, usually randomly distributed but occasionally aggregations are seen adjacent to the basal lamina. Golgi membranes and rough endoplasmic reticulum are not abundant, although the latter may occur in the form of parallel rows of cisternae beneath the level of the nucleus. Lysosomal, autophagic, and multi-vesicular bodies are also seen (Fig. 5). Concentric membranes of smooth endoplasmic reticulum also are observed within the basal cytoplasm of the Sertoli cell, often associated with or surrounding large lipid inclusions (Fig. 11). Earlier ultrastructural studies referred to these structures as lamellar bodies (6,59), but subsequently it was noted that these membranes were connected or perforated by many small annuli resembling the size and shape of nuclear pores (79,96), suggesting an origin from the nuclear membrane. More recent studies have suggested that they are similar to annulate lamellae found in a wide variety of other tissues (54,76). Smooth endoplasmic reticulum in the form of small vesicles or anastomosing tubules is always in plentiful supply throughout the Sertoli cell cytoplasm (Figs. 5 and 11). An unusual type of inclusion body found within the human Sertoli cell is the Charcot-Böttcher crystal (6,15,79,102) usually 10 to 12 μm in length and 1 to 2 μm in width. These crystalline inclusions are found in an infranuclear position, however their origin and function within the Sertoli cell is not clear. Similar crystalloid bodies have been noted in the Sertoli cells of the pig and koala (53,56,57,104). Lipid inclusions form a major component of the human Sertoli cell cytoplasm (Fig. 4) and marked variation in the lipid content of Sertoli cells is seen when examining individual Sertoli cells, or comparing the structure of Sertoli cells of different mammalian species (44). Although the size and number of Sertoli cell lipid inclusions has been demonstrated to undergo cyclic variation in relation to the spermatogenic cycle of the rat testis (67,72,84) this phenomenon has not been noted in the monkey or human Sertoli cells (36,96).

Variable amounts of glycogen, free ribosomes, lipofuscin pigments, and residual bodies may be observed deep within the Sertoli cell cytoplasm, although their precise role in the cell is not well understood. The cytoplasmic matrix of the human Sertoli cell contains microtubules and an extensive network of filaments throughout the basal and apical regions of the cell (44).

A 150 to 250 mμ wide zone consisting of fine filaments completely envelopes the Sertoli cell nucleus. Microtubules are commonly observed within the columnar trunk of the Sertoli cell cytoplasm wherein they probably assist in molding

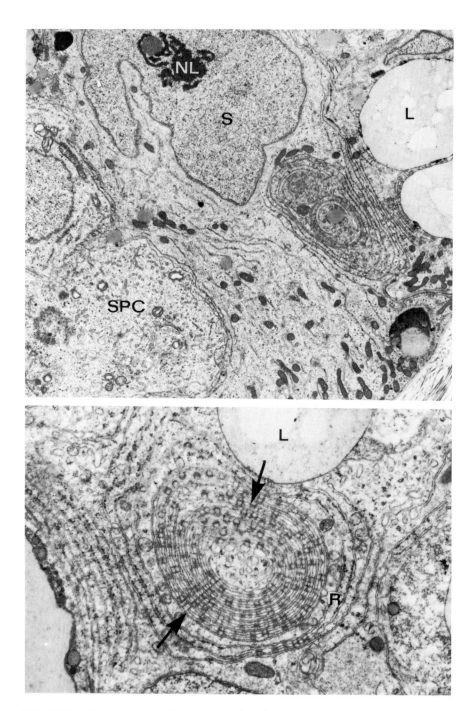

FIG. 11. Top: Electronmicrograph of a human Sertoli cell illustrating the pleomorphic nucleus (S), containing a complex nucleolar structure (NL). The Sertoli cell cytoplasm exhibits lipid inclusions (L) and a large multilayered membranous body surrounding a small lipid droplet. ×5,300. **Bottom:** At higher magnification, these Sertoli cell organelles resemble annulate lamellae, consisting of concentric smooth cisternae apparently connected by annular structures (arrows), similar to nuclear membrane pores. Rough endoplasmic reticulum (R) and part of a lipid droplet (L) are illustrated. ×17,000.

the shape of the thin lateral cytoplasmic processes which surround the germ cells.

Inter-Sertoli Cell Junctions

A remarkable specialization of the surface of the lateral aspects of the Sertoli cell near its base provides areas of adhesion and communication between the apposed plasma membranes of neighboring Sertoli cells. An extensive surface area of each Sertoli cell at or beneath the level of the nucleus contributes to a unique type of junctional complex, consisting of a number of components: (a) small gap junctions bordering an intercellular space narrowed to approximately 20Å, (b) subsurface smooth cisternae which run parallel to the plasma membrane demarcating a cytoplasmic zone containing bundles of cytoplasmic filaments, (c) obliteration of the intercellular space by many points of fusion of the adjacent cell membranes, forming occluding junctions (40,44,49,51,77,107). These junctional complexes found between Sertoli cells constitute the blood-testis barrier which functionally divides the seminiferous epithelium into two compartments. The basal compartment is adjacent to the basal lamina with the adluminal compartment occupying the central epithelial regions beyond the Sertoli cell junctional complexes. This highly selective permeability barrier excludes various blood-borne substances from entering the adluminal compartment of the seminiferous tubule (71,98,99,100) (see Chapter 8). The discovery of the blood-testis barrier was based upon many physiological experiments (9,66,70,83,87,106, 108,109) culminating in experimental studies in which electron-dense extracellular tracers were introduced into the testicular vascular system and it was shown that the intercellular penetration of these marker substances was abruptly restricted by the inter-Sertoli cell junctional complexes (4,36,39,40,49). Recent studies have shown that the creation of a basal epithelial compartment by the Sertoli cell is associated with pubertal development, when junctional complexes first appear between Sertoli cells, fluid secretion by the epithelium begins, and the meiotic maturation process commences (51,107). Spermatogonia and leptotene primary spermatocytes reside within the basal compartment, the subsequent maturation of the germ cells taking place within the specialized physiological milieu provided by the adluminal compartment (36,38,40,93,94). It is thought that blood-borne molecules therefore have direct access to the cells within the basal compartment, but in order to penetrate more deeply into the seminiferous epithelium, the occluding Sertoli cell junctions make it obligatory for these molecules to pass through the Sertoli cell.

Examination of freeze-fracture preparations of the surface of cleaved Sertoli cell membranes have shown that the points of membrane fusion consist of lengths of occluding junctions arranged in up to 50 parallel ridges of intramembranous particles. These rows form an impressive meshwork of tiny compartments which surround the Sertoli cell near its base (23,43,44,77,81). Interconnections between the many parallel rows are rarely seen, consistent with the view that this arrangement is the typical surface topography of epithelial cells continually altering their shape (64). Inter-Sertoli cell junctions are highly resistant to splitting or disruption as indicated by their ability to withstand exposure to hypertonic solutions that readily dissociate the junctional complexes within many other epithelial tissues (5,35,51,52,85). For this reason it is believed that the adluminal compartment of the seminiferous epithelium provides a unique micro-environ-ment supporting the development of spermatogenesis. Luminal movement of maturing spermatocytes arising within the basal compartment probably involves transient breakdown and reconstitution of the inter-Sertoli cell junctions (38, 44,92,94) and some studies have suggested that small lengths of disconnected junctions may accompany the mobile germ cells or are recycled through the columnar cytoplasm of the Sertoli cell (88,89,92,93).

The cytoplasm of the Sertoli cell immediately adjacent to the cell membrane of spermatids also shows specialization particularly near the head of the sperma-tid. Cisternae running parallel to the cell membrane demarcate a thin band of cytoplasm containing bundles of microfilaments similar to those adjacent to the inter-Sertoli cell junctions (Fig. 9). Desmosomes or other typical gap junc-tions (42) have not been observed between adjacent Sertoli cells in the adluminal region of the seminiferous epithelium (44). Although structures resembling inter-cellular junctions have been demonstrated between germ cells and Sertoli cells in the rat, dog, and human testis (2,23,77), it is not known if they represent sites of true cell contacts or communication.

PERITUBULAR TISSUE

The lamina propria surrounding the seminiferous tubule is responsible for the contractile activity of the tubules (18,60,73,90) and in the human consists of 5 to 6 layers of tissue attaining a width not normally exceeding 5 μm (Fig. 1). It commences with the thin basement membrane closely apposed to the basal surface of the Sertoli cells and spermatogonia. A layer of collagen fibers lies external to the basal lamina, followed by one or more layers of thin attenuated modified smooth muscle cells termed myoid cells. The surfaces of the myoid cells are frequently covered with a thin layer of basement membrane-like material in some areas composed of microfibrils and glycoprotein-type material containing elastin-type substances (8,11,12,30,31,90) (Figs. 4 and 5). The myoid cells contain pinocytotic vesicles, rough endoplasmic reticulum, and many cytoplasmic fila-ments, and although junctional complexes are not present between myoid cells, the extremities of adjacent cells often overlap, forming a narrowed intercellular space (8,11,40). The multiple layered arrangement of the lamina propria is sug-gestive of a barrier which may partially restrict the passage of molecules from the vascular system into the seminiferous epithelium, and in some rodents this appears to be the case (40,48,49). However, in monkeys the ultrastructure of the lamina propria is similar to the human, and extracellular tracers freely diffuse through the peritubular tissues indicating that it does not contribute to the maintenance of the blood-testis barrier (36,38).

INTERSTITIAL TISSUE

The convoluted loops of the human seminiferous tubules are supported by a loose connective tissue, richly supplied by a vascular network. Fibroblasts, macrophages, mast cells, small unmyelinated nerves, lymphatic vessels, and the clusters of Leydig or interstitial cells (74) are found within the intertubular tissue (Fig. 1). Fawcett et al. (43,50) have provided a detailed description of the morphology of the interstitial tissue, describing four basic patterns based upon the abundance of Leydig cells and the relationship between the relative volumes of intertubular lymphatics and connective tissues. In the human testis (16,25) the Leydig cells are large polyhedral cells with a characteristically basophilic cytoplasm. Lymphatics appear as irregularly shaped vessels 30 to 50 μm in diameter bounded by a thin delicate endothelium. The loose connective tissue may be readily distinguished from the lymphatic vessels since the former exhibits a finely granular matrix containing collagen fibers, whilst the latter exhibits a moderately dense fine precipitate, probably representing lymphatic fluid proteins (50). Slender cytoplasmic processes of connective tissue cells and endothelial cells within the interstitial tissue adopt a winding course to form interconnections between the seminiferous tubules which resemble an irregular labyrinth arrangement. Often large aggregations of Leydig cells are seen in proximity to blood vessels where many of the cells are closely packed, but over most of their opposing surfaces, contact is not observed (Fig. 12). Small points of adhesion are observed between adjacent Leydig cells, forming gap junctions 1–2 μm in diameter (Fig. 13). Occluding junctions between neighboring Leydig cells have not been observed (16,81). No variation in electron-density between Leydig cells of the perfused human testis was noted, in agreement with previous descriptions by Christensen and Gillim (17) who suggested that any variations in density represent artefacts of fixation associated with immersion fixation, giving rise to "dark and light" Leydig cells. The nuclei of human Leydig cells are usually ovoid, exhibiting a conspicuous nucleolus and many small patches of heterochromatin adherent to the inner aspect of the nuclear membrane (Figs. 12 and 13). A rich supply of anastomosing tubules of smooth endoplasmic reticulum fills the Leydig cell cytoplasm which also contains variable amounts of lipid droplets and lipofuscin pigments. Mitochondria are numerous, containing lamellar and tubular cristae, the latter typical of cells with steroidogenic capacity. Rough endoplasmic reticulum and Golgi membranes are also present (Fig. 13) but are not especially abundant. Marked variations occur in the relative proportions of most Leydig cell organelles suggesting different functional abilities; however, stereological measurements of cytoplasmic organelles in relation to androgen status are not available. Leydig cells from men treated with human chorionic

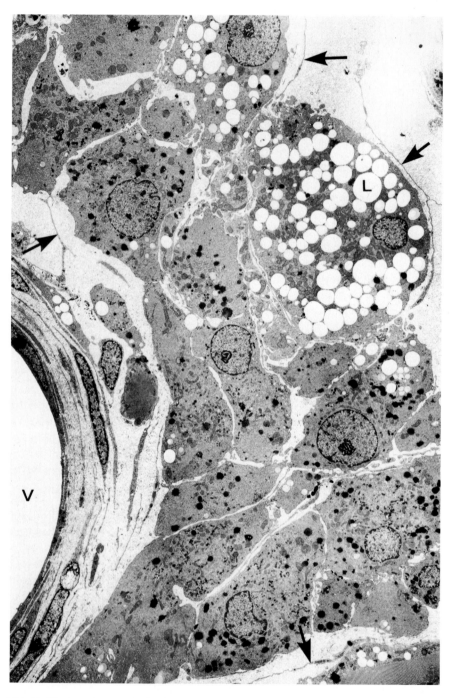

FIG. 12. Electronmicrograph of a cluster of human Leydig cells surrounding a venule (V) within the intertubular tissue of the testis. Delicate cytoplasmic processes of fibroblasts (arrows) surround the Leydig cells, and some Leydig cells contain abundant supplies of lipid (L). ×2,000.

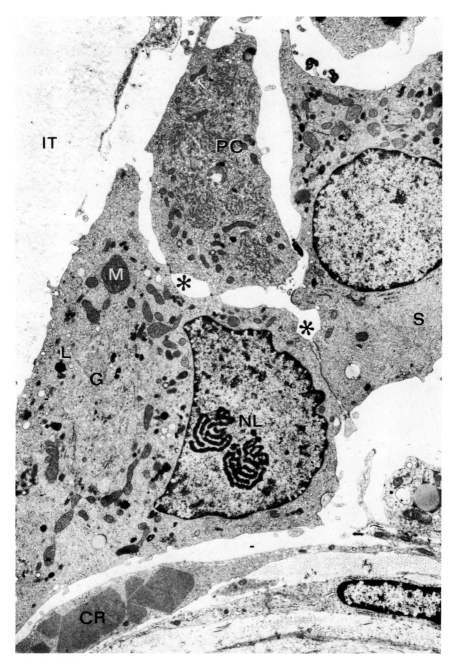

FIG. 13. Electronmicrograph of human Leydig cells within the interstitial connective tissue (IT) illustrating the complex nucleolus (NL) within the nucleus. Adjacent Leydig cell plasma membranes may form regions exhibiting gap junctions (asterisks) and the cytoplasm may contain smooth endoplasmic reticulum (S), mitochondria (M) lipofuscin bodies (L), Golgi membranes (G), paracrystalline inclusions (PC), and crystals of Reinke (CR). ×6,000.

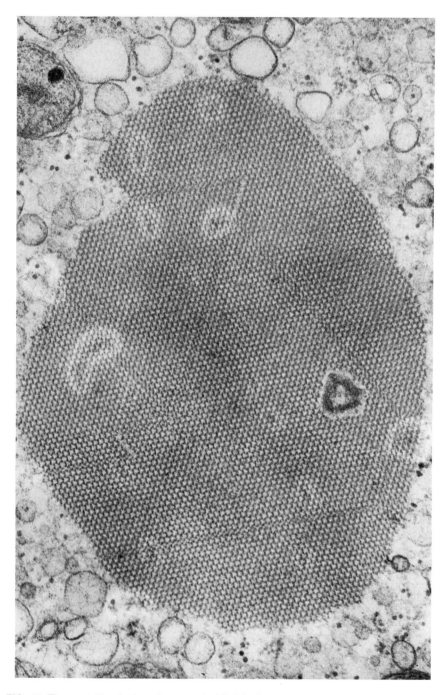

FIG. 14. The crystalline lattice of a crystal of Reinke in a Leydig cell is illustrated. ×47,400.

gonadotrophin show an increase in smooth endoplasmic reticulum, mitochondria, and the Golgi complex consistent with increased testosterone secretion (24,25). Human Leydig cells also contain crystals of Reinke (16,24,25,26,80, 86,112,113) ranging in size from 3 to 20 μm. They occur as polygonal, pyramidal, or rod-shaped inclusions (Fig. 13) and ultrastructural studies have shown that they consist of a complex crystalline latticework of 50Å thick filaments in hexagonal configurations approximately 190Å in width (Fig. 14) (16,25,45,47,80). Reinke crystals are not limited by a membrane and thus their subunits appear exposed to the surrounding cytoplasm. The crystals are composed chiefly of protein (65) and it has been suggested that they are assembled from many smaller para-crystalline inclusions commonly dispersed through the Leydig cell cytoplasm (Fig. 13) (25,32,33,47,80,101,113). Although crystals of Reinke apparently increase in abundance within the aging testis (16) their functional significance is unknown. A commonly held view is that Reinke crystals are unique to the human Leydig cell (7,16,17,37,80,101); however, the atrophied Leydig cells within the regressed testis of the seasonally breeding rodent *Rattus fuscipes* develop large crystalline inclusions very similar in shape and latticework arrangement to the crystals of Reinke (69). Since these crystals were only observed in association with temporary cessation of spermatogenesis and lowered plasma androgen levels, it is possible that these inclusions appear within the Leydig cell during phases of lowered steroid production. However, the functional significance of the crystals of Reinke of human Leydig cells must await further studies of their chemical composition in relation to normal and abnormal testicular function.

REFERENCES

1. Afzelius, B., Eliasson, R., Johnsen, Ø., and Lindholmer, C. (1975): Lack of dynein arms in immotile human spermatozoa. *J. Cell Biol.,* 66:225–232.
2. Altorfer, J., Fukuda, T., and Hedinger, C. (1974): Desmosomes in human seminiferous epithelium. An electron microscopic study. *Virchows Arch. (Zellpathol.)* 16:181–194.
3. André, J. (1962): Contribution à la connaissance du chondriome. Étude de ses modifications ultrastructurales pendant la spermatogénèse. *J. Ultrastruct. Res.,* (Suppl. 3), 1–185.
4. Aoki, A. and Fawcett, D. W. (1975): Impermeability of Sertoli cell junctions to prolonged exposure to peroxidase. *Andrologia,* 7:63–76.
5. Barr, L., Dewey, M. M., and Berger, W. (1965): Propagation of action potentials and structure of the nexus in cardiac muscle. *J. Gen. Physiol.,* 48:797.
6. Bawa, S. R. (1963): Fine structure of the Sertoli cell of the human testis. *J. Ultrastruct. Res.,* 9:459–474.
7. Bloom, W. and Fawcett, D. W. (1975): Male reproductive system, In: *A Textbook of Histology,* Chapt. 32. Saunders, Philadelphia.
8. Böck, P., Breitenecker, G., and Lunglmayr, G. (1972): Kontraktile Fibroblasten (Myofibroblasten) in der lamina propria der Hodenkanälchen vom Menschen. *Z. Zellforsch. Mikrosk. Anat.,* 133:519–527.
9. Bouffard, G. (1906): Injection des couleurs de benzidine aux animaux normaux. *Ann. Inst. Pasteur Lille,* 20:539–546.
10. Brökelmann, J. (1963): Fine structure of germ cells and Sertoli cells during the cycle of the seminiferous epithelium in the rat. *Z. Zellforsch. Mikrosk. Anat.,* 59:820–850.

11. Bustos-Obregón, E., and Holstein, A. F. (1973): On structural patterns of the lamina propria of human seminiferous tubules. *Z. Zellforsch. Mikrosk. Anat.,* 141:413–425.
12. Cavallotti, C., Carpino, F., Familiari, G., Re, M., and Vicari, A. (1977): Myosin-like microfilaments in the human normal and pathological testis. *Acta Anat.,* 99:220–227.
13. Cavicchia, J. C., and Dym, M (1977): Relative volume of Sertoli cells in monkey seminiferous epithelium: A stereological analysis. *Am. J. Anat.,* 150:501–507.
14. Chang, M. C., and Hunter, R. H. F. (1975): Capacitation of mammalian sperm: biological and experimental aspects. In: *Handbook of Physiology,* Vol. 5, Sect. 7, edited by D. W. Hamilton and R. O. Greep, pp. 339–351. Williams & Wilkins, Baltimore.
15. Chemes, H. E., Dym, M., Fawcett, D. W., Javadpour, N. J., and Sherins, R. J. (1977): Pathophysiological observations of Sertoli cells in patients with germinal aplasia or severe germ cell depletion. Ultrastructural findings and hormone levels. *Biol. Reprod.,* 17:108–123.
16. Christensen, A. K. (1975): Leydig cells. In: *Handbook of Physiology,* Section 7: Endocrinology, Vol. V, Male Reproductive System, edited by D. W. Hamilton and R. O. Greep, pp. 57–94. Williams & Wilkins, Baltimore.
17. Christensen, A. K., and Gillim, S. W. (1969): The correlation of fine structure and function in steroid-secreting cells, with emphasis on those of the gonads. In: *The Gonads,* edited by K. W. McKerns, pp. 415–418. Appleton-Century-Crofts, New York.
18. Clermont, Y. (1958): Contractile elements in the limiting membrane of the seminiferous tubules of the rat. *Exp. Cell Res.,* 15:438–440.
19. Clermont, Y. (1972): Kinetics of spermatogenesis in mammals: Seminiferous epithelium cycle and spermatogonial renewal. *Physiol. Rev.,* 52:198–236.
20. Clermont, Y. (1966): Renewal of spermatogonia in man. *Am. J. Anat.,* 118:509–524.
21. Clermont, Y. (1963): The cycle of the seminiferous epithelium in man. *Am. J. Anat.,* 112:35–51.
22. Clermont, Y. and Bustos-Obregón, E. (1968): Re-examination of spermatogonial renewal in the rat by means of seminiferous tubules mounted "in toto." *Am. J. Anat.,* 122:122–137.
23. Connell, C. J. (1978): A freeze-fracture and lanthanum tracer study of the complex junction between Sertoli cells of the canine testis. *J. Cell Biol.,* 76:57–75.
24. de Kretser, D. M. (1967*a*): Changes in the fine structure of the human testicular interstitial cells after treatment with human gonadotrophins. *Z. Zellforsch. Mikrosk. Anat.,* 83:344–358.
25. de Kretser, D. M. (1967): The fine structure of the testicular interstitial cells in men of normal androgenic status. *Z. Zellforsch. Mikrosk. Anat.,* 80:594–609.
26. de Kretser, D. M. (1968): Crystals of Reinke in the nuclei of human testicular interstitial cells, *Experientia,* 24:587–588.
27. de Kretser, D. M. (1969): Studies on the structure and function of the human testis. M. D. Thesis, Monash University, Clayton, Victoria, Australia.
28. de Kretser, D. M. (1969): Ultrastructural features of human spermiogenesis. *Z. Zellforsch.,* 98:477–505.
29. de Kretser, D. M., and Burger, H. G. (1972): Ultrastructural studies of the human Sertoli cell in normal men and males with hypogonadotrophic hypogonadism before and after gonadotrophic treatment. In: *Gonadotrophins,* edited by B. B. Saxena, C. G. Beling, and H. M. Gandy, pp. 640–656. Wiley-Interscience, New York.
30. de Kretser, D. M., Kerr, J. B., and Paulsen, C. A. (1975): The peritubular tissue in the normal and pathological human testis: an ultrastructural study. *Biol. Reprod.,* 12:317–324.
31. De Menezes, A. P. (1977): Elastic tissue in the limiting membrane of the human seminiferous tubule. *Am. J. Anat.,* 150:349–374.
32. Dessolle, N. (1967): Données ultrastructurales sur le noyan des cellules interstitielles du testicle humain azoospermique. *C.R. Acad. Sci. (Paris) Ser. D.,* 264:1018–1021.
33. Dessolle, N. (1967): Ultrastructure des cellules interstitielles du testicule humain dans un cas d'aspermatogénèse. *C.R. Assoc. Anat.,* 138:403–414.
34. Dietert, S. E. (1966): Fine structure of the formation and fate of the residual bodies of mouse spermatozoa with evidence for the participation of lysosomes. *J. Morphol.,* 120:317–346.
35. Dreifuss, J. J., Girardier, L., and Forsmann, W. G. (1966): Étude de la propagation de l'excitation dans le ventricule de rat du moyen de solutions hypertoniques. *Pfluegers Arch.,* 292:13–33.
36. Dym, M. (1973): The fine structure of the monkey *(Macaca)* Sertoli cell and its role in maintaining the blood-testis barrier. *Anat. Rec.,* 175:639–656.

37. Dym, M. (1977): The male reproductive system. In: *Histology,* edited by R. O. Greep and L. Weiss, pp. 979–1038. McGraw-Hill, New York.
38. Dym, M., and Cavvichia, J. C. (1977): Further observations on the blood-testis barrier in monkeys. *Biol. Reprod.,* 17:390–403.
39. Dym, M., and Fawcett, D. W. (1971): Further observations on the numbers of spermatogonia, spermatocytes and spermatids connected by intercellular bridges in the mammalian testis. *Biol. Reprod.,* 4:195–215.
40. Dym, M., and Fawcett, D. W. (1970): The blood-testis barrier in the rat and the physiological compartmentation of the seminiferous epithelium. *Biol. Reprod.,* 3:308–326.
41. Elftman, H. (1963): Sertoli cells and testis structure. *Am. J. Anat.,* 113:25–33.
42. Farquhar, M. G., and Palade, G. E. (1963): Junctional complexes in various epithelia. *J. Cell Biol.,* 17:375–412.
43. Fawcett, D. W. (1973): Observations on the organisation of the interstitial tissue of the testis and on the occluding cell junctions in the seminiferous epithelium. In: *Advances in the Biosciences,* Vol. 10, edited by R. Raspé, pp. 83–99. Pergamon Press, Vieweg.
44. Fawcett, D. W. (1975): Ultrastructure and function of the Sertoli cell. In: *Handbook of Physiology,* Section 7: Endocrinology, Vol. V., Male Reproductive System, edited by D. W. Hamilton and R. O. Greep, pp. 21–55. Williams &Wilkins, Baltimore.
45. Fawcett, D. W. and Burgos, M. H. (1956): Observations on the cytomorphosis of the germinal and interstitial cells of the human testes. In: *Ciba Colloquia on Ageing,* Vol. 2, edited by G. E. W. Wolstenholme, pp. 86–99. Churchill, London.
46. Fawcett, D. W., and Burgos, M. H. (1956): The fine structure of Sertoli cells in the human testis. *Anat. Rec.,* 124:401–402.
47. Fawcett, D. W. and Burgos, M. H. (1960): Studies on the fine structure of the mammalian testis. II. The human interstitial tissue. *Am. J. Anat.,* 107:245–269.
48. Fawcett, D. W., Heidger, P. M., and Leak, L. V. (1969): Lymph vascular system of the interstitial tissue of the testis as revealed by electron microscopy. *J. Reprod. Fert.,* 19:109–119.
49. Fawcett, D. W., Leak, L. V., and Heidger, P. M. (1970): Electron microscopic observations on the structural components of the blood-testis barrier. *J. Reprod. Fert.* (Suppl.), 10:105–122.
50. Fawcett, D. W., Neaves, W. B., and Flores, M. N. (1973): Comparative observations on intertubular lymphatics and the organisation of the interstitial tissue of the mammalian testis. *Biol. Reprod.,* 9:500–532.
51. Gilula, N. B., Fawcett, D. W., and Aoki, A. (1976): The Sertoli cell occluding junctions and gap junctions in mature and developing mammalian testis. *Dev. Biol.,* 50:142–168.
52. Goodenough, D. A., and Gilula, N. B. (1974): The splitting of hepatocyte gap junctions and zonulae occludentes with hypertonic disaccharides. *J. Cell Biol.,* 61:575–590.
53. Greenwood, A. W. (1923): Marsupial spermatogenesis. *Q. J. Microsc. Sci.,* 67:203–218.
54. Gulyas, B. J. (1971): The rabbit zygote: formation of annulate lamellae. *J. Ultrastruct. Res.,* 35:112–126.
55. Hansson, V., Purvis, K., Ritzén, E. M., and French, F. S. (1978): Hormonal regulation of Sertoli cell function in the rat. *Ann. Biol. Anim. Biochem. Biophys.,* 18:565–572.
56. Harding, H. R. (1979): Affinities of the Koala on the basis of sperm ultrastructure. In: *Proceedings: 21st Annual Meeting Australian Mammalian Society,* p. 45.
57. Harding, H. R., Carrick, F. N., and Shorey, C. D. (1978): Unusual features of spermiogenesis and the Sertoli cell in the koala (Phascolarctos cinereus). In: *Proceedings: 10th Conference Australian Society of Reproductive Biology,* p. 53.
58. Heller, C. G. and Clermont, Y. (1964): Kinetics of the germinal epithelium in man. *Recent Prog. Horm. Res.,* 20:545–575.
59. Horstmann, E. (1961): Elektronenmikroskopische Untersuchungen zur Spermiohistogenese beim Menschen. *Z. Zellforsch, Mikrosk. Anat.,* 54:68–89.
60. Hovatta, O. (1972): Contractility and structure of adult rat seminiferous tubule in organ culture. *Z. Zellforsch. Mikrosk. Anat.,* 130:171–179.
61. Huckins, C. (1971): Cell cycle properties of differentiating spermatogonia in adult Sprague Dawley rats. *Cell Tissue Kinet.,* 4:139–154.
62. Huckins, C. (1971): The spermatogonial stem cell population in adult rats. II. A radioautographic analysis of their cell cycle properties. *Cell Tissue Kinet.,* 4:313–334.

63. Huckins, C. (1971): The spermatogonial stem cell population in adult rats. III. Evidence for a long-cycling population. *Cell Tissue Kinet.* 4:335–349.
64. Hull, B. E. and Staehlin, L. A. (1976): Functional significance of the variations in the geometrical organisation of tight junction networks. *J. Cell Biol.,* 68:688–704.
65. Janko, A. B. and Sandberg, E. C. (1970): Histochemical evidence for the protein nature of the Reinke crystalloid. *Obstet. Gynecol.,* 35:493–503.
66. Johnson, M. H. and Setchell, B. P. (1968): Protein and immunoglobulin content of rete testis fluid of rams. *J. Reprod. Fert.,* 17:403–406.
67. Kerr, J. B., and de Kretser, D. M. (1975): Cyclic variations in Sertoli cell lipid content throughout the spermatogenic cycle in the rat. *J. Reprod. Fert.,* 43:1–8.
68. Kerr, J. B., and Dixon, K. E. (1974): An ultrastructural study of germ plasm in spermatogenesis of *Xenopus laevis. J. Embryol. Exp. Morphol.,* 32:573–592.
69. Kerr, J. B., Keogh, E. J., Hudson, B., Whipp, G. T., and de Kretser, D. M. (1980): Alterations in spermatogenic activity and hormonal status in a seasonally breeding rat, *Rattus fuscipes. Gen. Comp. Endocrinol.,* 40:78–88.
70. Kormano, M. (1967): Dye permeability and alkaline phosphatase activity of testicular capillaries in the postnatal rat. *Histochemie,* 9:327–338.
71. Koskimies, A. I., Kormano, M., and Alfthan, O. (1973): Proteins of the seminiferous tubule fluid in man—evidence for a blood-testis barrier. *J. Reprod. Fert.,* 32:79–86.
72. Lacy, D. (1960): Light and electron microscopy and its use in the study of factors influencing spermatogenesis in the rat. *J. R. Microsc. Soc.,* 79:209–225.
73. Lacy, D., and Rotblat, J. (1960): Study of normal and irradiated boundary tissue of the seminiferous tubules of the rat. *Exp. Cell Res.,* 21:49–70.
74. Leydig, F. (1850): Zur anatomie der männlichen geschlechtsorgane und analdrüsen der saügethiere. *Wissenschaft Zool.,* 2:1–66.
75. Lubarsch, O. (1896): Über das Vorkommen Krystallinischer und Krystalloider Bildungen in den Zellen des menschlichen Hodens. *Virchows Arch. (Pathol. Anat.),* 145:316–338.
76. Maul, G. G. (1970): On the relationship between the golgi apparatus and annulate lamellae. *J. Ultrastruct. Res.,* 30:368–384.
77. McGinley, D., Posalaky, Z., and Porvaknik, M. (1977): Intercellular junctional complexes of the rat seminiferous tubules: a freeze-fracture study. *Anat. Rec.,* 189:211–232.
78. Means, A. R., Fakunding, J. L., Huckins, C., Tindall, D. J., and Vitale, R. (1976): Follicle-stimulating hormone, the Sertoli cell and spermatogenesis. *Rec. Prog. Horm. Res.,* 32:477–527.
79. Nagano, T. (1966): Some observations on the fine structure of the Sertoli cell in the human testis. *Z. Zellforsch, Mikrosk. Anat.,* 73:89–106.
80. Nagano, T., and Ohtsuki, I. (1971): Reinvestigation of the fine structure of Reinke's crystals in the human testicular interstitial cell. *J. Cell Biol.,* 51:148–161.
81. Nagano, T., and Suzuki, F. (1976): Freeze-fracture observations on the intercellular junctions of Sertoli cells and of Leydig cells in the human testis. *Cell Tissue Res.,* 166:37–48.
82. Nicander, L. (1967): An electron microscopical study of cell contacts in the seminiferous tubules of some mammals. *Z. Zellforsch. Mikrosk. Anat.,* 83:375–397.
83. Pari, G. (1910): Über die Verwendbarkeit vitaler Karmineinspritzungen für die pathologische Anatomie. *Frank. Z. Pathol.,* 4:1–29.
84. Posalaki, Z., Szabó, D., Bácsi, E., and Ökros, I. (1968): Hydrolytic enzymes during spermatogenesis in rat. An electron microscopic and histochemical study. *J. Histochem. Cytochem.,* 16:249–262.
85. Rapoport, S. I., and Thompson, H. K. (1973): Osmotic opening of the blood-brain barrier in the monkey without associated neurological deficits. *Science,* 180:971.
86. Reinke, F. (1896): Beiträge zue histologie des Menschen. *Arch. Mikrosk. Anat.,* 47:34–44.
87. Ribbert, H. (1904): Die Abscheidung intravenös injizierten gelösten Karmins in den Geweben. *Z. Allg. Physiol.,* 4:201–214.
88. Ross, M. H. (1976): The Sertoli cell junctional specialisations during spermiogenesis and at spermiation. *Am. J. Anat.,* 186:79–103.
89. Ross, M. H., and Dobler, J. (1975): The Sertoli cell junctional specialisations and their relationship to the germinal epithelium as observed after efferent duct ligation. *Anat. Rec.,* 183:267–292.

90. Ross, M. H., and Long, I.R. (1966): Contractile cells in human seminiferous tubules. *Science,* 153:1271–1273.
91. Rowley, M. J., Berlin, J. D., and Heller C. G. (1971): The ultrastructure of four types of human spermatogonia. *Z. Zellforsch.,* 112:139–157.
92. Russell, L. D. (1977): Movement of spermatocytes from the basal to the adluminal compartment of the rat testis. *Am. J. Anat.,* 148:313–328.
93. Russell, L. D. (1977): Observations on rat Sertoli ectoplasmic ('junctional') specializations in their association with germ cells of the rat testis. *Tissue & Cell.,* 9:475–498.
94. Russell, L. D. (1978): The blood-testis barrier and its formation relative to spermatocyte maturation in the adult rat: a lanthanum tracer study. *Anat. Rec.,* 190:99–112.
95. Sachs, L. (1954): Sex linkage and the sex chromosome in man. *Ann. Eugen. (Lond),* 18:255–261.
96. Schulze, C. (1974): On the morphology of the human Sertoli cell. *Cell Tissue Res.,* 153:339–355.
97. Schulze, C., Holstein, A. F., Schirren, C., and Körner, F. (1976): On the morphology of the human Sertoli cells under normal conditions and in patients with impaired fertility. *Andrologia,* 8:167–178.
98. Setchell, B. P. (1969): Do Sertoli cells secrete fluid into the seminiferous tubules? *J. Reprod. Fert.,* 19:391–392.
99. Setchell, B. P. (1967): The blood-testicular fluid barrier in sheep. *J. Physiol.,* 189:63P–65P.
100. Setchell, B. P., Voglmayr, J. K., and Waites, G. M. H. (1969): A blood-testis barrier restricting passage from blood into rete testis fluid but not into lymph. *J. Physiol.,* 200:73–85.
101. Sohval, A. R., Gabrilove, J. L., and Churg, J. (1973): Ultrastructure of Leydig cell paracrystalline inclusions, possibly related to Reinke crystals, in the normal human testis. *Z. Zellforsch. Mikrosk. Anat.,* 142:13–26.
102. Sohval, A. R., Suzuki, Y., Gabrilove, J. L., and Churg, J. (1971): Ultrastructure of crystalloids in spermatogonia and Sertoli cells of normal human testis. *J. Ultrastruct. Res.,* 34:83–102.
103. Solari, A. J., and Tres, L. L. (1967): The ultrastructure of the human sex vesicle. *Chromosoma (Berlin),* 22:16–31.
104. Toyama, Y. (1975): Ultrastructural study of crystalloids in Sertoli cells of the normal, intersex and experimental cryptorchid swine. *Cell Tissue Res.,* 158:205–213.
105. Tres, L. L., and Solari, A. J. (1968): The ultrastructure of the nuclei and the behaviour of the sex chromosomes of human spermatogonia. *Z Zellforsch.,* 91:75–89.
106. Tuck, R. R., Setchell, B. P., and Waites, G. M. H. (1970): The composition of fluid collected by micropuncture and catheterization from the seminiferous tubules and rete testis of rats. *Pfluegers Arch.,* 378:225–243.
107. Vitale, R., Fawcett, D. W., and Dym, M. (1973): The normal development of the blood-testis barrier and the effects of climiphene and estrogen treatment. *Anat. Rec.,* 176:333–344.
108. Voglmayr, J. K., Waites, G. M. H., and Setchell, B. P. (1966): Studies on spermatozoa and fluid collected directly from the testis of the conscious ram. *Nature,* 210:861–863.
109. Waites, G. M. H., and Setchell, B. P. (1969): Some physiological aspects of the function of the testis. In: *The Gonads,* edited by K. W. McKerns, pp. 649–714. Appleton-Century-Crofts, New York.
110. Wettstein, R., and Sotelo, J. R. (1967): Electron microscope serial reconstruction of the spermatocyte I nuclei at pachytene. *J. Microsc.,* 6:557–576.
111. Woollam, D. H. M., and Ford, E. H. R. (1964): The fine structure of the mammalian chromosome in meiotic prophase with special reference to the synaptinemal complex. *J. Anat. (Lond),* 98:163–173.
112. Yamada, E. (1965): Some observations on the fine structure of the interstitial cell in the human testis as revealed by electron microscopy. *Gunma Symp. Endocrinol.,* 2:1–17.
113. Yamada, E. (1962): Some observations on the fine structure of the interstitial cell in the human testis. In: *Proceedings: 5th International Congress of Electron Microscopy,* Vol. 2, edited by S. Bresse, p. 1. Academic Press, New York.

The Testis, edited by H. Burger and D. de Kretser.
Raven Press, New York © 1981.

8

The Sertoli Cell

*E. Martin Ritzén, **Vidar Hansson, and †Frank S. French

*Pediatric Endocrinology Unit, Karolinska Sjukhuset, Stockholm, Sweden, **Institute of
Pathology, Rikshospitalet, Oslo, Norway, †Department of Pediatrics, School of Medicine,
University of North Carolina, Chapel Hill, North Carolina.*

The epithelium of the seminiferous tubule is made up of two fundamentally
very different cell populations; one is very stable, showing no proliferation at
all in the adult, the other proliferates rapidly and migrates between the stable
cells toward the lumen of the tubule. The fact that such a system is found
throughout the animal kingdom indicates that it is of great importance for
securing reproduction. The "mobile phase," the germ cells, has been amply
studied for a long time, while the "stationary phase," the Sertoli cells, has
received little attention. However, in the last few years, considerable new information has emerged concerning the "supportive" cells of the seminiferous epithelium. Progress has been made in several fields, including embryology, morphology, physiology, and pathology. Some of this newly gained knowledge will be
discussed in this chapter.

EMBRYOLOGY OF THE SERTOLI CELL

In certain respects, the Sertoli cell seems to express its most diversified activities
during fetal life. In the last few years, several secretory products of the fetal
Sertoli cells have been shown to direct not only the development of the testis
itself, but also the differentiation of the internal genital ducts. It is also a characteristic feature of the Sertoli cell that its functions vary markedly with the
stage of development, before as well as after birth. Therefore, a discrete function
of the prenatal Sertoli cell might not be traced in the postnatal period, and
vice versa.

The differentiation of the early gonad into a testis is the story of the maturing
Sertoli cell. Recent experiments by Wachtel et al. (127) have clearly demonstrated
the decisive importance of a cell surface component, the so-called H-Y antigen,
for testicular development. In the presence of H-Y antigen, cells of the mesenchymatous medullary gonadal blastema differentiate into primitive Sertoli cells,

which then form cell cords, embodying the germ cells that migrate to the gonadal fold from the yolk sac (134). The primitive Sertoli cells have long been thought to originate from the coelomic epithelium of the gonadal ridge. However, this assumption has recently been challenged by Jost el al. (52). These authors found morphological indications for a mesenchymal origin of the Sertoli cells, differentiating from blastema cells surrounding the germ cells. The "classical" and the "mesenchymatous" theories have to some extent been combined by Wartenberg (130), who divides the early Sertoli cells into "dark" and "light" types (see also Chapter 3). The latter are supposed to derive from the coelomic epithelium, the former from the central gonadal blastema. This hypothesis has not yet been proved. Another possibility is that the two types represent different developmental stages of one and the same cell strain.

The first sign of differentiation of the primitive gonad into a testis is the formation of cords of primitive Sertoli cells that encompass the germ cells (52). The organization of the blastema cells into cords starts in the center of the gonad, close to the mesonephric tubules (52), which indicates that the latter structures may be inducing testicular organization. Furthermore, the rete testis, developing from the mesonephric tubules, also secretes a diffusible substance that induces meiosis in both the fetal testis and the ovary, the so called meiosis-inducing substance, MIS, (4). After cord formation, there is evidence that the Sertoli cell takes an active part in regulation both of germ cell divisions and somatic sex differentiation.

The male gonad secretes a meiosis-preventing substance (MPS), that can arrest the female germ cells within the meiotic prophase (5). The Sertoli cell origin of MPS is not yet proved, although Wartenberg (130) has suggested that the "light" and "dark" Sertoli cells secrete meiosis-preventing and -inducing substances, respectively.

Once the Sertoli cells have gained full control of the germ cells by completely surrounding them, it is obvious that the future development of spermatogenesis will be dependent on normal Sertoli cell function. There is no evidence indicating hormonal control of the embryological differentiation of the seminiferous tubules. The major stimuli for adult Sertoli cells, androgens, and follicle stimulating hormone (FSH), are not produced in the fetus at the time of differentiation of the seminiferous tubules; neither fetal pituitary cells nor Leydig cells are differentiated. Furthermore, apparently normal seminiferous tubules develop in the androgen insensitivity syndrome indicating that androgens are of little importance in this early development.

The fetal Sertoli cells also influence extratesticular differentiation. It has been shown that during a limited period, the fetal testis secretes a peptide hormone that specifically suppresses the development of the female internal genital organs (Müllerian inhibiting hormone, MIH) (51).

The various locally diffusible substances proposed in the differentiation of the mammalian testis are schematically illustrated in Fig. 1.

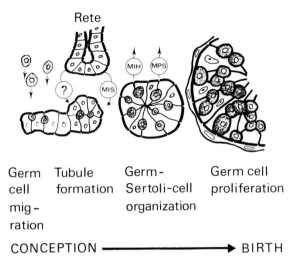

FIG. 1. Schematic presentation of some factors influencing testicular differentiation. The gonadal blastema cells attract germ cells (dotted cytoplasm) from the yolk sac region (132). These are embraced by the developing Sertoli cells, which then form cords under the influence of a hypothetical substance from the rete testis (mesonephric ducts). These latter structures probably also secrete a meiosis-inducing substance (MIS) (5). The fetal Sertoli cells secrete at least two active principles; the Müllerian inhibiting hormone (MIH) (51) and the meiosis-preventing substance (MPS, ref. 4).

SERTOLI CELL MATURATION

During embryological life, the Sertoli cell acquires several features that are later lost. This pattern is continued during postnatal life, up to adulthood. The most fundamental feature of these maturational changes may be the cessation of cell multiplication that occurs before puberty, in the rat at about 15 days of age (113). After that age, the Sertoli cells may change their metabolic activities under the influence of various factors, but do not multiply further.

Structural maturation of the Sertoli cells includes the formation of specialized inter-Sertoli cell tight junctions, which constitute a major component of the functional blood-testis barrier.

In the rat, this functional barrier develops at about 16 to 19 days of age (126) and is correlated to the morphological transition from gap junctions to typical occluding Sertoli junctions (29). Bressler (2) noted that in the mouse the development of these mature membrane structures seemed to be dependent on pituitary hormones.

Other known postnatal maturational changes of the Sertoli cells include secretion of fluid and androgen binding protein (ABP), steroid metabolism, FSH binding, and phosphodiesterase activity. The lumen of the seminiferous tubule is not formed until fluid production starts, which in the rat coincides with the formation of Sertoli cell junctions at about 16 to 19 days of age (126). Tindall et al. (121) observed that ABP secretion into the epididymis did not start until the age of 18 days. However, if ABP production is studied in organ culture *in vitro,* ABP secretion can be noted as early as 13 days of age. Measured in this way, there is a continuous increase in ABP production rate from 13 days (L. Hagenäs, E. M. Ritzén, and L. Plöen, *unpublished*) to adulthood (calculated per testis). However, the ABP secretion per unit of testis weight decreases owing to the changing ratio of Sertoli to germ cells (93).

Steroid metabolism is another feature of the rat Sertoli cell that changes rapidly in early life. The FSH-dependent ring A aromatase, that converts testosterone to estradiol, is very active in tissue cultured Sertoli cells from 5- to 20-day-old Wistar rats, but decreases rapidly thereafter (1). In the Sprague-Dawley rat, this enzyme activity is maximal at 5 to 10 days of age, but nondetectable at 20 days (10). Similarly, FSH stimulates 5α-reductase activity *in vitro* in Sertoli cells from 10 day old rats (131). In earlier experiments, Dorrington and Fritz (14) found higher 5α-reductase activity in isolated seminiferous tubules from immature (26–28 days) than from adult rats; in the latter case, however, part of the 5α-reductase was found in the spermatocytes.

The binding of FSH and its action on the Sertoli cells undergo dramatic changes during maturation. While the concentration of FSH receptors decreased with age, if expressed as binding per unit weight, Thanki and Steinberger (118) found a steadily increasing number of binding sites per rat testis, from "infancy" to adulthood. This means that after the Sertoli cells have ceased dividing at about 15 days of age (see above), there is a continuing maturational change that causes a sixfold increase in the total number of binding sites. In spite of the increase in FSH receptors, there is a marked fall in the FSH-stimulated cyclic AMP production even in the presence of a phosphodiesterase inhibitor (112) as measured *in vitro* in Sertoli cells obtained from rats of increasing age. Similarly, ABP production is stimulated by FSH in the immature but not the intact mature testis, *in vivo* (44), or *in vitro* (93). The latter observation has been interpreted as a refractoriness of the adult Sertoli cell, already maximally stimulated with FSH and resistant to further stimulation. However, recent experiments using an adenylyl cyclase assay have demonstrated an unchanged activity of this enzyme throughout sexual maturation (Jahnsen and Hansson, *unpublished*).

The maturational changes of the Sertoli cell, schematically illustrated in Fig. 2, should be related to the maturation of spermatogenesis that occurs at the same period. The first haploid cells, indicating meiosis, are found at 21 days of age in the Sprague-Dawley rat (8). This is just a few days after the Sertoli junctions have formed the functional blood-testis barrier and the lumen of the seminiferous tubule is opened by the initiation of fluid production by the Sertoli cells. At the same time, the FSH-dependent aromatase activity in Sertoli cells has decreased from very high levels to nearly zero, while the cyclic AMP and ABP response to FSH is at its maximum, and starting to fall. Considering

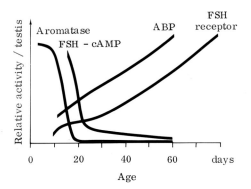

FIG. 2. Schematic illustration of some rat Sertoli cell functions that change rapidly during sexual maturation. Aromatase: The aromatizing enzyme that converts testosterone to estradiol. FSH-cAMP: The accumulation of cyclic AMP during FSH stimulation *in vitro*. ABP: Production of androgen binding protein. FSH receptor: The relative number of FSH receptors in the testis. For further explanations, see text.

the intimate relations of the germ cells to the surrounding Sertoli cells, and the correlation in time between the described changes in several parameters of Sertoli cell function and the initiation of spermatogenesis, it seems reasonable to assume that there are signals exchanged between them either in one direction or both.

STRUCTURAL RELATIONS OF SERTOLI CELLS TO NEIGHBORING CELLS

In any epithelium in the body, neighboring cells have structurally defined organelles, desmosomes, that seem to hold the cells together. This is also true for the Sertoli cells. However, the inter-Sertoli cell junctions were early found to be of two different types and structurally different from those of other epithelia (19,23,78); there was evidence of one "tight" and one less intimate junction. These structures have been the subject of numerous electron microscopic investigations. In the occluding tight junctions, the outer membranes of neighboring Sertoli cells are fused (reviewed by Fawcett, ref. 22). Furthermore, as revealed by freeze-fracture techniques, there are characteristic intramembranous granules organized in a linear or reticular pattern at the sites of occluding junctions (21,22,65,77). On the cytoplasmic side of these junctions, there are bundles of presumably contractile microfilaments, which have been shown to contain actin (122). Adjacent to the occluding junctions, cisternae of endoplasmic reticulum are present. There is general agreement that these occluding junctions constitute the most important part of the so called blood-testis barrier, that prevents passive diffusion of substances, including macromolecules and several small ions.

Each Sertoli cell reaches from the basal membrane to the tubule lumen, and is connected to the neighboring Sertoli cells by the occluding tight junctions.

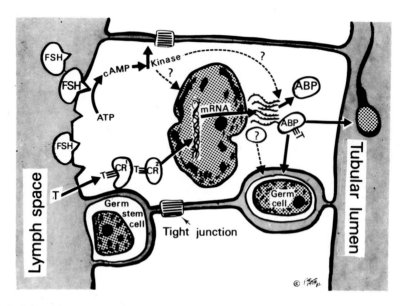

FIG. 3. Schematic representation of the seminiferous tubule wall and the current hypothesis on the mechanisms of hormonal action on Sertoli cells. The Sertoli cells completely encompass the postmeiotic germ cells, through the inter-Sertoli-cell tight junctions that form the main part of the blood-testis-barrier and thus creates the morphological basis for the specific tubule milieu. FSH is bound to receptors on the Sertoli cell membrane, thereby activating adenyl cyclase to produce cyclic AMP. This "second messenger" has multiple effects—one consists in increasing the activity of cAMP dependent protein kinase, which in its turn is assumed to be active in phosphorylation of proteins in the cytoplasm (and the nucleus?). One end effect of the FSH action is shown as the increased synthesis and secretion of the androgen binding protein, ABP. Testosterone (T) penetrates freely into the cell, where it is bound to a soluble receptor (CR[1]), either as such or after reduction to dihydrotestosterone. The receptor then undergoes an allosteric conformational change (CR[2]) and this complex is bound to the nuclear chromatin, inducing increased synthesis of specific messenger RNA (mRNA), ultimately causing an increased production of ABP. ABP is secreted into the tubular lumen, and presumably also into the Sertoli-germ cell intercellular space, together with other (unknown) substances influencing germ cell maturation. (From ref. 92).

In this way a basal compartment (between the tubule basal membrane and the occluding tight junctions) are formed (Fig. 3). Spermatogonia, that rest on the basal membrane between the Sertoli cells, occupy the basal compartment of the seminiferous epithelium together with the preleptotene and leptotene spermatocytes. Since all later stages of germ cell maturation are found within the adluminal compartment, the occluding junctions have to be opened up for the migrating spermatocytes and resealed behind them. It is important to point out that the initiation of meiosis thus occurs in a milieu similar to that of other cells in the body, while the progress of meiosis and further maturation of germ cells including spermiation takes place in a specific intratubular milieu that in certain respects is similar to the intracellular one (18).

It is to be stressed that Sertoli cells interconnected by the occluding junctions, form a continous epithelial layer preventing diffusion of substances into the intercellular spaces. This means that every substance of nutritional or regulatory character has to pass through the Sertoli cell cytoplasm to be available for germ cells residing within the adluminal compartment. This "nursing" character of the Sertoli cells is further stressed by the fact that spermatids before spermiation are situated in deep recesses of the Sertoli cell cytoplasm.

Typical nonoccluding gap junctions are found between Sertoli cells and spermatids (21,24,77,78,80,98,99). The latter gap junctions seem to function as anchoring devices (78,100), involved in the retraction of spermatids into the Sertoli cells during spermiogenesis. Furthermore, a third type of Sertoli cell-spermatid cell contact is described; projections of spermatid processes deep into the cytoplasm of the Sertoli cells.

Thus, there are at least two types of structural connections between Sertoli cells and late spermatids, which may form a basis for communication between the two cell types. However, such structures are conspicuously lacking at the border between Sertoli cells and primary or secondary spermatocytes (22). Exchange of signals between the two cell types thus has to rely on mechanisms that do not require direct membrane contact, but rather on transfer of substances that traverse the cell membranes or bind to cell surface receptors. There is no morphological evidence of pinocytotic activity in germ cells. On the other hand, Sertoli cells are known to exert a pronounced endocytotic activity incorporating degenerating germ cells and residual bodies into their cytoplasm. Although shared membranes or special junctions between Sertoli cells and the pre-spermatid germ cells seem to be lacking, the fact that late zygotene, pachytene, and secondary spermatocytes reside within the blood-testis barrier indicates that all nutrients or hormonal stimuli to these germ cells must pass through Sertoli cell cytoplasm. This, in turn, also indicates that not only nutrients, but also known and unknown hormonal stimuli may pass from one cell to the other. The nature of these presumptive factors is still largely unknown.

FINE STRUCTURE OF SERTOLI CELL CYTOPLASM AND NUCLEUS

Some features of the Sertoli cell fine structure have repeatedly been emphasized; the abundant rough and smooth endoplasmic reticulum, the Golgi apparatus, the electron dense vacuoles and inclusion bodies, the folded or indented nuclear membrane, and the prominent nucleolus. These and other findings have been reviewed elsewhere (106,108,115). Here only a few points that are of special interest for known or hypothetical specific Sertoli cell functions will be commented on and for more details Chapter 7 should be consulted.

The abundant smooth endoplasmic reticulum of the Sertoli cell is similar to what has been found in steroid synthesizing cells. It has been argued that this is in line with Sertoli cell synthesis of androgenic hormones, notably testosterone (57,58,60). Although some conversion of radioactive precursors to testosterone has been noted to occur in isolated seminiferous tubules, the amounts produced are very limited compared to the testosterone production in Leydig cells (69). Considering the fact that the seminiferous tubule is bathed in very high concentrations of easily accessible testosterone (38,128), the limited testosterone synthesis in the seminiferous tubules should be of minor importance. On the other hand, Sertoli cells in the young rat have been shown to metabolize androstenedione and testosterone actively to 5α-dihydrotestosterone and 3α,17β-androstanediol (15,133), and at an early age to estradiol (13). The smooth endoplasmic reticulum may be more involved in testosterone metabolism than synthesis.

The rough endoplasmic reticulum, and the prominent nucleolus may be looked upon as an indication of active protein synthesis. Since the adult Sertoli cell is not dividing, proteins must either be actively secreted, or degraded intracellularly. Sertoli cells are now known to secrete several proteins, as will be discussed below.

SECRETION OF PROTEINS FROM THE SERTOLI CELL

Androgen Binding Protein

The first secretory protein to be characterized and shown to derive from the Sertoli cell was the testicular androgen binding protein, ABP. Paradoxically, ABP was first identified in the epididymis (49,95) and only later found to derive from the testis (25,26), more specifically from the Sertoli cell (27,37,45,102). With the discovery of ABP and methods for its quantitation (90), a biochemical marker of Sertoli cell activity was available for study and new observations on the hormonal regulation of Sertoli cell function were subsequently made.

ABP has been detected at varying concentrations in several species; the rat (references above), guinea pig (B. Karpe, L. Hagenäs, and E. M. Ritzén, *unpublished*), and rabbit (11,89) show high concentrations of ABP in testis and epididymis. Moderate amounts are found in ram (50), bull (46), and mouse (E. M. Ritzén, *unpublished*). In the rhesus monkey, ABP has been detected at very low concentrations in some rete testis fluids but not in others (87). So far, conclusive evidence for human ABP is lacking, even though there are indications that human testis contains an androgen binding protein that seems to be different from the serum sex hormone binding globulin (TeBG) (3,124).

ABP has been well characterized in the rat (40,76,88) and the rabbit (131,132). In the rat, it was found to be a protein with a molecular weight of about 90,000 daltons that shows a high binding affinity to dihydrotestosterone and testosterone with a K_a of approximately 10^9 M. Other hormonal steroids showed little binding. It is secreted with the fluid from the seminiferous tubules through the rete testis and the efferent ducts into the epididymis, where it is degraded or taken up by the epithelial cells lining the convoluted epididymal duct.

The Sertoli cell origin of ABP was suggested when tubules depleted of germ cells by prenatal roentgen irradiation were still found to secrete ABP. Also, the peritubular interstitial fluid proved to contain little ABP compared to the rete testis fluid (37). Furthermore, Sertoli cell enriched cultures were shown to secrete ABP into the medium (27,28,102).

The testicular and epididymal ABP show great similarities to the TeBG found circulating in the blood of several species, including man (but excluding rat, mouse, guinea pig). A direct comparison between the two proteins was made by Hansson et al. (47) in the rabbit, a species that shows high concentrations of both ABP in rete testis fluid and TeBG in serum. After extensive purification, the only difference in their physical characteristics was a slightly different charge, when examined on an ion exchange or isoelectric focusing column. Four different guinea pigs, immunized against purified ABP, produced antisera that showed a complete cross reaction with rabbit TeBG. Thus, very similar, if not identical, glycoproteins seem to be produced by two different organs (testis and liver) under completely different regulatory control.

The purification of rat ABP and the subsequent development of a radioimmunoassay for rat ABP greatly increased the sensitivity of the ABP assay (33). These authors could then show that small amounts of ABP were detectable in peripheral blood of the rat. The blood ABP disappeared upon castration and could not be reinduced by hormonal treatment. This gave promise of a way of longitudinal monitoring of Sertoli cell function in rats by serial sampling of blood specimens. The validation of this approach has not yet been presented. However, it may be assumed that determinations of blood ABP will be of great importance in the future, since the secretion of ABP into the epididymis has previously been shown to correlate well with spermatogenesis (46).

Seven years after the detection of ABP, its physiological role is still obscure. Three possible functions may be discussed: as an *intracellular* carrier of testosterone or dihydrotestosterone in the Sertoli cell itself, as a large store of androgenic hormones in the seminiferous and epididymal tubules, or as a carrier of testosterone from the testis into the epididymis. These three possibilities will be discussed.

The Sertoli cell is dependent on high concentrations of testosterone for its normal function (see below) but also contains metabolizing enzymes for the same hormone. An androgen protective role has therefore been suggested for ABP (15). Similarly, ABP may secure the supply of androgens for the Sertoli cell from an extracellular store in the tubule fluid. The synthesis of testosterone in the Leydig cells may undergo rapid fluctuations, and the intratubular ABP may then serve as a readily available store of androgens. The concentration of ABP in the rat rete testis fluid is about 180 nmol/liter and total androgen concentrations (testosterone + dihydrotestosterone) about 120 nmol/liter. The concentration of free testosterone in the rete testis fluid is about 9 nmol/liter or 8% of the total assuming a K_d of about 10^{-8} at a 32°C. However, the seminiferous fluid may contribute with only 1/10 of the rete testis fluid (107) suggesting a much higher concentration of both ABP and testosterone in the seminiferous tubules. This concentration would be stabilized by the buffering function of the ABP. Furthermore, in the rat, specific androgen binding proteins are virtually absent in blood, which would further emphasize the storage effect of the intratubular ABP. Similar calculations were also made by Rommerts et al. (96) but they arrived at different conclusions. This may in part be explained by the erroneous assumption that the rat has the same high degree of protein binding of testosterone in serum as man.

Finally, ABP carries androgens from the rat testis into the epididymis. In the initial segment of the epididymal duct, there is an extensive resorption of fluid by the lining epithelial cells. Protein bound androgens would then be concentrated about 20 times to reach extreme concentrations (~2.4 μmol/liter). These androgens bathe the spermatozoa and the epididymal cells, and will eventually be resorbed. It is noteworthy, that the epithelium of the initial segment undergoes rapid hypoplasia after efferent duct ligation, indicating the loss of an essential factor normally supplied through the efferent ducts (L. Nicander, *personal communication*). Circulating testosterone is also rapidly taken up from the blood into the caput epididymis and bound to intraluminal ABP, as revealed by autoradiography (46).

The storage function of ABP may be illustrated by the close correlation between concentrations of ABP and testosterone in rete testis fluid of various species (94). Furthermore, a similar correlation between ABP and testosterone and dihydrotestosterone was found in rete testis fluids collected from individual rabbits (32). However, some species (man, monkey, swine, bull) seem to have low concentrations of ABP in their rete testis fluid. Thus, in these species, the androgen transport function of ABP does not seem to be essential.

Inhibin

The existence of a testicular substance, that after secretion into the blood stream was able to suppress the release of FSH from the pituitary, was postulated as early as in 1932 (64). Since then, numerous pieces of evidence have been accumulated supporting the original hypothesis (see Chapter 6), but it was not proved that Sertoli cells produced such a compound until very recently. In elegant experiments, Steinberger and Steinberger (114,116) showed that Sertoli cells in tissue culture secreted a factor that selectively inhibited the release of FSH by cultured anterior pituitary cells. It is still not excluded, however, that in addition other cell types in the testis may also produce substances with inhibin activity. It remains possible as well, that some other cells may enhance the production of inhibin by the Sertoli cells.

Other Secretory Proteins of Sertoli Cells

Some of the most potent regulators of gonadal differentiation in the embryo seem to derive from the Sertoli cells or their precursors, meiosis preventing substance and Müllerian inhibiting hormone. This has been reviewed above (pp. 171–172). A few other specific proteins have been identified as secretory products of Sertoli cells from postnatal testes.

Lacroix et al. (56) showed that the spent medium of cultures of immature Sertoli cells contained a specific protease, plasminogen activator. Like ABP, this activity was increased by addition of FSH or dibutyryl cyclic AMP to the medium during culture. The authors speculate that the protease may play a role in the opening of the occluding inter-Sertoli cell junctions, to allow passage of germ cells.

The above mentioned proteins have been identified as specific for Sertoli cells. However, Sertoli cells in culture secrete a large number of more or less "anonymous" proteins, the pattern of which has been discussed by Rommerts et al. (97). Among these, albumin-like proteins are in majority. It may be, that most of the proteins found in primary seminiferous fluid (54) are actually derived from the Sertoli cells.

SECRETION OF SEMINIFEROUS FLUID

Fluid production in the rat seminiferous tubule starts at about 18 days of age, when lumen formation is seen first by light microscopy. Waites (128) recently reviewed the current knowledge of the composition of this fluid. The most characteristic findings are the very high concentrations of potassium and bicarbonate, and low levels of sodium and chloride, compared to the blood plasma. In this respect, the seminiferous tubule fluid resembles intracellular ionic composition. The maintenance of this ionic gradient is a function of the Sertoli cell cytoplasm, and the occluding inter-Sertoli cell junctions. Several specific proteins (ABP, inhibin) and steroids (reviewed by Waites, ref. 128) are found in seminiferous tubule or rete testis fluid, and are believed to be carried into the epididymis.

The regulation of seminiferous fluid production is understood poorly. It has been reported that neither hypophysectomy nor gonadotrophins affected fluid production (107). Fluid production is grossly normal in the prenatally germ cell depleted testis (L. Hagenäs and E. M. Ritzén, *unpublished*), after nitrofurazone depletion of spermatogenesis in the adult rat (34) or after short-term experimental cryptorchidism. After prolonged cryptorchidism, fluid production is decreased (39,107). The ionic composition, on the other hand, was changed to a "blood pattern" in non-sperm-containing tubules of prenatally busulfan-treated testes, but was normal in adjacent sperm-containing tubules (59).

Considerably more information is available on the characterization of fluid collected from the rete testis rather than directly from the seminiferous tubules. However, Setchell (108) estimated that about nine-tenths of the rete fluid is actually secreted directly through the epithelium of the rete testis. This latter fluid resembles blood plasma in its ionic composition rather than the "primary" seminiferous tubule fluid, and it seems that the "primary" seminiferous tubule fluid must be analyzed if the Sertoli cell contribution to testicular fluid is to be understood. When considering the vast differences in ionic composition of the fluids on the opposite sides of the seminiferous epithelium, it seems natural to assume that this specific intratubular milieu is needed for normal maturation of the postmeiotic germ cells, and that interference with this ionic milieu would be disastrous for spermatogenesis. However, little is known about the ionic composition of the seminiferous fluid under various pathophysiological conditions.

HORMONAL REGULATION OF SERTOLI CELL FUNCTION

One of the major breakthroughs in research on the physiology of the seminiferous tubule function was the realization that many, if not all, of the hormonal effects on spermatogenesis are executed through the Sertoli cells. Studies on the function of the Sertoli cell in its natural environment, within the seminiferous epithelium, became possible with the discovery of a specific Sertoli cell marker, the androgen binding protein, ABP (see p. 178 above).

At an earlier stage, it was observed that the Sertoli cell of hypophysectomized rats responded morphologically to injection of FSH by hypertrophy and nuclear changes (74,75). Later, autoradiographic and electron microscopic studies using FSH labeled with radioactivity (12) or ferritin (6,7) showed that FSH accumulated on Sertoli cells, rather than germ cells. This was considered evidence for the hypothesis of a selective action of FSH on the Sertoli cells, but has recently been challenged by Orth and Christensen (79). The latter authors noted accumulation of radioactivity on the surface of spermatogonia as well as Sertoli cells after injection of ^{125}I-labeled hFSH. This is an important observation that needs to be confirmed by other methods before its significance can be evaluated.

Functional effects of FSH on Sertoli cells were also indicated by the observations that FSH stimulated RNA and protein synthesis in testes that had been depleted of most other cell types except Sertoli cells (reviewed by Means, ref. 66). However, it could be argued that these pathological testes had a different response from the normal organ. With the observation that FSH caused an increase in the production of the specific Sertoli cell protein ABP *in vivo* in the intact immature and in the hypophysectomized rat (45,101) as well as *in vitro* in organ cultures (91,93), and in isolated Sertoli cells from immature rats (15,27,111), it was concluded that the Sertoli cell is a major target for FSH in the testis (44). Subsequently, it was shown that isolated Sertoli cells in tissue culture respond to added FSH by increasing mitotic activity (30) and by increasing the secretion not only of ABP, but also of cyclic AMP (17), plasminogen activator (56), estradiol (1,10), and metabolites of androstenedione (133).

FSH is necessary for initiation of spermatogenesis in the immature rat, but once spermatogenesis is established, it can be maintained even in the hypophysectomized rat by large doses of testosterone or dihydrotestosterone (129). The maintenance of spermatogenesis by gonadotropin or androgen supplementation is paralleled by the effects of the same hormones on ABP production (41). This indicates that the only two hormones known to be of decisive importance for spermatogenesis exert at least part of their effects through the Sertoli cells.

Androgens alone can support spermatogenesis and ABP production in the adult hypophysectomized rat, if given immediately following hypophysectomy. However, if the androgen is given at a time when the seminiferous epithelium is regressed, there is little effect on spermatogenesis. Similarly, androgens given at this point cause little or no stimulation of ABP secretion by the Sertoli cells although they do respond to FSH alone (41). The effect of FSH administration on ABP synthesis in the hypophysectomized rat is dramatically enhanced in rats maintained on high doses of androgens (46). Under these conditions FSH and androgens act synergistically on the Sertoli cell. However, Tindall et al. (120) were not able to observe a synergistic effect when testosterone and FSH were given together for 4 days to rats hypophysectomized for 30 days. So far, no other hormones have been shown to enhance any Sertoli cell function. However, addition of serum increases the secretion of ABP by testicular minces *in vitro* (93), indicating that as yet unidentified factors may also be active.

Androgenic hormones alone can maintain ABP production and spermatogenesis. In accordance with this, cytoplasmic androgen receptors have been identified in testes (42,72,73) and in cultured Sertoli cells (104), and testosterone enhances ABP production *in vitro* (61). Androgen stimulation appears not to be obligatory for ABP production, since ABP is found in high concentrations in the testes of the androgen insensitive rat (Tfm rat) (43). However, efferent ducts and epididymides are lacking in these rats, and ABP may accumulate in the testis even if the production rate is low. Indeed, ABP production by testicular minces *in vitro* was found to be about one third of that of the control. The partial maintenance of ABP production by the Tfm rat testes could result from partial androgen sensitivity in combination with high local concentration of testosterone and normal FSH (84). However, the Tfm mouse which is believed to be totally androgen resistant (62) contains testicular ABP concentrations somewhat higher than the normal mouse (E. M. Ritzén, *unpublished*). The low overall ABP production by the mouse testis prevented a quantitative estimation of the production rate *in vitro*.

The acute intravenous administration of FSH to 14- to 16-day-old rats causes a rapid (within 2 hr) increase in the testicular content of ABP (55,67). However, this was also found to be the case after injection of LH or testosterone and it was suggested (119) that all these rapid effects on ABP accumulation were caused by testosterone (in the case of FSH by contamination of the preparation with LH). Furthermore, the same authors noted that addition of testosterone, Ca^{2+}, glycerol, and p-chloromercuriphenyl sulphonate to the homogenization buffer stabilized ABP, and increased its recovery. Thus, treatment which increases the concentrations of testosterone could increase the recovery of ABP, thereby appearing to stimulate ABP production. However, with the homogenization procedures used in our three laboratories, we have found only slight effects by addition of the substances mentioned, when tested under a great variety of experimental conditions. Kotite et al. (55) demonstrated an acute stimulation of ABP secretion by FSH even when ABP was stabilized by addition of testosterone to the homogenization buffer. The conclusion was that FSH induces a rapid increase in the production of ABP by the immature rat testis. A similar apparent increase in testicular ABP following LH treatment was abolished by homogenizing in the presence of excess testosterone indicating that LH does not rapidly stimulate ABP (N. I. Kotite, S. N. Nayfeh, and F. S. French, *unpublished data*).

Although the Sertoli cell has now convincingly been shown to be a target for androgens, it has been difficult to produce positive evidence against the hypothesis that some germ cells may also be androgen targets. The elegant experiments by Lyon et al. (62) speak against this theory. These authors made chimeric mice by fusing normal and Tfm blastocysts. Some of the resulting males proved to be fertile, and when mated with normal females they fathered female offspring that carried the Tfm gene. Since the Tfm gene is located on the X chromosome (63), this experiment showed that some spermatozoa had matured normally in spite of carrying the gene for androgen resistance. The most plausible theory to explain this would be that Sertoli cells and other somatic supporting cells, sensitive to androgens, had been nursing the germ cells.

The recent report by Grootegoed et al. (31) that nuclear androgen receptors could be demonstrated in Sertoli cells but not in germ cells (spermatocytes and round spermatids) also indicates that androgens, although important for spermatogenesis, do not act directly on the germ cells but rather through Sertoli cells. This conclusion is in conflict with the finding by Tsai et al. (125) that both Sertoli and germ cell nuclei contained acceptor sites for testicular androgen-receptor complexes. There are no structures described that could suggest a mechanism for intercellular passage of androgen-receptor complexes from Sertoli to germ cells. Furthermore, the postmeiotic genome is thought to be largely inactive (70).

It has repeatedly been pointed out that the Sertoli cell is more sensitive to FSH in the immature than the adult rat. As a matter of fact, it has not been shown that FSH is important for spermatogenesis in the adult, once fertility is well established. In the rat, prolonged treatment with a specific antiserum to FSH from 1 to 30 days of age markedly inhibited ABP secretion and spermatogenesis (20,85) while a similar treatment of the adult rat had little or no effect (18). Treatment with large doses of testosterone could not substitute for FSH in the immature rats. There may be important species differences in the requirement of FSH in the adult, since Moudgal (71) recently reported on preliminary studies in monkeys, where administration of FSH antiserum to adult animals seemed to induce sterility.

The strictly FSH dependent enzyme activity, aromatizing testosterone to estradiol in immature Sertoli cells (1) has recently been utilized to develop a sensitive and specific *in vitro* bioassay of FSH (10). Sertoli cell cultures from 10-day-old rats are exposed for 24 hr to medium containing FSH or the unknown sample, and the estradiol content of the spent media is measured by radioimmunoassay. By logarithmic transformation, a linear standard curve is obtained between 2 and 128 IU/liter, and all available FSH preparations showed parallel dose-response curves. The precision of the assay is good ($\lambda = 0.082$), the interassay coefficient of variation 17%. By comparison with radioimmunoassay (RIA) of FSH, the crude standard preparation LER 109 proved to give lower values for bioassay than for RIA while purified preparations of FSH gave values that were in good agreement, using the two methods. This indicates that even with the best available antisera and labeled FSH, the RIA method includes biologically nonactive material in the assay. Thus a specific reaction of the Sertoli cell to FSH could be utilized to develop an FSH bioassay that is of great use in validating RIA methods of measuring FSH.

Some of the present knowledge about the hormonal regulation of Sertoli cell function is schematically illustrated in Fig. 3.

CYCLIC ACTIVITY OF SERTOLI CELLS

In the previous sections of this chapter, it has been stressed that the Sertoli cell may have a regulatory role in the process of spermatogenesis. In that case, one should be able to detect some morphological or functional differences between Sertoli cells in different stages of spermatogenesis. This is actually the case. Tres and Kierszenbaum (123) pointed out that the endoplasmic reticulum is dilated in some Sertoli cells, not in others. The uptake of ^{3}H-uridine was slightly higher in the vacuolated type. Kerr and de Kretser (53) described cyclic variations in the Sertoli cell lipid content throughout the spermatogenic cycle in the rat.

The first evidence for a functional cyclic activity in Sertoli cells was recently reported by Parvinen et al. (81). In the rat, the spermatogenetic wave is organized along the seminiferous tubule, so that the individual stages can be identified and isolated by dissection of the living tubule under the microscope (83). When pools of tubule segments containing stages II–VI, VII–VIII, IX–XII, and XIII–XIV–I were incubated *in vitro* for 20 hr at 32°C, the stages VII–VIII were found to secrete 70% more ABP than the segments containing stages II–VI. Furthermore, when the 4 different pools of tubules were incubated with FSH in the presence of a phosphodiesterase inhibitor, there was a marked difference in the synthesis of cyclic AMP. In all pools, this effect of FSH was dose-dependent, but on different levels; stage II–VI showed 10 times higher cyclic AMP production than stage VII–VIII. Similarly, the concentration of FSH receptors in stages II–VI was twice that in stages VII–VIII. It was interesting that the concentration of receptors and the cyclic AMP response to FSH were inversely correlated to the secretion of ABP, indicating that the Sertoli cells most active in protein synthesis and secretion are the least sensitive to FSH stimulation. The observed variations in Sertoli cell activity in different stages of spermatogenesis may be interpreted as support of the controlling influence of Sertoli cells on spermatogenesis. However, it has not yet been disproved that the influence is in the other direction—that certain germ cells influence Sertoli cell functions.

The peak ABP production in stages VII–XII coincides with the occurrence of pachytene spermatocytes, which show the highest RNA synthesis (70,109). Parvinen and Söderström (82) also found that the combined (but not separate) addition of FSH and testosterone to segments of tubules *in vitro* caused an increased RNA synthesis in stage VII.

THE SERTOLI CELL IN CRYPTORCHIDISM

For a long time, the Sertoli cell was thought to be remarkably resistant to the increased temperature that caused a complete inhibition of spermatogenesis in the cryptorchid testis (9). This assumption was made when microscopy was the only tool by which Sertoli cells could be examined. However, with the advent of ABP as marker of Sertoli cell function, it was realized that this cell also was severely disturbed by the intraabdominal position (36,105). This was shown both when the cryptorchidism was induced in the adult rat and when descent was prevented by operation at 17 days of age, before spontaneous descent was completed (39,92).

In attempts to identify the mechanism behind this impairment of Sertoli cell function, several experiments were performed. The influence of the cryptorchidism on the hormonal milieu of the seminiferous tubule was examined by measuring the concentrations of androgens and FSH in the interstitial fluid surrounding the tubules (38). No evidence for hormone deficiency was found. On the contrary, both androgens and FSH were present at higher than normal amounts. Next, the androgen receptor content of cryptorchid testes of hypophysectomized rats were found to be the same as of noncryptorchid hypophysectomized rats. However, there was a dramatic decrease in the content of testicular receptors for FSH in the cryptorchid rats (39). To our knowledge, this is the first demonstration of an induced loss of FSH receptors in a pathological condition. It cannot yet be stated whether the loss of FSH receptors is primary or secondary to the impaired Sertoli cell function. The fact that secretion of ABP by Sertoli cells in culture is impaired by an elevation of the temperature from 32°C to 37°C, in the absence of any hormones, indicates that nonhormonal factors are involved (39). The blood-testis barrier is grossly unaffected by cryptorchidism (35). It is still too early to state whether the impaired spermatogenesis in cryptorchidism is primarily owing to impaired Sertoli cell function or to direct effects on germ cells.

It has been reported that in unilateral cryptorchidism in the rat ABP secretion is impaired even in the scrotal testis (105). This would be compatible with the frequent observation that in the human, fertility is impaired also in unilateral cryptorchidism. However, we have not been able to reproduce the findings mentioned above (L. Hagenäs and E. M. Ritzén, *unpublished*).

EFFECTS OF CERTAIN DRUGS ON SERTOLI CELLS

Although many drugs are known to interfere with spermatogenesis, little seems to be known about specific drug effects on Sertoli cells. One might expect that some of the antispermatogenic agents act not directly on germ cells but rather on one of the specific functions of the Sertoli cells.

Recent observations by Rich and de Kretser (86) indicate that this may indeed be the case. They found that treatment of adult rats with hydroxyurea or chronic feeding of a vitamin A deficient diet caused not only the previously known destruction of spermatogenesis, but also decreased ABP secretion, indicating impaired Sertoli cell function.

Hagenäs et al. (34) demonstrated how the mechanism of action of a specific drug, nitrofurazone, may be investigated with regard to Leydig cell, germ cell, and Sertoli cell function. The Sertoli cell function was evaluated by several parameters during 2 to 28 days of treatment with nitrofurazone; production of ABP and testicular fluid, maintenance of the blood-testis barrier, and concentration of FSH in serum, assuming a Sertoli cell origin of "inhibin" (116). Leydig cell function was followed by testosterone levels in serum and testosterone production *in vitro;* germ cells by light and electron microscopy. The secretion of ABP showed an initial drop, but after 28 days of treatment it was not significantly different from controls. Fluid production and barrier function (as judged by a simple lanthanum method) were normal. FSH levels were elevated from 10 days of treatment. The initial drop in ABP secretion was not a result of germ cell degeneration, since it was noticed also when rats that were depleted of germ cells by prenatal irradiation were treated with nitrofurazone. It was concluded that Sertoli cell function was close to normal after long-term treatment with the drug, although all germ cells except spermatogonia and some primary spermatocytes were absent. However, FSH levels were high. This dissociation between the secretion of two different Sertoli cell products, ABP and inhibin, is interesting. It may be interpreted as a relative damage to the Sertoli cell, affecting one parameter but not the other, but it may also indicate that a local positive feed-back is active between some germ cells and Sertoli cells, or that inhibin is made in both Sertoli cells and germ cells.

The possible use of Sertoli cell cultures for the purpose of screening for drugs active as male contraceptives does not yet seem to have been explored. By studying the effects of various drugs on ABP secretion, a rapid way of selecting those that would be suitable for further *in vivo* studies may be found. A drug with a selective inhibitory effect on Sertoli cells would certainly be a candidate for a future male contraceptive.

CONCLUDING REMARKS

Few cell types in the reproductive tract have come under attention as much as the Sertoli cell during the last few years. In the textbooks of the late 1960s, the Sertoli cell was described as a supporting cell for the seminiferous epithelium, without many specific features of its own. As late as 1974, Steinberger and Steinberger (117) concluded that "the role of hormones (if any) in regulating growth, differentiation and function of the Sertoli cells has not been demonstrated with certainty. In fact, the function or the role of Sertoli cells in testicular physiology remains to a great extent a mystery." The present review has briefly mentioned some of the new pieces of information gained in the last years. It has been shown that from the early embryonic stage, through prepubertal, pubertal to the adult ages, the Sertoli cell plays a key role in the development and function of the seminiferous tubule. The hormones known to be necessary for normal spermatogenesis seem to work through the Sertoli cells. A picture is emerging that shows the germ cell maturation in the seminiferous epithelium proceeds according to an intrinsic genetically determined timetable. However, in order to live through this maturation, they need a very specific milieu. This milieu is created by the Sertoli cell.

ACKNOWLEDGMENTS

The studies from our laboratories described in this review were supported by grants from the Swedish and Norwegian Medical Research Councils, the Nordic Insulin Foundation, the WHO expanded program on research on human fertility, the NIH, and the Population Council.

REFERENCES

1. Armstrong, D. T., and Dorrington, J. H. (1977): Estrogen biosynthesis in the ovaries and testes. In: *Advances in Sex Hormone Research, Regulatory Mechanisms Affecting Gonadal Hormone Action,* Vol. 3, edited by J. A. Thomas and R. L. Singhal, pp. 217–258. University Park Press, Baltimore.
2. Bressler, R. S. (1976): Dependence of Sertoli cell maturation on the pituitary gland in the mouse. *Am. J. Anat.,* 147:447–456.
3. Burke, W. R., Aten, R. F., Eisenfeld, A. J., and Lytton, B. (1977): Androgen binding in human testis. *J. Urol.,* 118:52–57.
4. Byskov, A. G. (1978): Regulation of initiation of meiosis in female gonads. In: *Endocrine Approach to Male Contraception,* edited by V. Hansson, E. M. Ritzén, K. Purvis, and F. S. French, pp. 29–38. Scriptor, Copenhagen.
5. Byskov, A. G., and Saxén, L. (1976): Induction of meiosis in fetal mouse testis in vitro. *Dev. Biol.,* 52:193–200.
6. Castro, A. E., Alonso, A., and Mancini, R. E. (1972): Localization of follicle-stimulating and luteinizing hormones in the rat testis using immunohistological tests. *J. Endocrinol.,* 52:129–136.
7. Castro, A. E., Seiguer, A. C., and Mancini, R. E. (1970): Electron microscopic study of the localization of the labeled gonadotropins in the Sertoli and Leydig cells of the rat testis. *Proc. Soc. Exp. Biol. Med.,* 133:582–586.
8. Clausen, O. P. F., Purvis, K., and Hansson, V. (1978): Quantitation of spermatogenesis by flow cytometric DNA measurements. In: *Endocrine Approach to Male Contraception,* edited by V. Hansson, E. M. Ritzén, K. Purvis, and F. S. French, pp. 513–522. Scriptor, Copenhagen.
9. Clegg, E. J. (1963): Studies on artificial cryptorchidism: Morphological and quantitative changes in the Sertoli cells of the rat testes. *J. Endocrinol.,* 26:567–574.
10. Damme, M.-P. van, Robertson, D. M., Marana, R., Ritzén, E. M., and Diczfalusy, E. (1979): A sensitive and specific in vitro bioassay method for the measurement of follicle-stimulating hormone activity. *Acta Endocrinol.,* 91:224–237.
11. Danzo, B. J., and Eller, B. D. (1978): Androgen metabolism by and binding to mature rabbit epididymal tissue: studies on cytosol. *J. Steroid Biochem.,* 9:209–217.
12. Desjardins, C., Zelernik, A. J., Midgley, A. R., Jr., and Reichert, L. E., Jr. (1974): In vitro

binding and autoradiographic localization of human chorionic gonadotropin and follicle stimulating hormone in rat testes during development. In: *Hormone Binding and Target Cell Activation in the Testis,* edited by M. L. Dufau and A. R. Means, pp. 221–235. Plenum Press, New York.

13. Dorrington, J. H., Armstrong, D. T. (1975): Follicle-stimulating hormone stimulates estradiol-17β synthesis in cultured Sertoli cells. *Proc. Natl. Acad. Sci. USA,* 72:2677–2681.
14. Dorrington, J. H., and Fritz, I. B. (1973): Metabolism of testosterone by preparations from the rat testis. *Biochem. Biophys. Res. Commun.,* 54:1425–1431.
15. Dorrington, J. H., and Fritz, I. B. (1975): Androgen synthesis and metabolism by preparations from the seminiferous tubule of the rat testis. In: *Hormonal Regulation of Spermatogenesis,* edited by F. S. French, V. Hansson, E. M. Ritzén, and S. N. Nayfeh, pp. 37–52. Plenum Press, New York.
16. Dorrington, J. H., and Fritz, I. B. (1975): Cellular localization of 5α-reductase and 3α-hydroxy-steroid dehydrogenase in the seminiferous tubule of the rat testis. *Endocrinology,* 96:879–889.
17. Dorrington, J. H., Roller, N. F., and Fritz, I. B. (1975): Effects of follicle-stimualting hormone on cultures of Sertoli cell preparations. *Mol. Cell. Endocrinol.,* 3:57–70.
18. Dym, M., and Cavicchia, J. C. (1977): Further observations on the blood-testis barrier in monkeys. *Biol. Reprod.,* 17:390–416.
19. Dym, M., and Fawcett, D. W. (1970): The blood-testis barrier in the rat and the physiological compartmentation of the seminiferous epithelium. *Biol. Reprod.,* 3:308–326.
20. Dym, M., Raj, H. G. M., and Chemes, H. E. (1977): Response of the testis to selective withdrawal of LH or FSH using antigonadotropic sera. In: *The Testis in Normal and Infertile Men,* edited by P. Troen and H. R. Nankin, pp. 97–124. Raven Press, New York.
21. Fawcett, D. W. (1974): Interactions between Sertoli cells and germ cells. In: *Male Fertility and Sterility,* edited by R. E. Mancini and L. Martini, pp. 13–36. Academic Press, New York.
22. Fawcett, D. W. (1975): Observations on the organization of the interstitial tissue of the testis and on the occluding cell functions in the seminiferous epithelium. In: *Advances in the Biosciences.* Schering Symposium on Contraception, Vol. 10, pp. 83–99. Pergamon Press, New York.
23. Fawcett, D. E., Leak, K. V., and Heidger, P. M., Jr. (1970): Electron microscopic observations on the structural components of the blood-testis barrier. *J. Reprod. Fertil.,* Suppl. 10:105–122.
24. Flickinger, C., and Fawcett, D. W. (1967): The functional specializations of Sertoli cells in the seminiferous epithelium. *Anat. Rec.,* 158:207–222.
25. French, F. S., and Ritzén, E. M. (1973): Androgen binding protein in efferent duct fluid of rat testis. *J. Reprod. Fertil.,* 32:479–483.
26. French, F. S., and Ritzén, E. M. (1973): A high affinity androgen binding protein (ABP) in rat testis: evidence for secretion into efferent duct fluid and absorption by epididymis. *Endocrinology,* 95:88–93.
27. Fritz, I. B., Kopec, B., Lam, K., and Vernon, R. G. (1974): Effects of FSH on levels of androgen binding protein in the testis. In: *Hormone Binding and Target Cell Activation in the Testis,* edited by M. L. Dufau and A. R. Means, pp. 311–327. Plenum Press, New York.
28. Fritz, I. B., Rommerts, F. G., Louis, B. G., and Dorrington, J. H. (1976): Regulation by FSH and dibutyryl cyclic AMP of the formation of androgen-binding protein in Sertoli cell-enriched cultures. *J. Reprod. Fertil.,* 46:17–24.
29. Gilula, N. B., Fawcett, D. W., and Aoki, A. (1976): The Sertoli cell occluding functions and gap functions in mature and developing mammalian testis. *Dev. Biol.,* 50:142–168.
30. Griswold, M. D., Solari, A., Tung, P. S., and Fritz, I. B. (1977): Stimulation by follicle-stimulating hormone of DNA synthesis and of mitosis in cultured Sertoli cells prepared from testes of immature rats. *Mol. Cell. Endocrinol.,* 7:151–165.
31. Grootegoed, J. A., Peters, M. J., Mulder, E., Rommerts, F. F. G., and Molen, H. J. van der (1977): Absence of a nuclear androgen receptor in isolated germinal cells of rat testis. *Mol. Cell. Endocrinol.,* 9:159–167.
32. Guerrero, R., Ritzén, E. M., Purvis, K., Hansson, V., and French, F. S. (1975): Concentration of steroid hormones and androgen binding protein (ABP) in rabbit efferent duct fluid. In: *Hormonal Regulation of Spermatogenesis,* edited by F. S. French, V. Hansson, E. M. Ritzén, and S. N. Nayfeh, pp. 213–221. Plenum Press, New York.
33. Gunsalus, G. L., Musto, N. A., and Bardin, C. W. (1978): Factors affecting blood levels of

androgen binding protein in the rat. In: *Endocrine Approach to Male Contraception*, edited by V. Hansson, E. M. Ritzén, K. Purvis, and F. S. French, pp. 482–493. Scriptor, Copenhagen.

34. Hagenäs, L., Plöen, L., and Ritzén, E. M. (1978): The effect of nitrofurazone on the endocrine, secretory and spermatogenetic functions of the rat testis. *Andrologia*, 10:107–126.
35. Hagenäs, L., Plöen, L., Ritzén, E. M., and Ekwall, H. (1977): Blood testis barrier: Maintained function of inter-Sertoli cell junctions in experimental cryptorchidism in the rat, as judged by a simple lanthanum-immersion technique. *Andrologia*, 9:250–254.
36. Hagenäs, L., and Ritzén, E. M. (1976): Impaired Sertoli cell function in experimental cryptorchidism in the rat. *Mol. Cell. Endocrinol.*, 4:25–34.
37. Hagenäs, L., Ritzén, E. M., Plöen, L., Hansson, V., French, F. S., and Nayfeh, S. N. (1975): Sertoli cell origin of testicular androgen-binding protein (ABP). *Mol. Cell. Endocrinol.*, 2:339–350.
38. Hagenäs, L., Ritzén, E. M., and Suginami, H. (1978): Hormonal milieu of the seminiferous tubules in the normal and cryptorchid rat. *Int. J. Androl.*, 1:477–484.
39. Hagenäs, L., Ritzén, E. M., Svensson, J., Hansson, V., and Purvis, K. (1978): Temperature dependence of Sertoli cell function. *Int. J. Androl.*, Suppl. 2:449–458.
40. Hansson, V. (1973): Further characterization of the 5α-dihydrotestosterone binding protein in the epididymal cytosol fraction. In vitro studies. *Steroids*, 20:575–596.
41. Hansson, V., Calandra, R., Purvis, K., Ritzén, E. M., and French, F. S. (1976): Hormonal regulation of spermatogenesis. *Vitam. Horm.*, 34:187–214.
42. Hansson, V., McLean, W. S., Smith, A. A., Tindall, D. J., Weddington, S. C., Nayfeh, S. N., French, F. S., and Ritzén, E. M. (1974): Androgen receptors in rat testis. *Steroids*, 23:823–832.
43. Hansson, V., Purvis, K., Attramadal, A., Torjesen, P., Andersen, D., and Ritzén, E. M. (1978): Sertoli cell function in the androgen insensitive (TFM) rat. *Int. J. Androl.*, 1:96–104.
44. Hansson, V., Purvis, K., Ritzén, E. M., and French, F. S. (1978): Hormonal regulation of Sertoli cell function in the rat. *Ann. Biol. Anim. Biochem. Biophys.*, 18:565–572.
45. Hansson, V., Reusch, E., Trygstad, O., Torgersen, O., Ritzén, E. M., and French, F. S. (1973): FSH stimulation of testicular androgen binding protein. *Nature [New Biol.]*, 246:56–58.
46. Hansson, V., Ritzén, E. M., French, F. S., and Nayfeh, S. N. (1975): Androgen transport and receptor mechanisms in testis and epididymis. In: *Handbook of Physiology*, Section 7: Endocrinology, Vol. V, edited by D. W. Hamilton and R. O. Greep, pp. 173–201. Williams & Wilkins, Baltimore.
47. Hansson, V., Ritzén, E. M., French, F. S., Weddington, S. C., and Nayfeh, S. N. (1975): Testicular androgen-binding protein (ABP): Comparison of ABP in rabbit testis and epididymis with a similar androgen-binding protein (TeBG) in rabbit serum. *Mol. Cell. Endocrinol.*, 3:1–20.
48. Hansson, V., Trygstad, O., French, F. S., McLean, W. S., Smith, A. A., Tindall, D. J., Weddington, S. C., Petrusz, P., Nayfeh, S. N., and Ritzén, E. M. (1974): Androgen transport and receptor mechanisms in testis and epididymis. *Nature (Lond)*, 250:387–391.
49. Hansson, V., and Tveter, K. J. (1971): Uptake and binding of ³H-labeled androgens in epididymis and ductus deferens of the rat. *Acta Endocrinol. (Kbh)*, 66:745–755.
50. Jegou, B. (1976): Étude des protéines de liaison des androgènes et le plasma sanguin de belier (Ile de France). Thèse, Université de P. et M. Curie, Paris IV.
51. Josso, N., Picard, J.-Y., and Tran, D. (1977): The antimüllerian hormone. *Recent Prog. Horm. Res.*, pp. 117–167.
52. Jost, A., Magre, S., Cressant, M., and Perlman, S. (1974): Sertoli cells and early testicular differentiation. In: *Male Fertility and Sterility*, edited by R. E. Mancini and L. Martini, pp. 1–11. Academic Press, New York.
53. Kerr, J. B., and Kretser, D. M. de (1975): Cyclic variations in the Sertoli cell lipid content throughout the spermatogenic cycle in the rat. *J. Reprod. Fertil.*, 43:1–8.
54. Koskimies, A. I., and Kormano, M. (1973): The proteins in the fluids from the seminiferous tubules in rete testis of the rat. *J. Reprod. Fertil.*, 34:433–444.
55. Kotite, N. J., Nayfeh, S. N., and French, F. S. (1978): FSH and androgen regulation of Sertoli cell function in the immature rat. *Biol. Reprod.*, 18:65–73.
56. Lacroix, M., Smith, F. E., and Fritz, I. B. (1977): Secretion of plasminogen activator by Sertoli cell enriched cultures. *Mol. Cell. Endocrinol.*, 9:227–236.

57. Lacy, D., and Pettitt, A. J. (1969): Transmission electron microscopy and the production of steroids by the Leydig and Sertoli cells of the human testis. *Micron,* 1:15–33.
58. Lacy, D., and Pettitt, J. A. (1970): Sites of hormone production in the mammalian testis, and their significance in the control of male fertility. *Br. Med. Bull.,* 26:87–91.
59. Levine, N., and Marsh, D. J. (1975): Micropuncture study of the fluid composition of the Sertoli cell-only seminiferous tubules in rats. *J. Reprod. Fertil.,* 43:547–549.
60. Lofts, B. (1972): The Sertoli cell. *Gen. Comp. Endocrinol.,* Suppl. 3:636–648.
61. Louis, B. G., and Fritz, I. B. (1977): Stimulation by androgens of the production of androgen binding protein by cultured Sertoli cells. *Mol. Cell. Endocrinol.,* 7:9–16.
62. Lyon, M. F., Glenister, P. H., and Lamoreux, M. L. (1975): Normal spermatozoa from androgen-resistant germ cells of chimaeric mice and the role of androgen in spermatogenesis. *Nature (Lond),* 258:620–622.
63. Lyon, M. F., and Hawks, S. G. (1970): X-linked gene for testicular feminization in the mouse. *Nature (Lond),* 227:1217–1219.
64. McCullagh, D. R. (1932): Dual endocrine activity of the testis. *Science,* 76:19–20.
65. McGinley, D., Posalaky, Z., and Porvaznik, M. (1977): Intercellular junctional complexes of the rat seminiferous tubules: A freeze-fracture study. *Anat. Rec.,* 189:211–232.
66. Means, A. R., and Huckins, C. (1974): Coupled events in the early biochemical actions of FSH on the Sertoli cells of the testis. In: *Hormone Binding and Target Cell Activation in the Testis,* edited by M. L. Dufau and A. R. Means, pp. 145–165. Plenum Press, New York.
67. Means, A. R., and Tindall, D. J. (1974): FSH-induction of androgen binding protein in testes of Sertoli cell-only rats. In: *Hormone Binding and Target Cell Activation in the Testis,* edited by M. L. Dufau and A. R. Means, pp. 383–398. Plenum Press, New York.
68. Merchant-Larios, H. (1975): The onset of testicular differentiation in the rat. An ultrastructural study. *Am. J. Anat.,* 145:319–330.
69. Molen, H. J. van der, Grootegoed, J. A., Greef-Bijleveld, M. J. de, Rommerts, F. F. G., and Vusse, G. J. van der (1975): Distribution of steroids, steroid production and steroid metabolizing enzymes in rat testis. In: *Hormonal Regulation of Spermatogenesis,* edited by F. S. French, V. Hansson, E. M. Ritzén, and S. N. Nayfeh, pp. 3–23. Plenum Press, New York.
70. Monesi, V., Geremia, R., D'Agostino, A., and Boitani, C. (1978): Biochemistry of male germ cell differentiation in mammals: RNA synthesis in meiotic and postmeiotic cells. *Curr. Top. Dev. Biol.,* 12:11–36.
71. Moudgal, N. R. (1978): Discussion remark. In: *Endocrine Approach to Male Contraception,* edited by V. Hansson, E. M. Ritzén, K. Purvis, and F. S. French, p. 188. Scriptor, Copenhagen.
72. Mulder, E., Peters, M. J., Beurden, W. M. O van, and Molen, H. J. van der (1974): A receptor for testosterone in mature rat testes. *FEBS Lett.,* 47:209–211.
73. Mulder, E., Peters, M. J., Vries, J. de, and Molen, H. J. van der (1975): Characterization of a nuclear receptor for testosterone in seminiferous tubules of mature rat testes. *Mol. Cell. Endocrinol.,* 2:171–182.
74. Murphy, H. D. (1965): Sertoli cell stimulation following intratesticular injections of FSH in the hypophysectomized rat. *Proc. Soc. Exp. Biol. Med.,* 118:1202–1205.
75. Murphy, H. D. (1965): Intratesticular assay of follicle stimulating hormone in hypophysectomized rat. *Proc. Soc. Exp. Biol. Med.,* 120;671–675.
76. Musto, N. A., Gunsalus, G. L., and Bardin, C. W. (1978): Further characterization of androgen binding protein in epididymis and blood. In: *Endocrine Approach to Male Contraception,* edited by V. Hansson, E. M. Ritzén, K. Purvis, and F. S. French, pp. 424–433. Scriptor, Copenhagen.
77. Nagano, T., and Suzuki, F. (1976): The postnatal development of the functional complexes of the mouse Sertoli cells as revealed by freeze-fracture. *Anat. Rec.,* 185:403–418.
78. Nicander, L. (1967): An electron microscopical study of cell contacts in the seminiferous tubules of some mammals. *Z. Zellforsch. Mikrosk. Anat.,* 83:375–397.
79. Orth, J., and Christensen, A. K. (1978): Autoradiographic localization of specifically bound ^{125}I-labeled follicle-stimulating hormone on spermatogonia of the rat testis. *Endocrinology,* 103:1944–1951.
80. Osman, D. I., and Plöen, L. (1978): The ultrastructure of Sertoli cells in the boar. *Int. J. Androl.,* 1:162–179.
81. Parvinen, M., Marana, R., Robertson, D. M., Hansson, V., and Ritzén, E. M. (1980): Functional cycle of rat Sertoli cells: Differential binding and action of FSH at various stages of the

spermatogenic cycle. In: *Testicular Development, Structure, and Function,* edited by A. Steinberger and E. Steinberger, pp. 425–432. Raven Press, New York.

82. Parvinen, M., and Söderström, K.-O. (1976): Effects of FSH and testosterone on the RNA synthesis in different stages of rat spermatogenesis. *J. Steroid Biochem.,* 7:1021–1023.

83. Parvinen, M., and Vanha-Perttula, T. (1972): Identification and enzyme quantitation of the stages of the seminiferous epithelial wave in the rat. *Anat. Rec.,* 174:435–449.

84. Purvis, K., Haug, E., Clausen, O. P. F., Naess, O., and Hansson, V. (1978): Endocrine status of the testicular feminized rat. *Mol. Cell. Endocrinol.,* 8:1053–1060.

85. Raj, H. G. M., and Dym, M. (1976): The effects of selective withdrawal of FSH or LH on spermatogenesis in the immature rat. *Biol. Reprod.,* 14:489–494.

86. Rich, K., and de Kretser, D. M. (1977): Effects of differing degrees of destruction of the rat seminiferous epithelium on levels of serum FSH and androgen binding protein. *Endocrinology,* 101:959–968.

87. Ritzén, E. M. (1978): Discussion remark. In: *Endocrine Approach to Male Contraception,* edited by V. Hansson, E. M. Ritzén, K. Purvis, and F. S. French, p. 433. Scriptor, Copenhagen.

88. Ritzén, E. M., Dobbins, M. C., Tindall, D. J., French, F. S., and Nayfeh, S. N. (1973): Characterization of an androgen binding protein (ABP) in rat testis and epididymis. *Steroids,* 21:593–607.

89. Ritzén, E. M., and French, F. S. (1974): Demonstration of an androgen binding protein (ABP) in rabbit testis: Secretion in efferent duct fluid and passage into epididymis. *J. Steroid Biochem.,* 5:151–154.

90. Ritzén, E. M., French, F. S., Weddington, S. C., Nayfeh, S. N., and Hansson, V. (1974): Steroid binding in polyacrylamide gels: Quantitation at steady state conditions. *J. Biol. Chem.,* 249:6597–6604.

91. Ritzén, E. M., Hagenäs, L., Hansson, V., and French, F. S. (1975): In vitro synthesis of testicular androgen binding protein (ABP): Stimulation by FSH and androgen. In: *Hormonal Regulation of Spermatogenesis,* edited by F. S. French, V. Hansson, E. M. Ritzén, and S. N. Nayfeh, pp. 353–366. Plenum Press, New York.

92. Ritzén, E. M., Hagenäs, L., Karpe, B., Plöen, L., and Hansson, V. (1979): Sertoli cell function in experimental cryptorchidism in the rat. In: *Pediatric and Adolescent Endocrinology,* Vol. 6, edited by Z. Laron, pp. 88–96. S. Karger, Basel.

93. Ritzén, E. M., Hagenäs, L., Plöen, L., French, F. S., and Hansson, V. (1977): In vitro synthesis of rat testicular androgen-binding protein (ABP). *Mol. Cell. Endocrinol.,* 8:335–346.

94. Ritzén, E. M., Hagenäs, L., Purvis, K., Guerrero, R., Johnsonbaugh, R. E., Dym, M., French, F. S., and Hansson, V. (1976): Androgens and androgen binding protein (ABP) in testicular fluids. In: *Maldescensus Testis,* edited by J. R. Bierich, K. Rager, and M. B. Ranke, pp. 79–87. Urban & Schwarzenberg, München-Wien-Baltimore.

95. Ritzén, E. M., Nayfeh, S. N., French, F. S., and Dobbins, M. C. (1971): Demonstration of androgen-binding components in rat epididymis cytosol and comparison with binding components in prostate and other tissues. *Endocrinology,* 89:143–151.

96. Rommerts, F. F. G., Grootegoed, J. A., and Molen, H. J. van der (1976): Physiological role for androgen binding protein-steroid complex in testis? *Steroids,* 28:43–49.

97. Rommerts, F. F. G., Krüger-Sewnarain, B. C., Woerkom-Blik, A. van, Grootegoed, J. A., and Molen, H. J. van der (1978): Secretion of proteins by Sertoli cell cultures: Effects of FSH, dibutyryl-cAMP and testosterone and correlation with secretion of estradiol and androgen binding protein. *Mol. Cell. Endocr.,* 10:39–55.

98. Ross, M. H. (1976): The Sertoli cell functional specialization during spermatogenesis and at spermiation. *Anat. Rec.,* 186:79–104.

99. Russell, L. (1977): Observations on rat Sertoli ectoplasmic ('junctional') specializations in their association with germ cells of the rat testis. *Tissue Cell,* 9:475–498.

100. Russell, L., and Clermont, Y. (1976): Anchoring device between Sertoli cells and late spermatids in rat seminiferous tubules. *Anat. Rec.,* 185:259–278.

101. Sanborn, B. M., Elkington, J. S. H., Chowdhury, M., Tcholakian, R. K., and Steinberger, E. (1975): Hormonal influences on the level of testicular androgen binding activity: Effect of FSH following hypophysectomy. *Endocrinology,* 96:304–312.

102. Sanborn, B. M., Elkington, J. S. H., Steinberger, A., and Steinberger, E. (1975): Androgen binding in the testis: In vitro production of androgen binding protein (ABP) by Sertoli cell cultures and measurement of nuclear bound androgen by a nuclear exchange assay. In:

Hormonal Regulation of Spermatogenesis, edited by F. S. French, V. Hansson, E. M. Ritzén, and S. N. Nayfeh, pp. 293–309. Plenum Press, New York.

103. Sanborn, B. M., Elkington, J. S. H., Tcholakian, R. K., and Steinberger, E. (1975): Some properties of androgen-binding activity in rat testis. *Mol. Cell. Endocrinol.,* 3:129–142.
104. Sanborn, B. M., Steinberger, A., Tcholakian, R. K., and Steinberger, E. (1977): Direct measurement of androgen receptors in cultured Sertoli cells. *Steroids,* 29:493–502.
105. Schenck, B., and Neumann, F. (1977): Sertoli cell function and unilateral cryptorchidism in rats. *Proc. Dtsch. Ges. Endokrinol. (Travemünde),* p. 55, (Abstract).
106. Schulze, C. (1974): On the morphology of the human Sertoli cell. *Cell Tis. Res.,* 153:339–355.
107. Setchell, B. P. (1970): The secretion of fluid by the testes of rats, rams and goats with some observations on the effect of age, cryptorchidism and hypophysectomy. *J. Reprod. Fertil.,* 23:79–85.
108. Setchell, B. P. (1974): Secretions of the testis and epididymis. *J. Reprod. Fertil.,* 37:165–177.
109. Söderström, K.-O., and Parvinen, M. (1976): RNA synthesis in different stages of rat seminiferous epithelial cycle. *Mol. Cell. Endocrinol.,* 5:181–199.
110. Solari, A. J., and Fritz, I. B. (1978): The ultrastructure of immature Sertoli cells. Maturation-like changes during culture and the maintenance of mitotic potentiality. *Biol. Reprod.,* 18:329–345.
111. Steinberger, A., Elkington, J. S. H., Sanborn, B. M., and Steinberger, E. (1975): Culture and FSH responses of Sertoli cells isolated from sexually mature rat testis. In: *Hormonal Regulation of Spermatogenesis,* edited by F. S. French, V. Hansson, E. M. Ritzén, and S. N. Nayfeh, pp. 399–411. Plenum Press, new York.
112. Steinberger, A., Hintz, M., and Heindel, J. J. (1978): Changes in cyclic AMP responses to FSH in isolated rat Sertoli cells during sexual maturation. *Biol. Reprod.,* 19:566–572.
113. Steinberger, A., and Steinberger, E. (1971): Replication pattern of Sertoli cells in maturing rat testis in vivo and in organ culture. *Biol. Reprod.,* 4:84–87.
114. Steinberger, A., and Steinberger, E. (1977): Inhibition of FSH by a Sertoli cell factor in vitro. In: *The Testis in Normal and Infertile Men,* edited by P. Troen and H. R. Nankin, pp. 271–279. Raven Press, New York.
115. Steinberger, A., and Steinberger, E. (1977): The Sertoli cells. In: *The Testis,* Vol. IV, edited by A. D. Johnson and W. R. Gomes, pp. 371–399. Academic Press, New York.
116. Steinberger, A., and Steinberger, E. (1976): Secretion of an FSH-inhibiting factor by cultured Sertoli cells. *Endocrinology,* 99:918–921.
117. Steinberger, E., and Steinberger, A. (1974): Hormonal control of testicular function in mammals. In: *Handbook of Physiology,* Section 7: Endocrinology. The Pituitary Gland and its Neuroendocrine Control, Vol. IV, Part 2, pp. 325–345. Williams & Wilkins, Baltimore.
118. Thanki, K. H., and Steinberger, A. (1978): Effect of age and hypophysectomy on FSH binding by rat testes. *Andrologia,* 10;195–202.
119. Tindall, D. J., and Means, A. R. (1976): Concerning the hormonal regulation of androgen binding protein in rat testis. *Endocrinology,* 99:809–818.
120. Tindall, D. J., Mena, C. R., and Means, A. R. (1978): Hormonal regulation of androgen binding protein in hypophysectomized rats. *Endocrinology,* 103:589–594.
121. Tindall, D. J., Schrader, W. T., and Means, A. R. (1974): The production of androgen binding protein by Sertoli cells. In: *Hormone Binding and Target Cell Activation in the Testis,* edited by M. L. Dufau and A. R. Means, pp. 167–175. Plenum Press, New York.
122. Toyama, Y. (1976): Actin-like filaments in the Sertoli cell junctional specializations in the swine and mouse testis. *Anat. Rec.,* 186:477–492.
123. Tres, L. L., and Kierszenbaum, A. L. (1975): Transcription during mammalian spermatogenesis with special reference to Sertoli cells. In: *Hormonal Regulation of Spermatogenesis,* edited by F. S. French, V. Hansson, E. M. Ritzén, and S. N. Nayfeh, pp. 455–478. Plenum Press, New York.
124. Troen, P. (1978): Discussion remark. In: *Endocrine Approach to Male Contraception,* edited by V. Hansson, E. M. Ritzén, K. Purvis, and F. S. French, pp. 432–433. Scriptor, Copenhagen.
125. Tsai, Y.-K., Sanborn, B. M., Steinberger, A., and Steinberger, E. (1977): The interaction of testicular androgen-receptor complex with rat germ cell and Sertoli cell chromatin. *Biochem. Biophys. Res. Commun.,* 75:366–372.
126. Vitale, R., Fawcett, D. W., and Dym, M. (1973): The normal development of the blood-

testis barrier and the effects of clomiphene and estrogen treatment. *Anat. Rec.,* 176:333–344.
127. Wachtel, S. S., Koo, G. C., and Ohno, S. (1977): H-Y antigen and male development. In: *The Testis in Normal and Infertile Men,* edited by P. Troen and H. R. Nankin, pp. 35–43. Raven Press, New York.
128. Waites, G. M. H. (1977): Fluid secretion. In: *The Testis,* Vol. IV, edited by A. D. Johnson and W. R. Gomes, pp. 91–123. Academic Press, New York.
129. Walsh, E. L., Cuyler, W. K., and McCullagh, D. R. (1934): Physiologic maintenance of male sex glands: Effect of androtin on hypophysectomized rats. *Am. J. Physiol.,* 107:508–512.
130. Wartenberg, H. (1978): Human testicular development and the role of the mesonephros in the origin of a dual Sertoli cell system. *Andrologia,* 10:1–21.
131. Weddington, S. C., Brandtzaeg, P., Sletten, K., Christensen, T., Hansson, V., French, F. S., Petrusz, P., Nayfeh, S. N., and Ritzén, E. M. (1975): Purification and characterization of rabbit testicular androgen binding protein (ABP). In: *Hormonal Regulation of Spermatogenesis,* edited by F. S. French, V. Hansson, E. M. Ritzén, and S. N. Nayfeh, pp. 433–451. Plenum Press, New York.
132. Weddington, S. C., McLean, W. S., Nayfeh, S. N., French, F. S., Hansson, V., and Ritzén, E. M. (1974): Androgen binding protein (ABP) in rabbit testis and epididymis. *Steroids,* 24:123–134.
133. Welsh, M. J., and Wiebe, J. P. (1976): Sertoli cells from immature rats: In vitro stimulation of steroid metabolism by FSH. *Biochem. Biophys. Res. Commun.,* 69:936–941.
134. Witschi, E. (1970): Embryology of the testis. In: *The Human Testis,* Vol. 10, edited by E. Rosenberg and C. A. Paulsen, pp. 3–10. Plenum Press, New York.

The Testis, edited by H. Burger and D. de Kretser.
Raven Press, New York © 1981.

9

Mechanism of Action of Gonadotrophins on the Testis

G. P. Risbridger, Y. M. Hodgson, and D. M. de Kretser

Department of Anatomy, Monash University, Melbourne, Victoria 3168, Australia

Although it was well known for many years that the gonadotrophic hormones follicle-stimulating hormone (FSH) and luteinizing hormone (LH) stimulated testicular function, it is only over the last decade that their basic mechanism of action has been unravelled. This was greatly facilitated by the advances made in the isolation and purification of the gonadotrophins and the techniques necessary to iodinate these hormones without grossly disturbing their biological activity (71). The availability of radioactively labelled gonadotrophins led to the identification of LH receptor sites on Leydig cells (32), and those for FSH on seminiferous tubules (66). More recently, evidence has accumulated to indicate a role for prolactin in gonadal function and this chapter will review briefly the action of these three gonadotrophic hormones on the testes.

ACTION OF LUTEINIZING HORMONE

Since the structure of human chorionic gonadotrophin (hCG) closely resembles that of LH, a considerable number of studies have utilized hCG instead of LH, since it is more readily available (4). However, caution should be exercised in the interpretation of the *in vivo* studies since the half-life of hCG is much greater than LH, allowing a more prolonged period of stimulation of target tissues (77,85).

Visualization of LH receptors employing autoradiography after *in vivo* (31) or *in vitro* exposure to iodinated hCG was followed by further biochemical evidence that the Leydig cells of the rat testes contained high-affinity (K_a 4 × 10^{10} M^{-1}) and low-capacity receptors for LH (14). More recently these observations have been extended to the human testis (58) and to those of subhuman primates (28). Using membrane fractions of purified Leydig cells, Mendelson et al. (69) confirmed the presence of membrane-associated LH receptors and subsequent studies have confirmed the concept that the interaction of LH with its receptors led to activation of the membrane-linked adenylate cyclase system leading to cyclic AMP formation (17). These observations explained the earlier findings of Sandler and Hall (86) that exogenously administered cyclic AMP could stimulate testosterone production by the testes. More recent data have shown that cyclic AMP could stimulate testosterone production by decapsulated testes (36) and that LH stimulated the activity of adenyl cyclase in Leydig cells (25). Furthermore, Catt and Dufau (16) presented evidence that occupation of only a small proportion of the LH receptors was necessary to stimulate testosterone production, thereby introducing the concept of spare receptors.

Despite these findings, the changes in endogenous levels of cyclic AMP in the testis did not completely support the proposal that cyclic AMP mediated the effects of LH on steroidogenesis. The results of the initial studies *(in vitro)* failed to demonstrate an increase in adenylate cyclase activity (i.e., an accumulation or a rise in the intracellular levels of cyclic AMP), in response to low doses of gonadotrophin, despite a stimulation of testosterone synthesis. Only at higher concentrations of hCG was a marked elevation of cyclic AMP observed with the associated induction of testosterone synthesis (69). The absence of evidence for a coupling of cyclic AMP formation and testosterone release at low concentrations of gonadotrophin stimulation raised the possibility that other membrane-associated responses could operate during the initial sequence of events of LH action. Dufau et al. (37) resolved this question in an elegant study based on the measurement of free and occupied cyclic AMP binding sites of the regulatory component of protein kinase. Their results provided the direct evidence for the intermediate role of cyclic AMP and protein kinase during the stimulation of steroidogenesis by low doses of gonadotrophin.

The subsequent mode of action of cyclic AMP as a mediator of steroidogenesis appears to involve the activation and dissociation of protein kinase. The Leydig cells of the rat testis have been shown to contain two forms of cyclic AMP-dependent protein kinase. The major protein kinase is a 6.2S form located in the cytosol and composed of two subunits when present in the inactive form— the regulatory and the catalytic subunits (27). Cyclic AMP binds to the regulatory subunit of protein kinase (78), causing a dissociation of the inactive complex and the activation of the enzyme by releasing the catalytic subunit (17).

The active catalytic subunit of protein kinase then initiates the phosphorylation of proteins that are believed to regulate the early steps in steroidogenesis (26), although the exact details of the events following the activation of protein kinase are not known. Nuclear events could be involved as LH stimulates the incorporation of labelled amino acids into specific proteins, and it appears that the continuous synthesis of a protein(s) with a short half-life is necessary for the action of LH (98). During the acute phase of protein hormone action, increased steroidogenesis is achieved through the phosphorylation and activation or modification of existing gene products. In contrast, the chronic actions of protein hormones appear to involve changes in nuclear activity and protein synthesis (17).

The fate of the hormone receptor complex itself has aroused interest in recent years. de Kretser, Catt, and Paulsen (32) reported the *in vitro* binding of ^{125}I-hLH to the cytoplasm of the interstitial cells and there is increasing evidence that the hormone receptor complexes are internalized, probably by the process of endocytosis (3). The role of hormone internalization is not clear and may indicate the hormone can act directly at intracellular sites, or it may represent a mechanism whereby the hormone-receptor complex is degraded. Huhtaniemi et al. (59) and Rajaniemi et al. (80) have demonstrated that hCG undergoes catabolic modifications leading to the cleavage of peptide fragments identical to hormone subunits and subsequent hydrolysis to amino acids. Therefore it is tempting to speculate that the removal of the receptor bound hormone from target cells proceeds by the internalization and subsequent degradation of the hormone-receptor complexes.

It is also likely that the process of internalization of the hormone-receptor complex is involved in the loss of LH receptors induced by the injection of high doses of hCG (38). It is well established that a marked loss of LH receptors follows a single injection of a large dose of hCG (88), ovine LH (56), and of luteinizing hormone-releasing hormone (LH-RH), the latter presumably by increasing endogenous LH levels (18). The loss of receptors is dose-dependent and reaches a nadir 24 hr after the injection, the receptor numbers gradually returning to normal after 6 to 7 days in adult (56) or immature rats (88). Similar losses of LH receptors have been shown to occur in the human testes after the injection of hCG (90).

Accompanying the loss of LH receptors, it was noted that the testis was refractory to further stimulation by hCG whether administered *in vitro* or *in vivo* (51,88). During this period of refractoriness or desensitization after an hCG injection, Hseuh et al. (57) demonstrated that further stimulation with hCG resulted in a poor cyclic AMP and testosterone response. Furthermore, they noted a return in responsivity during the gradual return of receptor numbers. However, the loss of receptors is not causally related to the refractoriness, since Haour and Saez (52) have shown that the receptor loss following hCG administration can be blocked by cycloheximide treatment, which did not alter the period of refractoriness to further hCG stimulation.

Further studies have shown that the failure of the testes to respond to restimulation is not determined by the poor rise in cyclic AMP, since no testosterone response could be elicited by exogenous dibutryl cyclic AMP or choleragen (95). The block in the response to hCG therefore must be located beyond cyclic AMP and more recent studies have demonstrated two lesions in the steroidogenic pathway (29). After very large doses of hCG given intravenously the *in vitro* response of pregnenolone to further hCG stimulation was completely abolished, indicating a loss of the processes necessary to maintain the cholesterol side chain cleavage system (95). With more moderate doses of hCG, the lesion induced in androgen biosynthesis occurred at the 17–20 lyase step, leading to the accumulation of progesterone, 17α-hydroxyprogesterone, pregnenolone, and 17α-hydroxypregnenolone (23). Dufau et al. (40) point out that the lesions observed in rats treated with intravenous hCG or LH-RH are similar to the enzyme inhibition produced in rodents by the direct effects of estrogens, which suppress the activity of 17α-hydroxylase and 17–20 lyase (38,97).

It is possible that local estrogen production in the testis is acutely increased by the injection of hCG or LH-RH, and therefore estrogen could play an important role in the regulation of 17–20 lyase and 17α-hydroxylase activities in the testis. Further support for this theory was suggested by the observation that testicular estradiol levels were acutely elevated 30 min after intravenous hCG, and by the ability of Tamoxifen (an estrogen antagonist) to prevent the refractoriness to hCG stimulation of the testes after an intravenous hCG injection (39).

More recent studies have followed the plasma response to hCG stimulation and add further to the complexity of the action of this hormone. In keeping with the results of *in vitro* stimulation, an acute rise in plasma testosterone occurs 2 hr after hCG in both the rat and in man (51,85), the magnitude being dependent on the magnitude of the dose of hCG used (77). At high doses (Fig. 1) the levels of testosterone decrease from the acute peak but remain significantly elevated at 24 hr rising to a second peak 48 to 72 hr after the initial injection. The magnitude of the response is again dose-dependent and after single injections of 6,000 IU hCG, testosterone levels in plasma are elevated

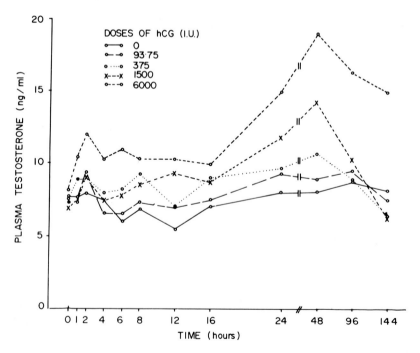

FIG. 1. The response of testosterone in normal men to increasing doses of hCG administered by intramuscular injection. Note the prolonged biphasic response. (From ref. 77, with permission.)

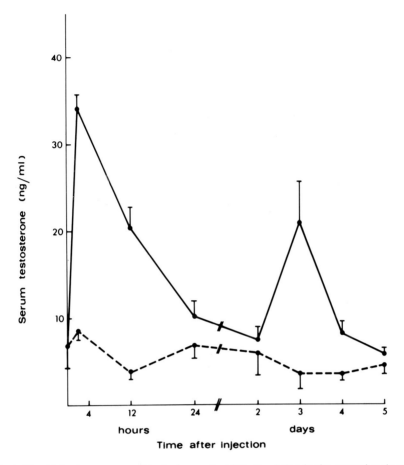

FIG. 2. The biphasic response of testosterone to hCG stimulation in the normal male rat is illustrated.

up to 7 days after the initial injection. Similar findings are seen in the rat (Fig. 2), in which the secondary response peaks 48 to 72 hr after the initial injection of hCG (51). Paradoxically, the second peak occurs at a time when refractoriness to further hCG stimulation is noted and when the hCG-induced steroidogenic lesions are supposedly operative. It is possible that the nadir between the initial and secondary responses represents the expression of these steroidogenic lesions and that the persistence of elevated plasma hCG levels (Fig. 3) enables a restimulation of the testis as it emerges from these steroid blockades (15,77). Measurement of plasma estradiol in men stimulated by large doses of hCG demonstrates peak levels at 24 hr after the injection (Fig. 4), corresponding to the nadir between the two testosterone responses (45,77). This rise in estradiol adds further evidence to the concept that an increase in testicular

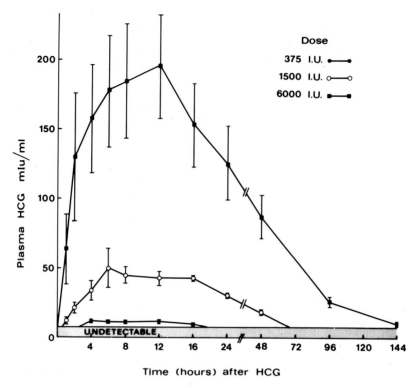

FIG. 3. The hCG levels in serum following graded doses of hCG are shown indicating the presence of detectable levels, up to 120 hr after the initial injection. (From ref. 77, with permission.)

estradiol levels after hCG administration may be the factor causing testicular refractoriness to further stimulation.

The ability of LH/hCG to regulate its own receptor has also been demonstrated in ovarian luteal tissues (24), but the exact physiological significance of this finding remains unclear. Tata (93) originally suggested that the ability of a hormone to regulate its own hormone receptor would provide a rapid means of regulating end organ sensitivity to the hormone. In the testis, the Leydig cell is known to possess approximately 15,000 LH receptors and occupancy of less than 1% of these was sufficient to evoke a maximum steroidogenic response *in vitro*. These latter observations led to the concept of "spare receptors" (16), although it is likely that rather than being redundant, these excess receptors enhance the sensitivity of the target cell to low concentrations of circulating hormone by increasing the probability that enough receptors will be occupied to initiate a steroidogenic response.

Some additional evidence in support of this concept can be obtained from the studies of LH receptors after testicular damage, since it has been demon-

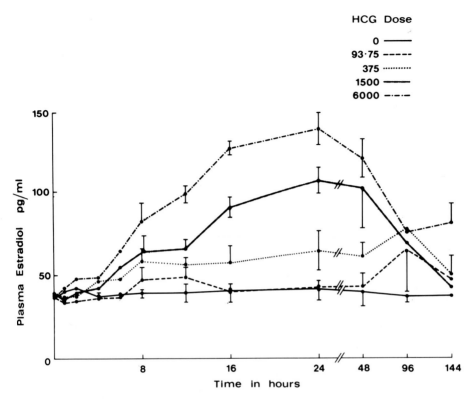

FIG. 4. Plasma estradiol levels rise in a dose-dependent pattern following single injections of hCG, peaking approximately 24 hr after administration. (From ref. 77, with permission.)

strated that a 50 to 60% loss of hCG binding occurs after spermatogenic damage induced by surgically induced cryptorchidism (33), fetal testicular irradiation (82), or efferent duct ligation (83). This loss of LH receptors is associated with a loss of sensitivity to hCG stimulation (Fig. 5), despite a large increase in the capacity of the testis to secrete testosterone *in vitro* (82) resulting from the hypertrophy of the Leydig cells that accompanies testicular damage (81).

The effects of chronic LH/hCG treatment have by comparison received little interest. Prolonged treatment with high doses of hCG results in changes in the fine structure of the interstitial cells of the testis (30,70). In both man and the guinea pig, the administration of hCG caused proliferation of the Leydig cells and an increase in the smooth endoplasmic reticulum and mitochondria and Golgi complexes. The striking increase in the volume of Leydig cell clusters during chronic stimulation with LH or hCG was previously documented and was generally assumed to result from an increase in the number and size of the Leydig cells (20,21). In the adult rat testis, Schoen (87) reported that the number of Leydig cells doubled after 2 weeks of daily hCG treatment (100

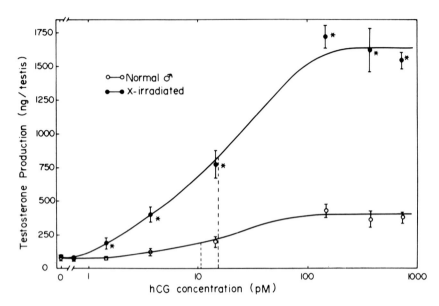

FIG. 5. The *in vitro* response of testosterone to hCG stimulation from normal rats and those with germ cell aplasia induced by fetal irradiation is shown. Note the increased capacity of the damaged testes for testosterone production. (From ref. 82, with permission.)

IU per day). Using morphometric methods, these results were confirmed by Christensen and Peacock (22), who concluded that an excess of hCG increased the number and size of the Leydig cells although the hyperplasia was more important than hypertrophy in the expansion of Leydig cell clusters.

In the human testis, however, Heller and Leach (53) reported that the administration of 4,000 IU of hCG two or three times a week for 6 to 16 weeks increased the size of the Leydig cells but did not produce any consistent increase in cell number. Similar findings were recorded by Neaves (73), who studied the striking change in the Leydig cell cluster over the seasonal cycle of the rock hyrax. He reported that the number of Leydig cells did not increase, although the size of the Leydig cell cluster increased by a factor of 2.5 as the animals came into the breeding season. It is not clear whether the conclusions presented in these studies differ from those in the rat because of species variation, the level of circulating hormone, or the methodology.

There is biochemical evidence that the Leydig cells of the human and the rat still respond to chronically elevated levels of hCG by an increase in testosterone production (30,31). Van der Vusse, Kalman, and van der Molen (99) have demonstrated that the production of testosterone by testicular homogenates *in vitro* is increased, and the activity of the enzyme 3β-hydroxysteroid dehydrogenase is enhanced. More recently van Nimmen et al. (100) have reported a drastic change in the pattern of metabolism of testicular steroids after prolonged hCG treatment, so that there is a depression of the normally active 7α-hydroxylation processes and an increase in the 5α-reduced metabolites.

Despite the acute regulatory effects of high doses of hCG that result in the autoregulation of testicular LH/hCG receptors and induce a period of refractoriness to further gonadotrophin stimulation, prolonged treatment with LH/hCG nevertheless causes hypertrophy of the Leydig cells and stimulates testosterone production. However, there are no data to indicate the role of the acute regulatory effects of hCG in situations where the trophic hormone is administered over long intervals of time and how these effects are balanced by the hypertrophy of existing Leydig cells and the recruitment of immature cells into the response.

FOLLICLE-STIMULATING HORMONE

The seminiferous epithelium is the primary site of action of FSH (66). From the autoradiographic studies of Orth and Christensen (75,76) the precise location of the FSH binding sites was shown to be on the spermatogonial cell membrane and the basal aspect of the Sertoli cell. Furthermore, the density of the FSH receptors was quite similar on the two cell types. Abou-Issa and Reichert (1) have previously described two classes of membrane-bound FSH receptors, but it is not clear at the present time whether the two classes are located on both cells or one type of site is specific to one type of cell.

The biochemical events that occur in response to the initial binding of FSH to the receptor are very similar to those described for LH (65,68). Again, the intracellular messenger is cyclic AMP and adenyl cyclase activity is stimulated when seminiferous tubule tissue is incubated with FSH *in vitro* (34).

The binding of FSH to receptors located on the plasma membrane of Sertoli cells results in the activation of adenyl cyclase and a decrease in the activity of cyclic AMP phosphodiesterase (42). The resultant elevation of intracellular cyclic AMP in turn activates cyclic AMP-dependent protein kinase (43). Rates of RNA and protein synthesis are elevated (68) and a number of specific proteins have been noted to be stimulated by FSH. They include the secretory protein androgen binding protein (ABP) as well as two intracellular proteins, protein kinase inhibitor (11) and γ-glutamyl transpeptidase (54). However, all of these effects have been demonstrated in immature testes and little if any effect on these parameters has been shown in adult testes (see chapter by Ritzén et al., *this volume*). Many of the effects of FSH are expressed through the receptors present on the Sertoli cell and the resultant changes in the function of isolated Sertoli cells are expressed as increases in mitotic activity (47), plasminogen activator (62), estradiol (35), and metabolites of androstenedione (101,102). Details of these actions on the Sertoli cell are considered more fully in Chapter 9.

The precise function of FSH in the process of spermatogenesis remains uncertain. Though it is generally accepted that the initiation of spermatogenic function requires FSH, Steinberger (92) has proposed that in the rat, only testosterone is required to maintain spermatogenesis. However, in man evidence exists to indicate that FSH may be important in the maintenance of spermatogenesis and this subject is considered more extensively in Chapter 6. It is clear that FSH cannot increase the rate of spermatogenesis and Means and Huckins (67) have proposed that the germ cell stimulation occurs at the spermatogonial level in keeping with the demonstration of FSH receptors on those cells (76). Their data suggest that FSH decreased the degeneration of spermatogonia as they commence the spermatogenic process and may thereby cause an increased sperm output.

Johnson and Ewing (60) demonstrated that FSH significantly increased the testosterone secretion by perfused rabbit testes exposed to LH, which suggested that FSH played an indirect role in the process of steroidogenesis. From other studies (41,63), it appeared that FSH could augment the action of LH on plasma testosterone levels. More recently attention has focused on the way in which FSH may affect LH action during puberty in the male rat. Odell and co-workers (74) had offered the hypothesis that one factor in sexual maturation was the FSH induction of testicular sensitivity to LH. In a comprehensive study, Ketel-slegers et al. (61) recorded the changes in the number of testicular LH and FSH receptors during sexual maturation and related them to circulating levels of gonadotrophins and testosterone. Their data showed that the sharp rise in plasma FSH levels was coincident with the development of testicular LH receptors and was followed by a rise in plasma testosterone. These temporal relationships are therefore consistent with the view that FSH initiates the increase in LH receptors and induced testicular sensitivity to LH in the immature rat and thus FSH may play a prominent role in steroidogenesis during puberty.

As in the case of other protein hormones, FSH also has the ability to regulate the number of its own receptors; Gnanaprakasam et al. (46) recently demonstrated the loss of FSH receptors in testicular tissue following a large injection of FSH. However, extensive studies of this phenomenon and the resultant effects on target tissues are not available. It is to be noted that as in the case of LH receptors, testicular damage results in a loss of FSH binding as shown by the studies of Hagenas et al. (49). This phenomenon is not the result of the elevated levels of FSH but probably due to local factors, since the abdominal testis following unilateral cryptorchidism shows the loss in FSH binding but this finding is not seen in the scrotal testis of the same rats (84).

PROLACTIN

Autoradiographic studies both *in vivo* and *in vitro* have demonstrated the presence of prolactin (PRL) binding to the prostate and the testis (27,79). These findings were confirmed by the *in vitro* binding of labeled PRL to subcellular fractions of testicular tissue, where it appeared that prolactin bound primarily to the Leydig cells (2,19). Recently immunohistochemical evidence has demonstrated that PRL binds to intracellular sites in the ventral prostate gland (103), but a similar phenomenon has not yet been reported in Leydig cells.

Despite the demonstration of specific testicular receptors for PRL, the mode of action of this hormone in maintaining gonadal function is not clearly understood. Three animal models have been used to elucidate the role of PRL: (a) hamsters with testicular regression induced by short photoperiod; (b) hereditary dwarf mice; (c) hypophysectomized rats. In all three models there is a deficiency in plasma gonadotrophins (10,96), prolactin (6), and testosterone (9), and testicular atrophy occurs (5,55). More recently it was demonstrated that these changes are also accompanied by a loss of LH binding to the testicular tissue (12,13).

The effects of PRL treatment on testicular function in the hamster are to stimulate testicular growth and restore plasma testosterone levels and LH receptor numbers (9,12). The administration of PRL to dwarf mice stimulates spermatogenesis (8), enhances the testicular response to hCG stimulation *in vitro* (10), and increases testicular LH binding (13). Similarly in the hypophysectomized rat treated with PRL, in the presence of LH, spermatogenesis is stimulated (104), plasma testosterone levels are restored, and the incorporation of labeled acetate into testosterone is promoted (48). PRL also increased testicular LH binding in hypophysectomized rats (105). Furthermore, McNeilly et al. (64) showed that in rats bearing pituitary grafts under the kidney capsule the elevated prolactin levels stimulated increased testicular LH receptors in the hypophysectomized animals.

Collectively these results suggest that PRL may act on the testis by augmenting the effect of LH on testicular function. For example, PRL may act directly on the Leydig cells to increase the ability of this tissue to bind LH and hence respond to gonadotrophin stimulation. There is also evidence that PRL increases the gonadal stores of cholesterol esters (7) and, in this manner, may augment the steroidogenic response to LH.

Recent observations have documented an antigonadal action of PRL, since hyperprolactinemia induced hypogonadism in men (94). Hyperprolactinemia interferes with gonadal function, and Fang et al. (44) observed testicular atrophy in rats bearing prolactin secreting tumours. In these animals, testosterone levels were significantly depressed whereas serum LH levels were elevated, and the authors suggested that the excessive prolactin was responsible for the observed hypogonadism.

In concluding this section of the action of gonadotrophins on the testis, it is noteworthy that although the mode of action of LH has been studied more fully than that of other gonadotrophins, there are still many aspects of LH action that remain unknown. Extensive biochemical investigations in the last 5 years have focused on the phenomenon of hormone-receptor regulation, and the associated changes in steroidogenesis. Only recently have investigations considered fundamental questions such as how LH or hCG reaches the Leydig cells from the blood stream, and how LH acts to increase the activity of the rate-limiting step in steroidogenesis.

In order to answer these and similar questions, we need to combine our knowledge of the biochemical effects of LH on the Leydig cells with the structural organization of Leydig cells themselves and their relationship with the other components of the testis. For example, Sharpe (89) had demonstrated that an hCG-induced accumulation of interstitial fluid precedes the negative effects of hCG on Leydig cell function by increasing the transport of hCG to the Leydig cells; he therefore suggests that interstitial fluid may play an important role in the normal transport of LH to the Leydig cells. Furthermore, the sensitivity of isolated Leydig cells to hCG differed significantly from that of decapsulated testis preparations (91). Hall et al. (50) have considered the way in which LH may increase the transport of cholesterol to the side-chain cleavage enzyme in the mitochondria. Previous evidence from studies on the adrenal gland have suggested that the intracellular transport of cholesterol involves the contractile activity of the microfilaments and that this process is accelerated by ACTH (72). The more recent studies of Hall et al. (50) on the steroidogenic response of Leydig cells to LH have suggested that LH and cyclic AMP stimulate side-chain cleavage of cholesterol and therefore steroidogenesis by a mechanism involving actin, presumably in microfilaments. The responding microfilaments may then promote transport of cholesterol to mitochondria.

Therefore, it may be important to remind ourselves of the structural and functional organization of various components of the testis while interpreting data concerned with discrete steps in the action of gonadotrophins on the testis.

REFERENCES

1. Abou-Issa, H., and Reichert, L. (1976): Properties of follitropin-receptor interaction. *J. Biol. Chem.,* 521:3326–3337.
2. Aragona, C., and Freisen, H. G. (1975): Specific prolactin binding sites in the prostate and testis of rats. *Endocrinology,* 97:677–684.
3. Ascoli, M., and Puett, D. (1978): Degradation of receptor-bound human chorio-gonadotropin by murine Leydig tumor cells. *J. Biol. Chem.,* 253:4892–4899.
4. Bahl, O. P. (1977): Human chorionic gonadotropin, its receptor and mechanism of action. *Fed. Proc.,* 36:2119–2127.
5. Bartke, A. (1964): Histology of the anterior hypophysis, thyroid and gonads of two types of dwarf mice. *Anat. Rec.,* 149:225–236.
6. Bartke, A. (1966): Influence of prolactin on male fertility in dwarf mice. *J. Endocrinol.,* 35:419–420.
7. Bartke, A. (1971): Effects of prolactin and luteinizing hormone on the cholesterol stores in the mouse testis. *J. Endocrinol.,* 49:317–324.
8. Bartke, A., and Lloyd, C. W. (1970): Influence of prolactin and pituitary isografts on spermatogenesis in dwarf mice and hypophysectomized rats. *J. Endocrinol.,* 46:321–329.
9. Bartke, A., Croft, B. T., and Dalterio, S. (1975): Prolactin restores plasma testosterone levels and stimulates testicular growth in hamsters exposed to short day lengths. *Endocrinology,* 97:1601–1604.
10. Bartke, A., Goldman, B. D., Bex, F., and Dalterio, S. (1977): Effects of prolactin (Prl) on pituitary and testicular function in mice with hereditary Prl deficiency. *Endocrinology,* 101:1760–1766.
11. Beale, E. G., Dedman, J. R., and Means, A. R. (1977): Isolation and regulation of the protein kinase inhibitor and the calcium-dependent cyclic nucleotide phosphodiesterase regulator in the Sertoli cell-enriched testis. *Endocrinology,* 101:1621–1634.
12. Bex, F., Bartke, A., Goldman, B. D., and Dalterio, S. (1978): Prolactin, growth hormone, luteinizing hormone receptors and seasonal changes in testicular activity in the golden hamster. *Endocrinology,* 103:2069–2080.

13. Bohnet, H. G., and Freisen, H. G. (1976): Effect of prolactin and growth hormone on prolactin and LH receptors in the dwarf mouse. *J. Reprod. Fert.,* 48:307–311.
14. Catt, K. J., Dufau, M. L., and Tsuruhara, T. (1971): Studies on a radioligand-receptor assay system for LH and chorionic gonadotropin. *J. Clin. Endocrinol. Metab.,* 32:860–863.
15. Catt, K. J., and Dufau, M. L. (1973): Interactions of LH and HCG with testicular gonadotropin receptors. *Adv. Exp. Med. Biol.,* 36:379–418.
16. Catt, K. J., and Dufau, M. L. (1973): Spare gonadotrophin receptors in rat testis. *Nature New. Biol.,* 244:219–221.
17. Catt, K. J., and Dufau, M. L. (1976): Basic concepts of the mechanism of action of peptide hormones. *Biol. Reprod.,* 14:1–15.
18. Catt, K. J., Baukal, A. J., Davies, T. F., and Dufau, M. L. (1979): Luteinizing hormone releasing hormone-induced regulation of gonadotropin and prolactin receptors in the rat testis. *Endocrinology,* 104:17–25.
19. Charreau, E. H., Attramadal, A., Torjesen, P. A., Purvis, K., Calandra, R., and Hansson, V. (1977): Prolactin binding in rat testis: Specific receptors in interstitial cells. *Mol. Cell. Endocrinol.,* 6:303–307.
20. Chemes, H. E., Rivarola, M. A., and Bergada, C. (1976): Effect of HCG on the interstitial cells and androgen production in the immature rat testis. *J. Reprod. Fert.,* 46:279–282.
21. Christensen, A. K. (1975): Leydig cells. In: *Handbook of Physiology, Sec. 7, Vol. 5,* edited by R. O. Greep and E. B. Astwood, pp. 57–94. Williams & Wilkins, Baltimore.
22. Christensen, A. K., and Peacock, K. C. (1980): Increase in Leydig cell number in testes of adult rats treated chronically with an excess of human chorionic gonadotropin. *Biol. Reprod.,* 22:383–391.
23. Cigorraga, S. B., Dufau, M. L., and Catt, K. J. (1978): Regulation of luteinizing hormone receptors and steroidogenesis in gonadotropin-desensitized Leydig cells. *J. Biol. Chem.,* 253:4297–4304.
24. Conti, M., Harwood, J. P., Dufau, M. L., and Catt, K. J. (1977): Effect of gonadotropin-induced receptor regulation in biological responses of isolated rat luteal cells. *J. Biol. Chem.,* 252:8869–8874.
25. Cooke, B. A., Van Beurden, W. M. O., Rommerts, F. F. G., and Van der Molen, H. J. (1972): Effects of trophic hormones on 3'5' cyclic AMP levels in rat testis interstitial tissue and seminiferous tubules. *FEBS Lett.,* 25:83–86.
26. Cooke, B. A., Lindh, M. L., and Janszen, F. H. A. (1976): Correlation of protein kinase activation and testosterone production after stimulation of Leydig cells with luteinizing hormone. *Biochem. J.,* 160:439–446.
27. Costlow, M. E., and McGuire, W. L. (1977): Autoradiographic localization of the binding of ^{125}I-labelled prolactin to rat tissues *in vitro. J. Endocrinol.,* 75:221–226.
28. Davies, T. F., Walsh, P. C., Hodgen, G. D., Dufau, M. L., and Catt, K. J. (1979): Characterization of primate luteinizing hormone receptor in testis homogenates and Leydig cells. *J. Clin. Endocrinol. Metab.,* 48:680–685.
29. De Jong, F. H., Hey, A. H., and Van der Molen, H. J. (1974): Oestradiol 17-β and testosterone in rat testis tissue: Effect of gonadotrophins, localization and production *in vitro. J. Endocrinol.,* 60:409–419.
30. de Kretser, D. M. (1967): Changes in the fine structure of the human testicular interstitial cells after treatment with human gonadotrophins. *Z. Zellforsch.,* 83:344–358.
31. de Kretser, D. M., Catt, K. J., Burger, H. G., and Smith, G. C. (1969): Radioautographic studies on the localization of ^{125}I-labelled human luteinizing and growth hormone in immature male rats. *J. Endocrinol.,* 43:105–111.
32. de Kretser, D. M., Catt, K. J., and Paulsen, C. A. (1971): Studies on the *in vitro* testicular binding of iodinated luteinizing hormone in rats. *Endocrinology,* 88:332–337.
33. de Kretser, D. M., Sharpe, R. M., and Swanston, I. A. (1979): Alterations in steroidogenesis and human chorionic gonadotropin binding in the cryptorchid rat testis. *Endocrinology,* 105:135–138.
34. Dorrington, J. H., Vernon, R. G., and Fritz, I. B. (1972): The effect of gonadotropins on the 3'5'-cyclic AMP levels of seminiferous tubules. *Biochem. Biophys. Res. Commun.,* 46:1523–1528.
35. Dorrington, J. H., and Armstrong, D. T. (1974): FSH stimulates estradiol-17β synthesis in cultured Sertoli cells. *Proc. Natl. Acad. Sci. USA,* 72:2677–2681.
36. Dufau, M. L., Catt, K. J., and Tsuruhara, T. (1971): Gonadotrophin stimulation of testosterone production by the rat testis *in vitro. Biochim. Biophys. Acta,* 252:574–579.

37. Dufau, M. L., Tsuruhara, T., Horner, K. A., Podesta, E., and Catt, K. J. (1977): Intermediate role of adenosine 3′5′-cyclic monophosphate and protein kinase during gonadotrophin-induced steroidogenesis in testicular interstitial cells. *Proc. Natl. Acad. Sci. USA,* 74:3419–3423.

38. Dufau, M. L., Hsueh, A. J., Cigorraga, S., Baukal, A. J. and Catt, K. J. (1978): Inhibition of Leydig cell function through hormonal regulatory mechanisms. *Int. J. Androl. (Suppl. 2),* 193–239.

39. Dufau, M. L., Cigorraga, S. B., Baukal, A. J., Bator, J. M., Sorrell, S. H., Neubauer, J. F., and Catt, K. J. (1979*a*): Steroid biosynthetic lesions in gonadotropin-desensitized Leydig cells. *J. Steroid Biochem.,* 11:193–199.

40. Dufau, M. L., Cigorraga, S. B., Baukal, A. J., Sorrell, S. H., Bator, J. M., Neubauer, J. F., and Catt, K. J. (1979*b*): Androgen biosynthesis in Leydig cells after testicular desensitization by luteinizing hormone-releasing hormone and human chorionic gonadotropin. *Endocrinology,* 105:1314–1321.

41. El Safoury, S., and Bartke, A. (1974): Effects of FSH and LH on plasma testosterone levels in hypophysectomized and intact immature and adult male rats. *J. Endocrinol.,* 61:193–198.

42. Fakunding, J. L., Tindall, D. J., Dedman, J. R., Mena, C., and Means, A. R. (1976): Biochemical actions of FSH in the Sertoli cell of the rat testis. *Endocrinology,* 98:392–402.

43. Fakunding, J. L., and Means, A. R. (1977): Characterization and follicle-stimulating hormone activation of Sertoli cell cyclic AMP-dependent protein kinases. *Endocrinology,* 101:1358–1368.

44. Fang, V. S., Refetoff, S., and Rosenfield, R. L. (1974): Hypogonadism induced by a transplantable, prolactin-producing tumor in male rats: Hormonal and morphological studies. *Endocrinology,* 95:991–998.

45. Forest, M. G., Lecoq, A., and Saez, J. M. (1979): Kinetics of human chorionic gonadotropin-induced steroidogenic response of the human testis. II. Plasma 17α-hydroxyprogesterone, Δ⁴-androstenedione, estrone and 17β-estradiol: Evidence for the action of human chorionic gonadotropin on intermediate enzymes implicated in steroid biosynthesis. *J. Clin. Endocrinol. Metab.,* 49:284–291.

46. Gnanaprakasam, M. S., Chen, C. J. H., Sutherland, J. G., and Bhalla, V. K. (1979): Receptor depletion and replenishment processes: *In vivo* regulation of gonadotropin receptors by luteinizing hormone, follicle-stimulating hormone and ethanol in rat testis. *Biol. Reprod.,* 20:991–1000.

47. Griswold, M. D., Solari, A., Tung, P. S., and Fritz, I. B. (1977): Stimulation by follicle-stimulating hormone of DNA synthesis and of mitosis in cultured Sertoli cells prepared from testes of immature rats. *Mol. Cell. Endocrinol.,* 7:151–165.

48. Hafiez, A. A., Bartke, A., and Lloyd, D. W. (1972): The role of prolactin in the regulation of testis function: The synergistic effects of prolactin and luteinizing hormone on the incorporation of ¹⁴C-acetate into testosterone and cholesterol by testes from hypophysectomized rats *in vitro. J. Endocrinol.,* 63:223–230.

49. Hägenas, L., Ritzen, E. M., Svensson, J., Hansson, V., and Purvis, K. (1978): Temperature dependence of Sertoli cell function. *Int. J. Androl. (Suppl. 2),* 2:449–456.

50. Hall, P. F., Charponnier, C. Nakamura, M., and Gabbiani, G. (1979): The role of microfilaments in the response of Leydig cells to luteinizing hormone. *J. Steroid Biochem.,* 11:1361–1366.

51. Haour, F., and Saez, J. M. (1977): hCG-dependent regulation of gonadotropin receptor sites: Negative control in testicular Leydig cells. *Mol. Cell. Endocrinol.,* 7:17–24.

52. Haour, F. P., Sanchez, P., Cathiard, A. M., and Saez, J. M. (1978): Gonadotropin receptor regulation in hypophysectomized rat Leydig cells. *Biochem. Biophys. Res. Commun.,* 81:547–551.

53. Heller, C. G., and Leach, D. R. (1971): Quantification of Leydig cells and measurement of Leydig-cell size following administration of human chorionic gonadotrophin to normal men. *J. Reprod. Fert.,* 25:185–192.

54. Hodgen, G. D., and Sherins, R. J. (1973): Enzymes as markers of testicular growth and development in the rat. *Endocrinology,* 93:985–989.

55. Hoffman, R. A., and Reiter, R. J. (1965): Pineal gland: Influence on gonads of male hamsters. *Science,* 148:1609–1610.

56. Hseuh, A. J. W., Dufau, M. L., and Catt, K. J. (1976): Regulation of luteinizing hormone receptors in testicular interstitial cells by gonadotropin. *Biochem. Biophys. Res. Commun.,* 72:1145–1152.

57. Hseuh, A. J. W., Dufau, M. L., and Catt, K. J. (1977): Gonadotropin-induced regulation of

LH receptors and desensitization of testicular 3'5'-cyclic AMP and testosterone responses. *Proc. Natl. Acad. Sci. USA,* 74:592–595.

58. Hsu, A., Stratico, D., and Hosaka, M. (1978): Studies of the human testis: X. Properties of human chorionic gonadotrophin receptor in adult testis and relation to intratesticular testosterone concentration. *J. Clin. Endocrinol. Metab.,* 47:529–536.

59. Huhtaniemi, I., Rajaniemi, H., Martikainen, H., and Tikkala, L. (1978): Autoregulation of LH/HCG receptors and catabolism of HCG in rat testis. *Int. J. Androl. (Suppl. 2),* 1:276–286.

60. Johnson, B. H., and Ewing, L. L. (1971): Follicle-stimulating hormone and the regulation of testosterone secretion in rabbit testes. *Science,* 173:635–637.

61. Ketelslegers, J. M., Hetzel, W. D., Sherins, R. J., and Catt, K. J. (1978): Developmental changes in testicular gonadotropin receptors: Plasma gonadotropins and plasma testosterone in the rat. *Endocrinology,* 103:212–222.

62. Lacroix, M., Smith, F. E., and Fritz, I. B. (1977): Secretion of plasminogen activator by Sertoli cell enriched cultures. *Mol. Cell Endocrinol.,* 9:227–236.

63. Lostroh, A. J. (1969): Regulation by FSH and ICSH (LH) of reproductive function in the immature male rat. *Endocrinology,* 85:438–445.

64. McNeilly, A. S., de Kretser, D. M., and Sharpe, R. M. (1979): Modulation of prolactin, luteinizing hormone (LH) and follicle-stimulating hormone (FSH) secretion by LHRH and bromocriptine (CB154) in the hypophysectomized pituitary-grafted male rat and its effect on testicular LH receptors and testosterone output. *Biol. Reprod.,* 21:141–147.

65. Means, A. R. (1975): Biochemical effects of FSH on the testis. In: *Handbook of Physiology, Sect. 7, Vol. 5,* edited by R. O. Greep and D. W. Hamilton, pp. 203–218. Williams & Wilkins, Baltimore.

66. Means, A. R., and Vaitukaitis, J. (1972): Peptide hormone receptors: Specific binding of ^{3}H-FSH to testis. *Endocrinology,* 90:39–46.

67. Means, A. R., and Huckins, C. (1974): Coupled events in the early biochemical actions of FSH on the Sertoli cell of the testis. In: *Hormone Binding and Target Cell Activation in the Testis,* edited by M. L. Dufau and A. R. Means, pp. 145–165. Plenum Press, New York.

68. Means, A. R., Fakunding, J. L., Huckins, C., Tindall, D. J., and Vitale, R. (1976): Follicle-stimulating hormone, the Sertoli cell and spermatogenesis. *Rec. Prog. Horm. Res.,* 32:477–525.

69. Mendelson, C., Dufau, M. L., and Catt, K. J. (1975): Gonadotropin binding and stimulation of cyclic adenosine 3'5'-monophosphate and testosterone production in isolated Leydig cells. *J. Biol. Chem.,* 250:8818–8823.

70. Merkow, L., Acevedo, H. F., Slifkin, M., and Pardo, M. (1968): Studies on the interstitial cells of the testis. II. The ultrastructure in the adult guinea pig and the effect of stimulation with human chorionic gonadotropin. *Am. J. Pathol.,* 53:989–1007.

71. Miyachi, Y., Vaitukaitis, J. L., Nieschlag, E., and Lipsett, M. B. (1972): Enzymatic radio-iodination of gonadotropins. *J. Clin. Endocrinol. Metab.,* 34:23–28.

72. Mrotek, J., and Hall, P. F. (1975): The influence of cytochalasin B on the response of adrenal tumor cells to ACTH and cyclic AMP. *Biochem. Biophys. Res. Commun.,* 64:891–896.

73. Neaves, W. B. (1973): Changes in testicular Leydig cells and in plasma testosterone levels among seasonally-breeding rock hyrax. *Biol. Reprod.,* 8:451–466.

74. Odell, W. D., Swerdloff, R. S., Jacobs, H. S., and Hescox, M. A. (1973): FSH induction of sensitivity to LH: One cause of sexual maturation in the male rat. *Endocrinology,* 92:160–165.

75. Orth, J., and Christensen, A. K. (1977): Localization of ^{125}I-labelled FSH in the testes of hypophysectomized rats by autoradiography at the light and electron microscope levels. *Endocrinology,* 101:262–278.

76. Orth, J., and Christensen, A. K. (1978): Autoradiographic localization of specifically bound ^{125}I-labelled follicle-stimulating hormone on spermatogonia of the rat testis. *Endocrinology,* 103:1944–1951.

77. Padron, R. S., Wischusen, J., Hudson, B., Burger, H. G., and de Kretser, D. M. (1980): Prolonged biphasic response of plasma testosterone to single intramuscular injections of human chorionic gonadotrophin. *J. Clin. Endocrinol. Metab.,* 50:1100–1104.

78. Podesta, E. J., Dufau, M. L., Solano, A. R., and Catt, K. J. (1978): Hormonal activation of protein kinase in isolated Leydig cells: Electrophoretic analysis of cyclic AMP receptors. *J. Biol. Chem.,* 253:8994–9001.

79. Rajaniemi, H. J. Oksanen, A., and Vanha-Perttula, T. (1974): Distribution of ^{125}I-prolactin in mice and rat. Studies on whole body and microautoradiography. *Horm. Res.,* 5:6–20.
80. Rajaniemi, H. J., Manninen, M., and Huhtaniemi, I. (1979): Catabolism of human (^{125}I)-iodo-chorionic gonadotropin in rat testis. *Endocrinology,* 105:1208–1214.
81. Rich, K. A., Kerr, J. B., and de Kretser, D. M. (1979): Evidence for Leydig cell dysfunction in rats with seminiferous tubule damage. *Mol. Cell. Endocrinol.,* 13:123–135.
82. Rich, K. A., and de Kretser, D. M. (1979): Effect of fetal irradiation on testicular receptors and testosterone response to gonadotrophin stimulation in adult rats. *Int. J. Androl.,* 2:343–352.
83. Risbridger, G. P., Kerr, J. B., and de Kretser, D. M. (1980): An assessment of Leydig cell function after bilateral or unilateral efferent duct ligation: Further evidence for local control of Leydig cell function. *Endocrinology (submitted).*
84. Risbridger, G. P., Kerr, J. B., and de Kretser, D. M. (1980): An evaluation of Leydig cell function and gonadotropin binding in unilateral and bilateral cryptorchidism: Evidence for local control of Leydig cell function by the seminiferous tubule. *Biol. Reprod. (in press).*
85. Saez, J. M., and Forest, M. G. (1979): Kinetics of human chorionic gonadotropin-induced steroidogenic response of the human testis. I. Plasma testosterone: Implications for human chorionic gonadotropin stimulation test. *J. Clin. Endocrinol. Metab.,* 49:278–283.
86. Sandler, R., and Hall, P. F. (1966): Stimulation *in vitro* by adenosine-3'-5'-cyclic monophosphate of steroidogenesis in rat testis. *Endocrinology,* 79:647–649.
87. Schoen, E. J. (1964): Effect of local irradiation on androgen biosynthesis. *Endocrinology,* 75:56–65.
88. Sharpe, R. M. (1976): hCG-induced decrease in availability of rat testis receptors. *Nature,* 264:644–646.
89. Sharpe, R. M. (1980): The temporal relationship between interstitial fluid accumulation and changes in gonadotrophin receptor numbers and steroidogenesis in the rat testes. *Biol. Reprod. (in press).*
90. Sharpe, R. M., Wu, F. C. W., and Hargreave, T. B. (1980): Binding of human chorionic gonadotrophin to testicular biopsy tissue from infertile men and the effect of prior treatment with human chorionic gonadotrophin. *J. Endocrinol. (in press).*
91. Sharpe, R. M., and McNeilly, A. S. (1980): Differences between dispersed Leydig cells and intact testes in their sensitivity to gonadotrophin-stimulation *in vitro* after alteration of LH-receptor numbers. *Mol. Cell. Endocrinol.,* 18:75–86.
92. Steinberger, E. (1971): Hormonal control of mammalian spermatogenesis. *Physiol. Rev.,* 51:1–22.
93. Tata, J. R. (1975): Hormonal regulation of hormone receptors. *Nature,* 257:740–741.
94. Thorner, M. O., Edwards, C. R. W., Hanker, J. P. Abraham, G., and Besser, G. M. (1977): Prolactin and gonadotropin interaction in the male. In: *The Testis in Normal and Infertile Men,* edited by P. Troen and H. R. Nankin, pp. 351–366. Raven Press, New York.
95. Tsuruhara, T., Dufau, M. L., Cigorraga, S., and Catt, K. J. (1977): Hormonal regulation of testicular luteinizing hormone receptors. *J. Biol. Chem.,* 252:9002–9009.
96. Turek, F. W., Elliot, J. A., Alvis, J. D., and Menaker, M. (1975): The interaction of castration and photoperiod in the regulation of hypophyseal and serum gonadotropin levels in the male golden hamster. *Endocrinology,* 96:854–860.
97. Van Beurden, W. M. O., Roodnat, B., and Van der Molen, H. J. (1978): Effect of oestrogen and FSH on LH stimulation of steroid production by testis Leydig cells from immature rats. *Int. J. Androl. (Suppl. 2),* 1:374–382.
98. Van der Molen, H. J., Beurden, W. M. O., Blankenstein, M. A., De Boer, W., Cooke, B. A., Grootgoed, J. A., Janzen, F. H. A., De Jong, F. H., Mulder, E., and Rommerts, G. (1979): The testis: Biochemical action of trophic hormones and steroids on steroid production and spermatogenesis. *J. Steroid Biochem.,* 11:13–18.
99. Van der Vusse, G. J., Kalkman, M. L., and Van der Molen, H. J. (1975): Endogenous steroid production in preparations of rat testis after long-term treatment with HCG. *J. Steroid Biochem.,* 6:357–359.
100. Van Nimmen, D., Eechaute, W., Lacroix, E., Demeester, G., and Leusen, I. (1979): (4-C[14])-testosterone metabolism and steroid production by incubated whole testes, seminiferous tubules and interstitial tissue from rats. *J. Steroid Biochem.,* 10:505–511.
101. Welsh, M. J., and Wiebe, J. P. (1976): Sertoli cells from immature rats: *In vitro* stimulation of steroid metabolism. *Biochem. Biophys. Res. Commun.,* 69:936–941.

102. Welsh, M. J., and Wiebe, J. P. (1978): Sertoli call capacity to metabolize C_{19} steroids: Variation with age and the effect of FSH. *Endocrinology,* 103:838–844.
103. Witorsch, R. J., and Smith, J. P. (1977): Evidence for androgen-dependent intracellular binding in rat ventral prostate gland. *Endocrinology,* 101: 929–938.
104. Woods, M. C., and Simpson, M. E. (1961): Pituitary control of the testis of the hypophysecto-mized rat. *Endocrinology,* 69:91–125.
105. Zipf, W. B., Payne, A. H., and Kelch, R. P. (1978): Prolactin, growth hormone and luteinizing hormone in the maintenance of testicular luteinizing hormone receptors. *Endocrinology,* 103:595–600.

The Testis, edited by H. Burger and D. de Kretser.
Raven Press, New York © 1981.

10

Testicular Steroidogenesis

H. J. van der Molen and F. F. G. Rommerts

*Department of Biochemistry (Division of Chemical Endocrinology), Medical Faculty,
Erasmus University Rotterdam, Rotterdam, The Netherlands*

A discussion of all metabolic reactions and compounds required for testicular steroidogenesis would involve the description of a very large number of steroids and enzymes which have been detected in testis tissue. Several excellent comprehensive reviews offer many details of testicular steroids and steroidogenesis (36,37,40,54,155). In the present chapter we will discuss the main pathways of testicular metabolism of those steroids that have important biological functions. This concerns mainly the steroids and enzyme activities involved in formation and degradation of testicular pregnenolone, testosterone, dihydrotestosterone, and estradiol. Most of the data to be presented have been obtained with testis tissues of rats, but results of other species (mainly man) will be mentioned when the differences may be physiologically important. If steroid production is considered to be an important aspect of testis function it should not be overlooked that the testis may be equally, if not more, important in the production of spermatozoa.

Until a few years ago biochemists in contrast to histologists hardly paid attention to the fact that the testis was composed of many different cell types. Only a few investigations were carried out on isolated tissue compartments (seminiferous tubules and interstitial tissue). Recently techniques for isolation of different cell types have been applied to testis tissue and as a result new insights have been obtained into the cellular localization of steroid metabolizing enzymes and into changes of these enzyme activities during development of the testis. It is now clearly established that *de novo* steroid biosynthesis occurs mainly in the interstitial Leydig cells whereas spermatogenesis occurs in the seminiferous tubules.

The presence of enzyme activities in a particular tissue or cell type is one of the factors that determine conversion rates. The rate of enzyme reactions *in vivo*, however, will depend also on the presence of proper substrates, cofactors, etc. In this respect, it is important to mention that many observations on steroid metabolism have been made using radioactive substrates. The estimation of radioactivity in intermediates and end products after incubation with radioactive precursors may yield information on possible pathways used for biosynthesis of end products, but data on incorporation of radioactivity in such experiments will at best (under steady state conditions) give an impression about rates of conversion of the radioactive substrate, but will not yield information on the quantitative contribution of a specific pathway. The quantitative significance of pathways for endogenous steroid production can only be established when the endogenous amounts and the pool sizes of substances serving as intermediates in these pathways are also measured. The increasing sensitivity of techniques including radioimmunoassay and mass spectrometry for estimating steroids have made it possible, however, to measure the contribution of several pathways by measuring endogenous steroid levels and production rates in isolated testis cells. The biological significance of the steroids produced will depend on many factors such as the inherent biological activity of the steroid, the amount of steroid produced, the rate of secretion of the steroid into one of the three draining systems of the testis (blood, lymph, tubular fluid) or the transfer to other testicular cell types, degradation of the produced steroid (either in the testis or after secretion), etc.

It will not be attempted to discuss all these aspects within the context of this chapter, but the discussion will be restricted to the most significant new information on steroidogenic pathways in the testis, contributions of different testicular cell types to steroid production and the changes in steroidogenesis during development or in pathological situations.

PATHWAYS OF STEROIDOGENESIS

The qualitative pattern of the pathways and intermediates in steroid production in the testis of the human (as well as of most other mammals) resembles those in other steroid producing tissues, viz., the ovaries, adrenals, and placenta. Cholesterol appears to be the obligatory precursor which can be converted intramitochondrially to pregnenolone, which in turn is further metabolized extramitochondrially to several other steroids via different pathways. The most important reactions will be discussed in the following paragraphs.

Conversion of Cholesterol to Pregnenolone

Early experiments with labelled cholesterol and acetate (94) have shown that cholesterol serving as precursor of testicular steroids is probably mainly synthesized in the testis itself from acetate, rather than being derived from dietary cholesterol in the blood. The testicular biosynthesis of cholesterol from acetate occurs in the endoplasmic reticulum and involves the "usual" intermediates in cholesterol formation, such as mevalonate, squalene, and lanosterol (29, 129,142). It is still not certain whether the testicular cholesterol required for steroidogenesis is stored in the testis as such or is derived from cholesterol-

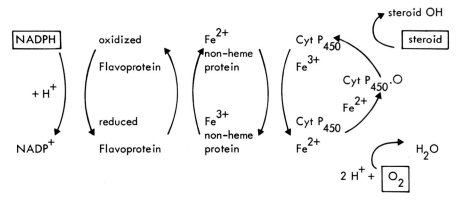

FIG. 1. Simplified metabolic interrelationships in the hydroxylation of steroids. NADPH and molecular oxygen are required in the hydroxylations of steroids.

esters. Normally, 95% or more of the cholesterol in the testis is present in an unesterified form (111,112,145) and newly synthesized cholesterol from acetate mixes with the pool(s) of free cholesterol. Production of testosterone may require hydrolysis of cholesterol-esters under the influence of luteinizing hormone. In this respect, it is important to realize that the cholesterol-ester content of testis tissue from different rodents can show large differences: in mouse testes 10 to 40% of the cholesterol occurs in esterified form (4,116), whereas in rat testes this may be only 2 to 5% (111,145).

The enzymatic steps involved in the removal of the cholesterol side-chain resulting in the formation of pregnenolone ("cholesterol side-chain cleavage activity") can be completely isolated in mitochondrial fractions of testicular Leydig cells (140,148,149). This cholesterol side-chain cleavage activity is probably located in the inner mitochondrial membrane (95,149,150) and requires nicotinamide adenine dinucleotide phosphate (NADPH), molecular oxygen, and an enzyme system containing cytochrome P-450, a flavoprotein, and a non-heme iron protein (33,82,87,88,140) for hydroxylation reactions (see Fig. 1) involved in removing the side-chain.

The production of pregnenolone and isocaproic-aldehyde from cholesterol is clearly established (33,89,140), but the exact nature of the intermediates involved in the *in vivo* conversion of cholesterol into pregnenolone is still not clear. Most information in this respect has been derived from experiments with adrenal cortex mitochondrial preparations (13,14,15,16,121) and it has been shown that cholesterol can be converted into metabolites of cholesterol which subsequently can be converted to pregnenolone. Such metabolites include 20α-OH-cholesterol, 22R-OH-cholesterol, and 20α,22R-dihydroxy-cholesterol. Some alternative pathways for the metabolism of cholesterol to pregnenolone, including Δ20-22 cholesterol and 20,22-epoxycholesterol as possible intermediates (14, 72,73,152) are shown in Fig. 2.

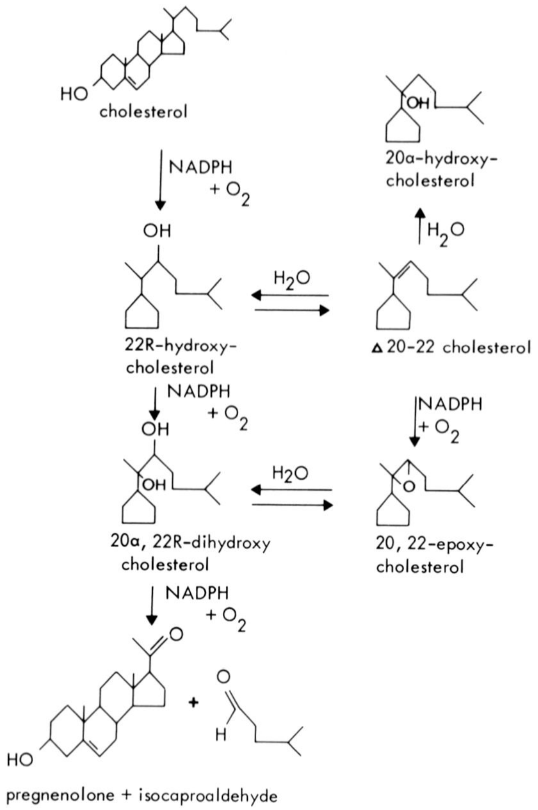

FIG. 2. Possible intermediates in the formation of pregnenolone from cholesterol.

The rate-limiting step in testicular steroid production, which is regulated by luteinizing hormone (LH), depends probably on the rate of association between cholesterol and the cholesterol side-chain cleavage cytochrome P-450 system in the mitochondria (82). Further metabolism of Δ5-pregnenolone will take place outside the mitochondria.

Conversion of Pregnenolone to Testosterone

In most mammals testosterone is considered to be the main biologically important steroid produced by the testis. Numerous *in vitro* and *in vivo* studies (2,8, 10,57,59,83,130,139,146) have shown that biosynthesis of testosterone from pregnenolone in testes of mammals can occur via several Δ5-intermediates (involving pregnenolone, 17α-hydroxy-pregnenolone, dehydroepiandrosterone and 5-androstene-3β,17β-diol) as well as via several Δ4-intermediates (progesterone, 17α-hydroxy-progesterone and 4-androstene-3,17-dione) (Fig. 3).

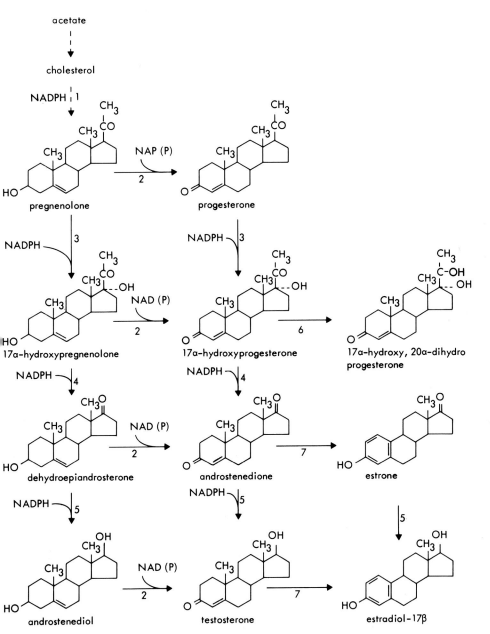

FIG. 3. Pathways involved in biosynthesis of testicular steroids from cholesterol. 1. cholesterol side-chain cleavage complex; 2. 3β-hydroxysteroid dehydrogenase; 3. 17α-hydroxylase; 4. steroid C_{17-20}-lyase; 5. 17β-hydroxysteroid dehydrogenase; 6. 20α-hydroxysteroid dehydrogenase; 7. aromatizing enzyme complex.

The testicular rate of conversion of pregnenolone through the $\Delta 4$- and $\Delta 5$-pathway is different in different animal species and probably the physiologically occurring pathways include several $\Delta 5$- as well as $\Delta 4$-steroids (20). In the human testis the $\Delta 5$-pathway appears to be the most significant (157).

In the human fetal testis it has been shown that pregnenolone and dehydro-epiandrosterone, but no progesterone, are present (58) and it was concluded that in human fetal testis testosterone formation may occur via pregnenolone, dehydroepiandrosterone, and androstenedione, and not via progesterone. Several other observations (2,59,83) are in agreement with the prevalence of this pathway in human fetal testis. For testosterone production in the rat testis, the $\Delta 4$-pathway via progesterone appears to be the most important (130).

Other Metabolites of Pregnenolone and Testosterone

Estimations of endogenous steroids in testis tissue have shown that greatly different amounts of different steroids can occur (91). For example in the immature rat testis 5α-androstane-$3\alpha,17\beta$-diol and 3α-hydroxy-5α-androstan-17-one (androsterone) are present in much larger amounts than testosterone, whereas the amount of testosterone is relatively increased in older rats (76; see also page 103). Similar observations have been made for the relative amounts of androstenedione and testosterone in bull testis, androstenedione being high in immature animals and testosterone being highest in mature animals (79). Similarly in the adult rat the testicular secretion of 7α-hydroxytestosterone can be as high as that of testosterone (76,77) and in the testis of the boar production of C_{19}-$\Delta 16$-steroids may be quantitatively more important than that of testosterone (11,48,50,127). It will not be attempted to give an exhaustive summary of all the metabolites of pregnenolone (and testosterone) that have been detected in testis tissue. Among these metabolites (see also Figs. 3 and 4) are 20α-hydroxy-4-pregnene-3-one, several pregnanes and 17α-hydroxypregnanes and several androstane steroids (91). Such metabolites are generally formed via an action of hydroxylases or dehydrogenases with NAD(P)H as cofactor. Some of the interconnections between the different metabolites are illustrated in Fig. 4.

The significance of these steroids and the importance of the enzyme activities involved in their formation will be considered only when they are involved in the regulation of the formation of the biologically active steroids (i.e., testosterone) or when they can be used as parameters for the normal or abnormal steroidogenic function of the testis. A still puzzling aspect of testicular steroidogenesis concerns the biosynthesis of estrogens. It is known that the testis of several animal species secretes estrogens. Exceptional in this respect is the production of large quantities of equilins, equilinins, and estriol by the stallion testis (8,102,103). In the human and the rat estradiol-17β is the main testicular estrogen (25,109) but the testicular contribution to the total estradiol-17β production appears to be small (in the order of 20-25%) as compared to the peripheral aromatization of androgens (158,159). In vitro experiments have shown that

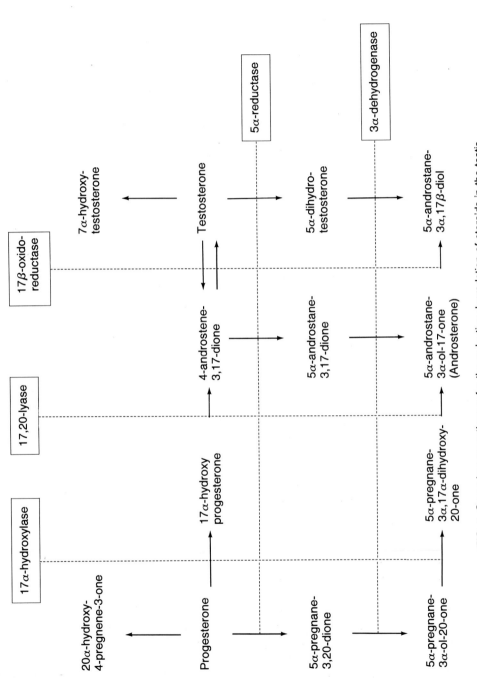

FIG. 4. Some known pathways for the reductive degradation of steroids in the testis.

androstenedione, testosterone, and 19-hydroxy-androstenedione can serve as substrates for testicular estradiol production, but little is known about the occurrence of possible intermediates in this conversion in the testis (8,102,103,109,113).

Several steroid-sulphates, including pregnenolone-sulphate, dehydroepiandrosterone-sulphate, and androsterone-sulphate have also been detected in testis tissue (75,108,126), and the presence of sulphokinase as well as sulphatase activities involved in the introduction and removal of the sulphate group has been described for the testis (100,107). However, there is no good evidence for a possible role of steroid-sulphates in the production of the biologically important steroids.

The significance of the information on metabolic pathways resulting in the production of biologically inactive steroids is obvious when it is realized that the net production of a biologically active steroid reflects the balance between its rate of synthesis and its rate of degradation. In this respect it has been suspected for several years that the observed differences in testicular testosterone production between immature and adult rats could reflect a difference in the capacity of the testis for conversion of testosterone (or its precursors) rather than a difference in testosterone synthesis (20,96). This has recently been substantiated by the estimation of the total amount of different endogenously produced steroids (119) which showed that the capacity of the immature (rat) testis to produce steroids is at least comparable to that of the adult testis.

Subcellular Aspects of Steroid Metabolism

The enzymes required for the conversion of cholesterol to pregnenolone are specifically localized in mitochondria, whereas the enzymes involved in the further conversion of pregnenolone occur mainly in the endoplasmic reticulum. Regulation of the rate of testicular steroidogenesis can depend on the subcellular localization of enzyme activities and steroid substrates. It has been shown, for example, that *in vitro* the endoplasmic reticulum of rat testes preferentially binds pregnenolone rather than progesterone. The enzyme activities for conversion of C_{21} to C_{19} steroids are present in the endoplasmic reticulum and it appeared that more testosterone is produced from pregnenolone than from progesterone (85,130,131).

It has been shown by several workers that the cholesterol side-chain cleaving enzyme complex can be quantitatively isolated in the mitochondrial fraction (33,87,88,138,140,148,150). This is supported by observations on the endogenous steroid production by isolated testicular mitochondria which show that the pregnenolone production by this fraction is of the same order of magnitude as the total steroid production by the total testis (66,148,150). Submitochondrially, the testicular cholesterol side-chain cleavage enzyme is probably mainly located in the inner membranes of the mitochondria (95,137,149).

The conversion of pregnenolone to testosterone, involving 3β-hydroxysteroid dehydrogenase, 17α-hydroxylase, 17α,20-lyase, and 17β-hydroxysteroid dehydrogenase, occurs mainly in the endoplasmic reticulum (61,62,139). However, the presence of part of the total testicular activity of these enzymes in mitochondria cannot be excluded (149). After subfractionation of the endoplasmic reticulum and correlation of the electronmicroscopic characteristics of the subfractions with the presence of steroid metabolizing enzymes (59,95,139,149), it was shown that enzymes for the conversion of pregnenolone to testosterone are mainly present in the smooth surfaced microsomal subfraction rather than the rough surfaced (ribosomal) microsomal subfraction.

Quantitatively the (rat) testis has an overcapacity for conversion of pregnenolone to C_{19} steroids because even in subcellular mitochondrial fractions containing less than 20% of the microsomes, 20 times more testosterone is produced than pregnenolone (21,148,150). These observations may explain why with rat Leydig cells the extracellular amount of C_{21} intermediates is normally small as compared to testosterone. However, in other species, for instance the rabbit, more extracellular C_{21} intermediates can be detected (24).

Testicular steroids may be secreted from the Leydig cells into three different extracellular fluids: blood, lymph, and tubular fluid. Blood is quantitatively the most important effluent system because the flow rate is more than 20 times that of lymph or tubular fluid. A good correlation exists between the testicular intracellular and extracellular testosterone concentrations and it appears that diffusion is the most important mechanism for secretion of steroids (37,106,151). No convincing evidence has been reported for the existence of steroid storage pools in subcellular granules or vesicles. The distribution of steroids between intra- and extracellular fluid is quantitatively mainly influenced by extracellular binding proteins and, in plasma, more than 90% of the testicular androgens are bound to proteins. Receptor proteins in the cell play a minor role in this respect because the binding capacity is relatively low.

REGULATION OF TESTICULAR STEROIDOGENESIS

In principle, steroid metabolism can be regulated by any of the known processes that can regulate biochemical reactions, such as availability of substrates and cofactors, induction, inhibition, stimulation of enzyme activities, compartmentalization of substrates and/or enzymes, etc. Not all of these possibilities have been investigated in detail, but from the available evidence it appears that enzyme induction or activation either under the influence of LH or during maturation of the testis is probably the most important biochemical mechanism in regulating testicular steroid production. In addition, there are indications that several steroids can inhibit certain testicular enzymes required for steroidogenesis. Because all of the latter observations have been obtained under *in vitro* conditions, it is not clear to what extent such effects are important for the regulation of testicular steroidogenesis *in vivo*.

Effect of Tropic Hormones

Hypophysectomy of male animals results in a regression of the testis, including a decreased testosterone production, resulting in decreased testicular and plasma testosterone levels. These effects of hypophysectomy can be counteracted by administration of tropic hormones with luteotropin-like activity (LH and hCG), and it is known that LH can stimulate testosterone production and secretion by testes in intact animals (36,38,92,101) as well as in isolated testicular tissue (21,25,77), isolated interstitial tissue (21,25,150), and purified Leydig cells (66,119,144).

The mechanism of action of LH in stimulating testicular testosterone production is discussed in detail in Chapter 9. During long term administration of LH increased activities of many of the enzymes involved in testosterone production from pregnenolone and in further metabolism of testosterone to androstane steroids have been observed (54,133,134,140). For example, the testicular conversion of testosterone to 5α-reduced metabolites appears to decrease concomitant with an increased conversion to 7α-hydroxytestosterone (77). Such long term effects probably reflect a growth effect of LH on the testis resulting in an increased activity of enzymes. No convincing studies are at present available that have estimated the long term effect of LH on specific activities of the enzymes involved per Leydig cell.

All of the described effects of tropic hormones appear to be specific for LH and hCG. There are some reports on possible effects of follitropin (FSH) (19) and prolactin (5,53) on testicular steroid metabolism, but it is not yet understood whether and how these hormones influence enzyme activities involved in testicular steroidogenesis.

Effects of Steroids

Results of *in vitro* incubations with testis tissue preparations show that several steroids can inhibit enzymes involved in steroidogenesis. Among those steroids are several that are produced also endogenously in the testis. Table 1 gives several examples of such *in vitro* inhibitions.

The potential physiological importance of such *in vitro* observations is still unclear (105), but some observed correlations between the changes in enzyme activities and levels of endogenous steroids (124) might reflect a causal relationship.

Estrogens could play an important role within the testis. The potential production of estradiol (E_2) in Sertoli cells is dependent on testosterone as substrate and the conversion is regulated by FSH (31,32). It has been shown that testicular 17α-steroid hydroxylase and $C_{17,20}$-lyase in Leydig cells are inhibited after administration of E_2 to male rats (68,74,144) and after long term estrogen administration to males (122). It may be possible therefore that E_2 is involved in an intratesticular feedback system between Leydig cells and Sertoli cells. However,

TABLE 1. *Some examples of in vitro inhibition of testicular steroid metabolism by steroids*

| | Inhibitors | |
Enzyme activity	Physiological steroids	Synthetic compounds
Cholesterol side-chain cleavage	pregnenolone (71)[e] testosterone (89)	amphenone B (49) aminoglutethimide (39)
Δ5,3β-Hydroxysteroid dehydrogenase	7α-OH-androstenedione (63,65) 7α-OH-testosterone (63,65) estradiol-17β (67)	cyanoketone (99)[a] WIN 24.540 (98)[b]
17α-Hydroxylase	17α-hydroxyprogesterone (96) estradiol-17β (74,122,144)	SU 8000 (18,47,135)[c] SU 10603 (18,47,135)[d]
C$_{17-20}$-Lyase	progesterone (81,84) 17α,20α-dihydroxypregn-4-en-3-one (24) estradiol-17β (68)	17β-ureido-1,4- androstadien-3-one (3,24)
17β-Hydroxysteroid dehydrogenase	7α-OH-androstenedione (63,65) testosterone (63) estradiol-17β (67)	
5α-Reductase	7α-OH-testosterone (124)	methyl-3-oxo-androst-4-ene- 17β-carboxylate (96)
7α-Hydroxylase	testosterone (63)	
3α-Hydroxysteroid dehydrogenase	testosterone (80,124) 7α-OH-testosterone (124)	
3β-Hydroxysteroid dehydrogenase aromatizing activity	testosterone (124)	1,4,6-androstatriene- 3,17-dione (132) 4-OH-4-androstene- 3,17-dione (12)

[a] Cyanoketone is: 2α-cyano-4,4,17α-trimethyl-17β-hydroxy-androst-5-en-3-one.
[b] WIN 25.540 is: 4α,5-epoxy-17β-hydroxy-androstane-2α-carbonitrile.
[c] SU 8000 is: 3-(6-chloro-3-methyl-2-indenyl)pyridine.
[d] SU 10603 is: 7-chloro-3,4-dihydro-2(3-pyridyl)-1-(2H)-naphtalenone.
[e] Numbers within parentheses are references.

the amount of estradiol secreted by the testis is small (20%) compared to the amount of estrogens synthesized peripherally (25).

In addition to the effects of physiologically occurring steroids on steroidogenesis, there are numerous synthetic compounds known to influence specific enzyme activities (see Table 1), and several of these compounds have been studied as potential specific inhibitors in studying steroidogenesis (35).

CONTRIBUTION OF DIFFERENT CELL TYPES TO TESTICULAR STEROIDOGENESIS

Steroid metabolizing enzymes required for the formation of pregnenolone and for the further conversion of pregnenolone to androstenedione are mainly, if not solely present in the testis Leydig cells. Some steroid metabolizing enzyme activities have, however, also been demonstrated in other testis cell types (Table 2). Quantitative information on steroid production can be obtained by measuring endogenous steroid levels and production rates in isolated testis cell types in the presence of physiological levels of trophic hormones. Initial studies (21) demonstrated that endogenous testosterone levels in interstitial tissue were 8 times higher than in seminiferous tubules and that testosterone levels after incubation *in vitro* increased in interstitial tissue but not in seminiferous tubules. The production rate of testosterone in homogenates of seminiferous tubules was shown to be about 500 times lower than the production rate in homogenates of interstitial tissue (148) and no convincing evidence for *de novo* testosterone synthesis in cell types other than the Leydig cells has been reported as yet. In contrast, suspensions of Leydig cells synthesize testosterone and respond to physiological amounts of LH (66).

All these data indicate that the Leydig cells are the main, if not the only, source of endogenous testosterone production. This does not rule out a function for the seminiferous tubular cells in utilizing steroids formed in the Leydig cells for further steroid synthesis. The transfer of various steroids (the exception being cholesterol) from the interstitial compartment to the seminiferous tubules has been demonstrated (106,151).

Steroid metabolizing enzymes present in the seminiferous tubules might thus act on steroids initially produced in the Leydig cells. The major importance of steroid metabolism in seminiferous tubules must be sought in the production of specific steroids which cannot or only in small amounts be produced in Leydig cells. Intratubular production of small amounts of steroids which can also be synthesized in Leydig cells is probably unimportant because of the quick equilibration of steroids between the different testis compartments (106,151).

Many approaches have been followed for investigations on steroid metabolism in seminiferous epithelium or isolated cell types. In most studies intact cells or homogenates have been incubated with radioactively labelled precursors and the percentage of label in various metabolites has been measured. Results of these studies can only give a rough impression of the actual steroid converting

TABLE 2. *Localization of steroid metabolizing enzymes in interstitial tissue (Leydig cells) and seminiferous tubules of rat testis*

Enzyme activity	Percent of enzyme activity present in		References
	Interstitial tissue	Seminiferous tubules	
Cholesterol side-chain cleavage	98	2	150
Δ5-3β-Hydroxysteroid dehydrogenase/ Δ5-Δ4-Isomerase complex	95–98	2–5	149
17α-Steroid hydroxylase	93–94	6–7	117,60
20α-Hydroxysteroid dehydrogenase	3	97	24,60
C_{17-20}-Steroid lyase	93–94	6–7	117,60
17β-Hydroxysteroid dehydrogenase	present	present	30,150,110
5α-Steroid reductase	>90% (immature) present (adult)	<10% (immature) present (adult)	147,30,42,136
3α(3β)-Hydroxysteroid dehydrogenase	>90% (immature) present (adult)	<10% (immature) present (adult)	147,30,42,136
Aromatase system	absent?	present	25,32

capacities under *in vivo* conditions because the endogenous concentrations of steroids are often unknown. Also, it is important to realize that studies with homogenates with added cofactors result in maximal enzyme activities which are not necessarily similar to the activities under *in vivo* conditions. In studies on the cellular localization of steroid metabolizing enzymes, it is important to characterize the purity of the tissue preparations very carefully. This is especially important when, e.g., in seminiferous tubules, enzymes are investigated which are also present in interstitial tissue in higher concentrations. Conclusions from studies on distribution of steroid-converting enzymes over the various compartments are therefore completely dependent on the specificity of the characterization of the tissue or cell preparations with suitable marker enzymes.

Considering these requirements, it has been possible to establish the tissue localization of some enzymes with reasonable specificity. From the results summarized in Table 2, it can be concluded that the enzymes required for generation of C_{19} steroids are almost exclusively present in interstitial tissue. The small amounts of these enzymes detected in preparations of isolated seminiferous tubules may be explained by contamination with small amounts of interstitial cells that could not be measured with marker enzymes. It can also be concluded from these data that some steroid biosynthetic enzymes may be excellent markers for interstitial tissue cells.

The presence of 3α-hydroxysteroid dehydrogenase and 5α-steroid reductase in seminiferous tubules of testes from adult animals has been observed by many investigators (30,34,42,86,147) and these enzymes may contribute to the formation of dihydrotestosterone and androstanediols. From studies with isolated cell types it can also be concluded that the distribution of the enzymes over cells within the tubules is not equal. 5α-Reductase appears to be present in Sertoli cells and spermatocytes whereas 3α-hydroxysteroid dehydrogenase appears to be localized mainly in Sertoli cells (30). Peritubular cells also appear capable of steroid metabolism (27). Nothing, however, is known about the relative importance of these tubular enzyme activities in comparison with the activities in interstitial tissue. In the immature rat it appears that these enzyme activities in Leydig cells are quantitatively more important than those in seminiferous tubules for the testicular reductions of androgens.

Two of the enzymes listed in Table 2, 20α-hydroxysteroid dehydrogenase and the aromatase enzyme complex, have been detected mainly in seminiferous tubules. The localization of 20α-hydroxysteroid dehydrogenase appears peculiar because the availability of substrate for this enzyme appears limited at least in the rat. This argument does not hold for the aromatase enzyme complex present in the seminiferous tubules, because testosterone and androstenedione are available as substrate for conversion to estrogens.

Testicular formation of estrogens has been shown to occur *in vivo* (25), in isolated tubules from adult rats (25), as well as in isolated Sertoli cells from immature rats if testosterone was added as substrate (32). It is not certain whether the aromatase is exclusively localized in Sertoli cells. It has been reported

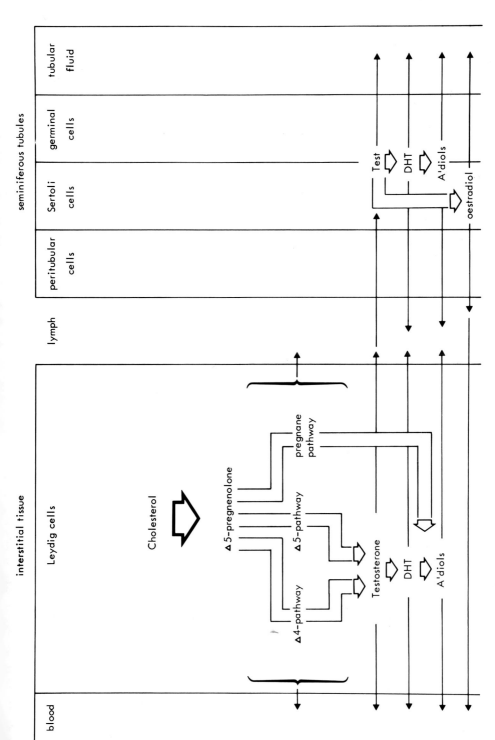

FIG. 5. Localization of steroid metabolic pathways and interactions between different tissue compartments in the testis.

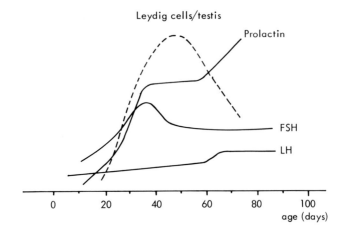

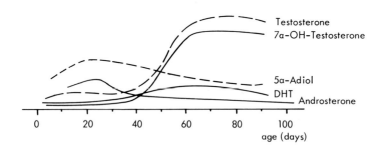

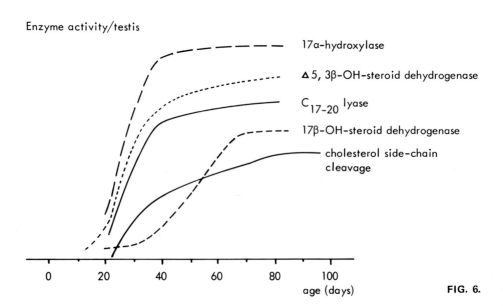

FIG. 6.

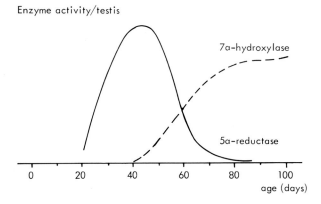

FIG. 6. Age-related changes in testicular Leydig cell content, circulating pituitary hormones, testicular steroid production, and some testis enzyme activities involved in steroid metabolism in the rat. Data obtained from results by different authors (17,41,43,44,46,69,70,76,78,90,92, 97,110,114,115,124,147,154) are expressed in arbitrary units.

that Leydig cells may be the site of estrogen biosynthesis in human testis (109) and in Leydig cell tumors (113). In the rat, however, it appears unlikely that estradiol is synthesized in Leydig cells because this could not be demonstrated in isolated interstitial tissue (25) and because 70% of the estrogen receptors are not occupied in isolated Leydig cells (23). Figure 5 gives a summary of the cellular localization of the most important steroid biosynthetic pathways and their interactions in the testis.

CHANGES IN STEROIDOGENESIS DURING TESTICULAR DEVELOPMENT

Testis development takes place continuously from the earliest appearance of the testis in the fetus, continuing after birth until completion after puberty. *De novo* steroidogenesis has been demonstrated in fetal rat testis from day 15 of gestation on and in the human testis starting at week 21 of gestation (1,156). Changes in the testicular steroidogenesis from this period up to maturity have been observed (7,69) and several factors, such as changes in sensitivity of the testis to trophic hormones, number of Leydig cells, and levels of gonadotrophins, as well as a continuous differentiation of Leydig cells, have been suggested to explain the variations observed.

In neonatal rat testis the number of Leydig cells increases from day 20 to day 50 without a concomitant increase in testosterone production, and androsterone and 5α-androstane-3α,17β-diol appear to be the main steroids produced during this period (69,119). It has been reported that steroidogenic pathways in immature testis from mice and rats may not require testosterone as an intermediate. Progesterone was found to be metabolized to hydroxypregnane compounds which were subsequently converted to androsterone and androstanediols (93, 143). It may be that this steroidogenic pathway prevents the exposure of the fetal rat to (too much) testosterone.

The cellular composition of the developing testis is continuously changing and it is therefore difficult to relate changes in steroid metabolism to specific cell types. Figure 6 gives a schematic impression of the changes with age of different enzymes involved in steroid metabolism and of changes in steroid production. Leydig cells are the most important cell type in this respect, because several steroid-metabolizing enzymes have histochemically been detected in these cells and because steroidogenesis has been shown to occur in Leydig cells isolated from immature rats (119). It was concluded from such studies with isolated cells that the total amount of secreted androgens (testosterone, dihydrotestosterone, androstanediols and androsterone) per Leydig cell is continuously decreasing during development of the testis (119). The increase in the testicular production of testosterone around day 40 can be explained by an increase in the number of Leydig cells and a drop in the steroid-metabolizing enzymes 5α-steroid reductase and the 3α-hydroxysteroid dehydrogenase and a change in the steroidogenic pathway (69,143,147). Developmental changes also occur in the seminiferous tubules. Preliminary results from *in vitro* studies (31) indicate that the activity of the aromatase system in immature rat Sertoli cells is very high in cells from 5-day-old animals and very low in cells from animals of more than 30 days old. The significance of these changes for *in vivo* testicular estradiol steroidogenesis is not clear because the Sertoli cells require endogenous testosterone as substrate and the testicular levels of this precursor are low during the period when the aromatase activity is high.

STEROIDOGENESIS IN ABNORMAL TESTES

The steroid producing capacity of the testis is mainly dependent on the number of Leydig cells present and the presence or absence of sufficient LH (see Chapter 6). The steroidogenic function of Leydig cells in many testicular disorders, such as germinal aplasia, Klinefelter's syndrome, and severe germinal arrest appears to be less affected than the spermatogenic function of the seminiferous tubules (125). A good example is cryptorchidism which is characterized by clear defects in spermatogenesis concomitant with no reduction or only a slight reduction in testosterone production (51,52,55,56,64). A few observations in the human suggest that disturbed spermatogenesis may be related to a defect of testicular steroidogenesis resulting in a decreased androgen production (104,123). A partial deficiency of 3β-hydroxysteroid dehydrogenase has been reported in this respect (123). However, several studies of oligospermic men have reported apparently normal levels of testosterone in peripheral blood, despite qualitative and/or quantitative changes in enzyme activities for testicular steroid production (26,118,141).

More specific abnormalities in testicular steroidogenesis have been detected in genetic defects classified as male pseudohermaphroditism (45,128,153). It appears that defects resulting in pseudohermaphroditism, such as Reifenstein syndrome and testicular feminization (9), are especially characterized by decreased activities of testicular 17β-hydroxysteroid dehydrogenase and 5α-steroid reductase, resulting in abnormally low testosterone productions (120,153). Testicular (Leydig cell) tumors in rats may have characteristics of normal Leydig cells synthesizing testosterone (22), but also estradiol-producing tumors have been observed and it is as yet difficult to make general statements on abnormalities of steroidogenesis in these tumor Leydig cells.

ACKNOWLEDGMENT

The authors wish to acknowledge the assistance of Ms. W. Bakhuizen in the preparation of this manuscript.

REFERENCES

1. Abramovich, D. R., Baker, T. G., and Neal, P. (1974): Effect of human chorionic gonadotrophin on testosterone secretion by the foetal human testis in organ culture. *J. Endocrinol.,* 60:179–185.
2. Acedevo, H. F., Axelrod, L. R., Ishikawa, E., and Takaki, F. (1963): Studies in fetal metabolism-II. Metabolism of progesterone-4-(C^{14}) and pregnenolone-7α-(H^3) in human fetal testes. *J. Clin. Endocrinol. Metab.,* 23:885–890.
3. Arth, G. E., Patchett, A. A., Jefopoulus, T., Bugianesi, R. L., Peterson, L. H., Ham, E. A., Kuehl Jr., F. A., and Brink, N. G. (1971): Steroidal androgen biosynthesis inhibitors. *J. Med. Chem.,* 14:675–681.
4. Bartke, A. (1971): Concentration of free and esterified cholesterol in the testes of immature and adult mice. *J. Reprod. Fert.,* 25:153–156.
5. Bartke, A., and Dalerio, S. (1976): Effects of prolactin on the sensitivity of the testis to LH. *Biol. Reprod.,* 15:90–93.
6. Bartke, A., Williams, K. I. H., and Dalterio, S. (1977): Effects of estrogens on testicular testosterone production in vitro. *Biol. Reprod.,* 17:645–649.
7. Becker, W. G., and Snipes, C. A. (1968): Shift with age in steady state concentrations of androstenedione and testosterone in incubations of guinea pig testis. *Biochem. J.,* 107:35–40.
8. Bedrak, E., and Samuels, L. T. (1969): Steroid biosynthesis by the equine testis. *Endocrinology,* 85:1186–1195.
9. Bell, J. B. G. (1975): Studies of in vitro steroid metabolism by testis tissue from "complete" and "incomplete" forms of testicular feminization. *Clin. Endocrinol.,* 4:343–356.
10. Bell, J. B. G., Vinson, G. P., Hopkin, D. J., and Lacy, D. (1968): Pathways of androgen biosynthesis from (7α-^{3}H)pregnenolone and (4-^{14}C)progesterone by rat testis interstitium in vitro. *Biochim. Biophys. Acta,* 164:412–420.
11. Booth, W. D. (1975): Changes with age in the occurrence of C-19 steroids in the testis and submaxillary gland of the boar. *J. Reprod. Fert.,* 42:459–472.
12. Brodie, A. M. H., Schwarzel, W. C., Shaikh, A. A., and Brodie, H. J. (1977): Effect of an aromatase inhibitor, 4-hydroxy-4-androstene-3,17-dione, on estrogen-dependent processes in reproduction and breast cancer. *Endocrinology,* 100:1684–1695.
13. Burstein, S., and Gut, M. (1971): Biosynthesis of pregnenolone. *Recent Prog. Horm. Res.,* 27:303–349.
14. Burstein, S., and Gut, M. (1976): Intermediates in the conversion of cholesterol to pregnenolone: Kinetics and mechanism. *Steroids,* 28:115–131.
15. Burstein, S., Kimball, H. L., and Gut, M. (1970): Transformation of labelled cholesterol 20α-hydroxycholesterol, (22R)-22-hydroxycholesterol and (22R)-20α,22-dihydroxycholesterol

by adrenal acetone-dried preparations from guinea pigs, cattle and man: II. Kinetic studies. *Steroids,* 15:809–857.

16. Burstein, S., Middleditch, B. S., and Gut, M. (1974): Enzymatic formation of (20R,22R)-20,22-dihydroxycholesterol from cholesterol and a mixture of 16_{o_2} and 18_{o_2}: Random incorporation of oxygen atoms. *Biochem. Biophys. Res. Commun.,* 61:692–697.

17. Chan, S. W. C., Leathem, J. H., and Esashi, T. (1977): Testicular metabolism and serum testosterone in aging male rats. *Endocrinology,* 101:128–133.

18. Chart, J. J., Gisoldi, E., Howic, N., and Gaunt, R. (1969): Effect of an adrenal 17α-hydroxylase inhibitor on gonad function. *Proc. Soc. Exp. Biol. Med.,* 130:870–873.

19. Chen, Y.-D. I., Payne, A. H., and Kelch, R. F. (1976): FSH stimulation of Leydig cell function in the hypophysectomized immature rat. *Proc. Soc. Exp. Biol. Med.,* 153:473–475.

20. Coffey, J. C., French, F. S., and Nayfeh, S. N. (1971): Metabolism of progesterone by rat testicular homogenates. IV. Further studies of testosterone formation in immature testis in vitro. *Endocrinology,* 89:865–872.

21. Cooke, B. A., de Jong, F. H., van der Molen, H. J., and Rommerts, F. F. G. (1972): Endogenous testosterone concentrations in rat testis interstitial tissue and seminiferous tubules during in vitro incubation. *Nature [New Biol.],* 237:255–256.

22. Cooke, B. A., Lindh, M. L., and Janszen, F. H. A. (1977): Effect of lutropin on phosphorylation of endogenous proteins in testis Leydig cells. *Biochem. J.,* 168:43–48.

23. De Boer, W., de Vries, J., Mulder, E., and van der Molen, H. J. (1977): Comparative study of nuclear binding sites for oestradiol in rat testicular and uterine tissue. *Biochem. J.,* 162:331–339.

24. De Bruijn, H. W., and van der Molen, H. J. (1974): An assessment of the possible role of 17α,20α-dihydroxy-4-pregnen-3-one in the regulation of testosterone synthesis by rat and rabbit testis. *J. Endocrinol.,* 61:401–410.

25. De Jong, F. H., Hey, A. H., and van der Molen, H. J. (1974): Oestradiol-17β and testosterone in rat testis tissue: Effect of gonadotrophins, localization and production in vitro. *J. Endocrinol.,* 60:409–419.

26. de Kretser, D. M., Burger, H. G., Fortune, D., Hudson, B., Long, A. R., Paulsen, C. A., and Taft, M. P. (1972): Hormonal, histological and chromosomal studies in adult males with testicular disorders. *J. Clin. Endocrinol. Metab.,* 35:392–401.

27. de Kretser, D. M., Catt, K. J., Dufau, M. L., and Hudson, B. (1971): Studies on rat testicular cells in tissue culture. *J. Reprod. Fert.,* 24:311–318.

28. De la Torre, B., Hedman, M., and Diczfalusy, E. (1977): Species differences in steroidogenesis following the in vitro incubation of decapsulated testes. *Acta Endocrinol. (Kbh),* 86:851–864.

29. Dennick, R. G. (1972): The intracellular organisation of cholesterol biosynthesis. A review. *Steroids Lipids Res.,* 3:236–256.

30. Dorrington, J. H., and Fritz, I. B. (1975): Cellular localization of 5α-reductase and 3α-hydroxysteroid dehydrogenase in the seminiferous tubule of the rat testis. *Endocrinology,* 96:879–889.

31. Dorrington, J. H., Fritz, I. B., and Armstrong, D. T. (1976): FSH control of estrogen synthesis by cultured Sertoli cells. *Vth International Congress of Endocrinology,* Hamburg, Abstract 768.

32. Dorrington, J. H., Fritz, I. B., and Armstrong, D. T. (1976): Site at which FSH regulates estradiol-17β biosynthesis in Sertoli cell preparations in culture. *Molec. Cell. Endocrinol.,* 16:117–122.

33. Drosdowsky, M., Menon, K. M. J., Forchielli, E., and Dorfman, R. I. (1965): Requirements of the cholesterol side-chain-cleaving enzyme system of rat-testis mitochondria. *Biochim. Biophys. Acta,* 104:229–236.

34. Dufau, M. L., de Kretser, D. M., and Hudson, B. (1971): Steroid metabolism by isolated rat seminiferous tubules in tissue culture. *Endocrinology,* 88:825–832.

35. Dupuy, G. M., Roberts, K. D., Bleau, G., and Chapdelaine, A. (1977): Inhibition of prostatic 5α-reductase and 3α-hydroxysteroid dehydrogenase by two antiandrogens. *J. Steroid Biochem.,* 8:1145–1152.

36. Eik-Nes, K. B. (1970): *The Androgens of the Testis.* Marcel Dekker, New York.

37. Eik-Nes, K. B. (1975): Biosynthesis and secretion of testicular steroids. In: *Handbook of Physiology,* Section 7: Endocrinology, Vol. V, edited by R. O. Greep and E. B. Astwood, pp. 95–115. American Physiological Society, Washington D.C.

38. El Safoury, S., and Bartke, A. (1974): Effects of follicle-stimulating hormone and luteinizing

hormone on plasma testosterone levels in hypophysectomized and in intact immature and adult male rats. *J. Endocrinol.,* 61:193–198.

39. El Safoury, S., and Bartke, A. (1974): Aminoglutethimide inhibits steroidogenesis in the rat testis. *Steroids,* 23:165–172.
40. Ewing, L. and Brown, B. L. (1977): Testicular steroidogenesis. In: *The Testis,* Vol. IV, edited by A. D. Johnson, W. R. Gomes, and N. L. VandeMark, pp. 239–287. Academic Press, New York.
41. Ficher, M., and Steinberger, E. (1971): In vitro progesterone metabolism by rat testicular tissue at different stages of development. *Acta Endocrinol.,* 68:285–292.
42. Folman, Y., Ahmad, N., Sowell, J. G., and Eik-Nes, K. B. (1973): Formation in vitro of 5α-dihydrotestosterone and other 5α-reduced metabolites of ³H-testosterone by the seminiferous tubules and interstitial tissue from immature and mature rat testes. *Endocrinology,* 92:41–47.
43. Forest, M. G., de Peretti, E., and Bertrans, J. (1976): Hypothalamic-pituitary-gonadal relationships in man from birth to puberty. *Clin. Endocrinol.,* 5:551–569.
44. Ghanadian, R., Lewis, J. G., and Chisholm, G. D. (1975): Serum testosterone and dihydrotestosterone changes with age in rat. *Steroids,* 25:753–762.
45. Givens, J. R., Wiser, W. L., Summit, R. L., Kerber, I. J., Andersen, R. N., Pittaway, D. E., and Fish, S. A. (1974): Familial male pseudohermaphroditism without gynecomastia due to deficient testicular 17-ketosteroid reductase activity. *N. Engl. J. Med.,* 291:938–944.
46. Goebelsmann, U., Hall, T. D., Paul, W. L., and Stanczyk, F. Z. (1975): In vitro steroid metabolic studies in testicular 17β-reduction deficiency. *J. Clin. Endocrinol. Metab.,* 41:1136–1143.
47. Goldman, A. S. (1971): Production of hypospadias in the rat by selective inhibition of fetal testicular 17α-hydroxylase and C_{17-20}-lyase. *Endocrinology,* 88:527–531.
48. Gower, D. B. (1972): 16-Unsaturated C_{19} steroids. A review of their chemistry, biochemistry and possible physiological role. *J. Steroid Biochem.,* 3:45–103.
49. Gower, D. B. (1974): Modifiers of steroid-hormone metabolism: A review of their chemistry, biochemistry and clinical applications. *J. Steroid Biochem.,* 5:501–523.
50. Gower, D. B., and Ahmad, N. (1967): Studies on the biosynthesis of 16-dehydrosteroids. The metabolism of (4-¹⁴C)-pregnenolone by boar adrenal and testis tissue in vitro. *Biochem. J.,* 104:550–556.
51. Gupta, D., Rager, K., Zarzycki, J., and Eichner, M. (1975): Levels of luteinizing hormone, follicle-stimulating hormone, testosterone and dihydrotestosterone in the circulation of sexually maturing intact male rats and after orchidectomy and experimental bilateral cryptorchidism. *J. Endocrinol.,* 66:183–193.
52. Gupta, D., and Rager, K. (1975): Plasma testosterone and dihydrotestosterone in male rats during sexual maturation and following orchidectomy and experimental bilateral cryptorchidism. *Steroids,* 25:33–42.
53. Hafiez, A. A., Bartke, A., and Lloyd, C. W. (1972): The role of prolactin in the regulation of testis function: The synergistic effects of prolactin and luteinizing hormone on the incorporation of 1-¹⁴C acetate into testosterone and cholesterol by testes from hypophysectomized rats in vitro. *J. Endocrinol.,* 53:223–230.
54. Hall, P. F. (1970): Endocrinology of the testis. In: *The Testis,* Vol. II, edited by A. D. Johnson, W. R. Gomes, and N. L. VandeMark, pp. 1–71. Academic Press, New York.
55. Hall, R. W., and Gomes, W. R. (1975): The effect of artificial cryptorchidism on serum oestrogen and testosterone levels in the adult male rat. *Acta Endocrinol.,* 80:583–591.
56. Hoschoian, J. C., and Andrada, J. A. (1975): Androgen biosynthesis in experimental cryptorchidism. *Fertil. Steril.,* 26:730–738.
57. Hoschoian, J. C., and Brownie, A. C. (1967): Pathways for androgen biosynthesis in monkey testis. *Steroids,* 1:49–69.
58. Huhtaniemi, I. (1977): Studies on steroidogenesis and its regulation in human fetal adrenal and testis. *J. Steroid Biochem.,* 8:491–497.
59. Ikonen, M., and Niemi, J. (1966): Metabolism of progesterone and 17α-hydroxypregnenolone by the human testis in vitro. *Nature,* 212:716–717.
60. Inano, H. (1974): Studies on enzyme reactions related to steroid biosynthesis-III. Distribution of the testicular enzymes related to androgen production between the seminiferous tubules and interstitial tissue. *J. Steroid Biochem.,* 5:145–149.
61. Inano, H., Inano, A., and Tamaoki, B. (1970): Studies on enzyme reactions related to steroid

biosynthesis-II. Submicrosomal distribution of the enzymes related to androgen production from pregnenolone and of the cytochrome P-450 in testicular gland of rat. *J. Steroid Biochem.,* 1:83–89.

62. Inano, H., Nakano, H., Shikita, M., and Tamaoki, B. (1967): The influence of various factors upon testicular enzymes related to steroidogenesis. *Biochim. Biophys. Acta,* 137:540–548.
63. Inano, H., Suzuki, K., Wakabayashi, K., and Tamaoki, B. I. (1973): Biological activities of 7α-hydroxylated C_{19}-steroids and changes in rat testicular 7α-hydroxylase activity with gonadal status. *Endocrinology,* 92:22–30.
64. Inano, H., and Tamaoki, B. I. (1968): Effect of experimental bilateral cryptorchidism on testicular enzymes related to androgen formation. *Endocrinology,* 83:1074–1082.
65. Inano, H., and Tamaoki, B. I. (1971): Regulation of testosterone biosynthesis in rat testes by 7α-hydroxylated C_{19}-steroids. *Biochim. Biophys. Acta,* 239:482–493.
66. Janszen, F. H. A., Cooke, B. A., van Driel, M. J. A., and van der Molen, H. J. (1976): Purification and characterization of Leydig cells from rat testes. *J. Endocrinol.,* 70:345–359.
67. Kaartinen, E., Laukkanen, M., and Saure, A. (1971): Metabolism of dehydroepiandrosterone by rat testicular homogenates: Kinetic study at different temperatures of direct effect of 17β-oestradiol. *Acta Endocrinol. (Kbh),* 66:50–64.
68. Kalla, N. R., Nisula, B. C., Menard, R. H., and Loriaux, D. (1977): Estrogen modulation of Leydig cell function. *59th Annual Meeting American Endocrine Society,* Abstract No. 52.
69. Knorr, D. W., Vanha-Perttula, T., and Lipsett, M. B. (1970): Structure and function of rat testis through pubescence. *Endocrinology,* 86:1298–1304.
70. Kobayashi, S., and Ishii, S. (1967): The effect of age on the activity of cholesterol side-chain cleavage in rat testis. *Endocrinol. Jap.,* 2:134–137.
71. Koritz, S. B., and Kumar, A. M. (1970): On the mechanism of action of the adrenocorticotrophic hormone. *J. Biol. Chem.,* 245:152–159.
72. Kraaipoel, R. J., Degenhart, H. J., and Leferink, J. G. (1975): Incorporation of $H_2{}^{18}O$ into $20\alpha,22R$-di-OH-cholesterol: Evidence for an epoxide-diol pathway in the adrenocorticol cholesterol side-chain cleavage mechanism. *FEBS Lett.,* 57:294–300.
73. Kraaipoel, R. J., Degenhart, H. J., Leferink, J. G., van Beek, V., de Leeuw-Boon, H., and Visser, H. K. A. (1975): Pregnenolone formation from cholesterol in bovine adrenal cortex mitochondria: proposal of a new mechanism. *FEBS Lett.,* 50:204–209.
74. Kremers, P., Tixhon, C., and Gielen, J. (1977): 17α-Hydroxylase and testosterone biosynthesis in rat testis. *J. Steroid Biochem.,* 8:873–878.
75. Laaitikainen, T., Laitinen, E. A., and Vihko, R. (1971): Secretion of free and sulphate-conjugated neutral steroids by the human testis. Effect of administration of human chorionic gonadotropin. *J. Clin. Endocrinol. Metab.,* 32:59–64.
76. Lacroix, E., Eechaute, W., and Leusen, I. (1975): Influence of age on the formation of 5α-androstanediol and 7α-hydroxytestosterone by incubated rat testes. *Steroids,* 25:649–661.
77. Lacroix, E., Eechaute, W., and Leusen, I. (1977): The influence on gonadotrophin (HCG) treatment on the steroidogenesis by incubated rat testis. *J. Steroid Biochem.,* 8:269–275.
78. Lee, V. K. W., de Kretser, D. M., Hudson, B., and Wang, C. (1975): Variations in serum FSH, LH and testosterone levels in male rats from birth to sexual maturity. *J. Reprod. Fert.,* 42:121–126.
79. Lindner, H. R. (1961): Androgens and related compounds in the spermatic vein blood of domestic animals: I. Neutral steroids secreted by the bull testis. *J. Endocrinol.,* 23:139–167.
80. Lloret, A. P., and Weisz, J. (1974): Metabolism of testosterone and 5α-dihydrotestosterone in vitro by the seminiferous tubules of the mature rat. *Endocrinology,* 95:1306–1316.
81. Mahajan, K., and Samuels, L. T. (1962): Inhibition of steroid 17-desmolase by progesterone. *Fed. Proc.,* 21:209 (Abstract).
82. Mason, J. I., Estabrook, R. W., and Purvis, J. L. (1973): Testicular cytochrome P-450 and iron-sulfur protein as related to steroid metabolism. *Ann. N.Y. Acad. Sci.,* 212:406–419.
83. Mathur, R. S., Wiqvist, N., and Diczfalusy, E. (1972): De novo synthesis of steroids and steroid sulphates by the testicles of the human foetus at midgestation. *Acta Endocrinol. (Kbh),* 71:792–800.
84. Matsumoto, K., Mahajan, D. K., and Samuels, L. T. (1974): The influence of progesterone on the conversion of 17-hydroxyprogesterone to testosterone in the mouse testis. *Endocrinology,* 94:808–814.
85. Matsumoto, K., and Samuels, L. T. (1969): Influence of steroid distribution between microsomes

and soluble fraction on steroid metabolism by microsomal enzymes. *Endocrinology,* 85:402–410.

86. Matsumoto, K., and Yamada, M. (1973): 5α-Reduction of testosterone in vitro by rat seminiferous tubules and whole testes at different stages of development. *Endocrinology,* 93:253–255.
87. Menard, R. H., Latif, S. A., and Purvis, J. L. (1975): The intratesticular localization of cytochrome P-450 and cytochrome P-450 dependent enzymes in the rat testis. *Endocrinology,* 97:1587–1592.
88. Menon, K. M. J., Dorfman, R. I., and Forchielli, E. (1967): Influence of gonadotrophins on the cholesterol side-chain cleavage reaction by rat-testis mitochondrial preparations. *Biochim. Biophys. Acta,* 148:486–494.
89. Menon, K. M. J., Drosdowsky, M., Dorfman, R. I., and Forchielli, E. (1965): Side-chain cleavage of cholesterol-26-^{14}C and 20α-hydroxycholesterol-22-^{14}C by rat testis mitochondrial preparations and the effect of gonadotrophin administration and hypophysectomy. *Steroids,* Suppl. 1:95–111.
90. Mills, N. C., Mills, T. M., and Means, A. R. (1977): Morphological and biochemical changes which occur during postnatal development and maturation of the rat testis. *Biol. Reprod.,* 17:124–130.
91. Mizutani, S., Tsujimura, T., Akashi, S., and Matsumoto, K. (1977): Lack of metabolism of progesterone, testosterone and pregnenolone to 5α-products in monkey and human testes compared with rodent testes. *J. Clin. Endocrinol. Metab.,* 44:1023–1031.
92. Moger, W. H. (1977): Serum 5-alpha-androstane-3-alpha, 17-beta-diol, androsterone, and testosterone concentrations in male rat—Influence of age and gonadotropin stimulation. *Endocrinology,* 100:1027–1032.
93. Moger, W. H., and Armstrong, D. T. (1974): Steroid metabolism by the immature rat testis. *Can. J. Biochem.,* 52:744–750.
94. Morris, M. D., and Chaikoff, I. L. (1959): The origin of cholesterol in liver, small intestine, adrenal gland, and testis of the rat: Dietary versus endogenous contributions. *J. Biol. Chem.,* 234:1095–1097.
95. Moyle, W. R., Jungas, R. L., and Greep, R. O. (1973): Metabolism of free and esterified cholesterol by Leydig-cell tumour mitochondria. *Biochem. J.,* 134:415–424.
96. Nayfeh, S. N., and Baggett, B. (1969): Metabolism of progesterone by rat testicular homogenates. III. Inhibitory effects of intermediates and other steroids. *Steroids,* 14:269–283.
97. Negro-Vilar, A., Krulich, L., and McCann, S. M. (1973): Changes in serum prolactin and gonadotropins during sexual development of the male rat. *Endocrinology,* 93:660–664.
98. Neumann, H. C., Potts, G. O., Ryan, W. R., and Stonner, F. W. (1970): Steroidal heterocycles. XIII. 4α,5-epoxy-5α-androst-2-eno-(2,3-d)isoxazoles and related compounds. *J. Med. Chem.,* 13:948–951.
99. Nevile, A. M., and Engel, L. L. (1968): Inhibition of α- and β-hydroxysteroid dehydrogenases and steroid Δ-isomerase by substrate analogues. *J. Clin. Endocrinol. Metab.,* 28:49–60.
100. Notation, A. D., and Ungar, F. (1972): Testis steroid sulfatase activity in rats treated with chorionic gonadotrophin. *Endocrinology,* 90:1537–1542.
101. Odell, W. D., Swerdloff, R. S., Bain, J., Wollesen, F., and Grover, P. K. (1974): The effect of sexual maturation on testicular response to LH stimulation of testosterone secretion in the intact rat. *Endocrinology,* 95:1380–1384.
102. Oh, R., and Tamaoki, B. (1970): Steroidogenesis in equine testis. *Acta Endocrinol. (Kbh),* 64:1–16.
103. Oh, R., and Tamaoki, B. (1973): Intermicrosomal distribution of aromatizing enzyme system in equine testicular tissue. *Acta Endocrinol. (Kbh),* 72:366–375.
104. Oshima, H., Nankin, H. R., Troën, P., Yoshida, K., and Ochi-ai, K. (1977): Leydig cell number and function in infertile men. In: *The Testis in Normal and Infertile Men,* edited by P. Troën and H. R. Nankin, pp. 445–455. Raven Press, New York.
105. Oshima, H., Paraska, L., Yoshida, K. I., and Troën, P. (1977): Studies of the human testis. VIII. Product activation of 17β-hydroxysteroid oxidoreductase for testosterone. *J. Clin. Endocrinol. Metab.,* 45:1097–1099.
106. Parvinen, M., Hurme, P., and Niemi, M. (1970): Penetration of exogenous testosterone, pregnenolone, progesterone and cholesterol into the seminiferous tubules of the rat. *Endocrinology,* 87:1082–1084.
107. Payne, A. H. (1972): Gonadal steroid sulfatase. V. Human testicular steroid sulfatase: Partial

characterization and possible regulation by free steroids. *Biochim. Biophys. Acta,* 258:473–483.

108. Payne, A. H., and Jaffe, R. B. (1970): Comparative roles of dehydroepiandrosterone sulfate and androstenediol sulfate as precursors of testicular androgens. *Endocrinology,* 87:316–322.

109. Payne, A. H., Kelch, R. P., Musich, S. S., and Halpern, M. E. (1976): Intratesticular site of aromatization in the human. *J. Clin. Endocrinol. Metab.,* 42:1081–1087.

110. Payne, A. H., Kelch, R. P., Murono, E. P., and Kerlan, J. T. (1977): Hypothalamic pituitary and testicular function during sexual maturation of the male rat. *J. Endocrinol.,* 72:17–26.

111. Pearlman, P. L. (1950): The functional significance of testis cholesterol in the rat: Effects of hypophysectomy and cryptorchidism. *Endocrinology,* 46:341–346.

112. Pearlman, P. L. (1950): The functional significance of testis cholesterol in the rat: Histochemical observations on testes following hypophysectomy and experimental cryptorchidism. *Endocrinology,* 46:347–352.

113. Pierrepoint, C. G., Griffiths, K., Grant, J. K., and Stewart, J. S. S. (1966): Neutral steroid sulphation and oestrogen biosynthesis by a feminizing Leydig cell tumour of the testis. *J. Endocrinol.,* 35:409–417.

114. Pirke, K. M., Doerr, P., Sintermann, R., and Vogt, H. J. (1977): Age-dependence of testosterone precursors in plasma of normal adult males. *Acta Endocrinol. (Kbh),* 86:415–429.

115. Podesta, E. J., and Rivarola, M. A. (1974): Concentration of androgens in whole testis seminiferous tubules and interstitial tissue of rats at different stages of development. *Endocrinology,* 95:455–461.

116. Pokel, J. D., Moyle, W. R., and Greep, R. O. (1972): Depletion of esterified cholesterol in mouse testis and Leydig cell tumors by luteinizing hormone. *Endocrinology,* 91:323–325.

117. Purvis, J. L., and Menard, R. H. (1975): Compartmentation of microsomal cytochrome P-450 and 17α-hydroxylase activity in the rat testis. In: *Hormonal Regulation of Spermatogenesis,* edited by F. S. French, V. Hansson, E. M. Ritzén, and S. N. Nayfeh, pp. 65–84. Plenum Press, New York.

118. Purvis, K., Brenner, P. L., Landgren, B. M., Cekan, Z., and Diczfalusy, E. (1975): Plasma levels of unconjugated steroids and gonadotrophins under normal and pathological conditions. *Clin. Endocrinol.,* 4:237–246.

119. Purvis, K., Clausen, O. P. F., and Hansson, V. (1978): Age-related changes in responsiveness of rat Leydig cell to hCG. *J. Reprod. Fert.,* 52:379–386.

120. Purvis, K., Haug, E., Clausen, O. P. F., Naess, O., and Hansson, V. (1977): Endocrine status of the testicular feminized male (tfm) rat. *Molec. Cell. Endocrinol.,* 8:317–334.

121. Roberts, K. D., Bandy, L., and Lieberman, S. (1969): The occurrence and metabolism of 20α-hydroxycholesterol in bovine adrenal preparations. *Biochemistry,* 8:1259–1270.

122. Rodriguez-Rigau, L. J., Tcholakian, R. K., Smith, K. D., and Steinberger, E. (1977): In vitro steroid metabolic studies in human testis. I. Effects of estrogen on progesterone metabolism. *Steroids,* 29:771–786.

123. Rodriguez-Rigau, L. J., Weiss, D. B., Smith, K. D., and Steinberger E. (1978): Suggestion of abnormal testicular steroidogenesis in some oligospermic men. *Acta Endocrinol. (Kbh),* 87:400–412.

124. Rosness, P. A., Sunde, A., and Eik-Nes, K. B. (1977): Production and effects of 7α-hydroxytestosterone on testosterone and dihydrotestosterone metabolism in rat testis. *Biochim. Biophys. Acta,* 488:55–68.

125. Ruder, H. J., Loriaux, D. L., Sherins, R. J., and Lipsett, M. B. (1974): Leydig cell function in men with disorders of spermatogenesis. *J. Clin. Endocrinol. Metab.,* 38:244–247.

126. Ruokonen, A., Laatikainen, T., Laitinen, E. A., and Vihko, R. (1972): Free and sulfate-conjugated neutral steroids in human testis tissue. *Biochemistry,* 11:1411–1416.

127. Ruokonen, A., and Vihko, R. (1974): Steroid metabolism in testis tissue: concentrations of unconjugated and sulfated neutral steroids in boar testis. *J. Steroid Biochem.,* 5:33–38.

128. Saez, J., de Peretti, M. E., Morera, A. M., David, M., and Bertrand, J. (1971): Familial male pseudohermaphroditism with gynecomastia due to a testicular 17-ketosteroid reductase defect. I. Studies in vivo. *J. Clin. Endocrinol. Metab.,* 32:604–610.

129. Salokangas, R. A., Rilling, H. C., and Samuels, L. T. (1964): Terpene metabolism in the rat testis-I. The conversion of isopentenylpyrophosphate to squalene and sterols. *Biochemistry,* 3:833–837.

130. Samuels, L. T., Bussman, L., Matsumoto, K., and Huseby, R. A. (1975): Organization of androgen biosynthesis in the testis. *J. Steroid Biochem.,* 6:291–296.
131. Samuels, L. T., and Matsumoto, K. (1974): Localization of enzymes involved in testosterone biosynthesis by the mouse testis. *Endocrinology,* 94:55–60.
132. Schwarzel, W. C., Kruggel, W. G., and Brodie, H. (1973): Studies on the mechanism of estrogen biosynthesis. VIII. The development of inhibitors of the enzyme system in human placenta. *Endocrinology,* 92:866–880.
133. Shikita, M., and Hall, P. F. (1967): Action of human chorionic gonadotrophin in vivo upon microsomal enzymes in testes of hypophysectomized rats. *Biochim. Biophys. Acta,* 141:433–435.
134. Shikita, M., and Hall, P. F. (1967): The action of human chorionic gonadotrophin in vivo upon microsomal enzymes of immature rat testis. *Biochim. Biophys. Acta,* 136:484–497.
135. Shikita, M., Ogiso, T., and Tamaoki, B. (1965): Effect of inhibitors on testicular microsomal steroid 17α-hydroxylase and 17α-hydroxypregnene C_{17-20}-lyase. *Biochim. Biophys. Acta,* 105:516–522.
136. Sowell, J. G., Folman, Y., and Eik-Nes, K. B. (1974): Androgen metabolism in rat testicular tissue. *Endocrinology,* 94:346–354.
137. Sulimovici, S., Bartoov, B., and Lunenfeld, B. (1973): Localization of 3β-hydroxysteroid dehydrogenase in the inner membrane subfraction of rat testis mitochondria. *Biochim. Biophys. Acta,* 321:27–40.
138. Sulimovici, S., and Boyd, G. S. (1969): The cholesterol side-chain cleavage enzymes in steroid-hormone producing tissues. *Vitam. Horm.,* 27:199–234.
139. Tamaoki, B. (1973): Steroidogenesis and cell structure, biochemical pursuit of sites of steroid biosynthesis. *J. Steroid Biochem.,* 4:89–118.
140. Toren, D., Menon, K. M., Forchielli, E., and Dorfman, R. I. (1964): In vitro enzymatic cleavage of the cholesterol side-chain cleavage in rat testis preparations. *Steroids,* 3:381–390.
141. Troën, P., Yanaihara, T., Nankin, H., Tominaga, T., and Lever, H. (1970): Assessment of gonadotropin therapy in infertile males. In: *The Human Testis,* edited by E. Rosemberg and C. A. Paulsen, pp. 591–604. Plenum Press, New York.
142. Tsai, S. C., Ying, B. P., and Gaylor, J. (1964): Testicular sterols. I. Incorporation of mevalonate and acetate into sterols by testicular tissue from rats. *Arch. Biochem. Biophys.,* 105:329–338.
143. Tsujimura, T., Mizutani, S., and Matsumoto, K. (1975): Pathway from progesterone to 5α-reduced C_{19} steroids not involving androstenedione and testosterone in immature mouse testes in vitro. *Endocrinology,* 96:515–518.
144. Van Beurden, W. M. O., Roodnat, B., and van der Molen, H. J. (1978): Effects of oestrogens and FSH on LH stimulation of steroid production by testis Leydig cells from immature rats. *Int. J. Androl.,* Suppl. 2:374–383.
145. Van der Molen, H. J., Bijleveld, M. J., van der Vusse, G. J., and Cooke, B. A. (1972): Effect of gonadotrophins on cholesterol and cholesterol esters as precursors of steroid production in the testis. *J. Endocrinol.,* 57:vi–vii.
146. Van der Molen, H. J., and Eik-Nes, K. B. (1971): Biosynthesis and secretion of steroids by the canine testis. *Biochim. Biophys. Acta,* 248:343–362.
147. Van der Molen, H. J., Grootegoed, J. A., de Greef-Bijleveld, M. J., Rommerts, F. F. G., and van der Vusse, G. J. (1975): Distribution of steroids, steroid production and steroid-metabolizing enzymes in rat testis. In: *Hormonal Regulation of Spermatogenesis,* edited by F. S. French, V. Hansson, E. M. Ritzén, and S. N. Nayfeh, pp. 3–23. Plenum Press, New York.
148. Van der Vusse, G. J., Kalkman, M. L., and van der Molen, H. J. (1973): Endogenous production of steroids by subcellular fractions from total rat testis and from isolated interstitial tissue and seminiferous tubules. *Biochim. Biophys. Acta,* 297:179–185.
149. Van der Vusse, G. J., Kalkman, M. L., and van der Molen, H. J. (1974): 3β-Hydroxysteroid dehydrogenase in rat testis tissue. Inter- and subcellular localization and inhibition by cyanoketone and nagarse. *Biochim. Biophys. Acta,* 348:404–414.
150. Van der Vusse, G. J., Kalkman, M. L., and van der Molen, H. J. (1975): Endogenous steroid production in cellular and subcellular fractions of rat testis after prolonged treatment with gonadotropins. *Biochim. Biophys. Acta,* 380:473–485.
151. Van Doorn, L. G., de Bruijn, H. W. A., Galjaard, H., and van der Molen, H. J. (1974): Intercellular transport of steroids in the infused rabbit testis. *Biol. Reprod.,* 10:47–53.

152. Van Lier, J. E., Rousseau, J., Langlois, R., and Fisher, G. J. (1977): Mechanism of cholesterol side-chain cleavage. II. The enzymic hydroperoxide-glycol rearrangement of the epimeric 20-hydroperoxycholesterols in ^{18}O-enriched water. *Biochim. Biophys. Acta,* 487:395–399.
153. Virdis, R., Saenger, P., Senior, P., and New, M. I. (1978): Endocrine studies in a pubertal male pseudohermaphrodite with 17-ketosteroid reductase deficiency. *Acta Endocrinol. (Kbh),* 87:212–224.
154. Wiebe, J. P. (1976): Steroidogenesis in rat Leydig cells: Changes in activity of 5-ane and 5-ene 3β-hydroxysteroid dehydrogenases during sexual maturation. *Endocrinology,* 98:505–513.
155. Wilson, J. D. (1975): Metabolism of testicular androgens. In: *Handbook of Physiology,* Section 7: Endocrinology, Vol. V, edited by R. O. Greep and E. B. Astwood, pp. 491–508. American Physiological Society, Washington D.C.
156. Wilson, J. D., and Siiteri, P. K. (1973): Developmental pattern of testosterone synthesis in the fetal gonad of the rabbit. *Endocrinology,* 92:1182–1191.
157. Yanaihara, T., and Troën, P. (1972): Studies of the human testis. I. Biosynthetic pathways for androgen formation in human testicular tissue in vitro. *J. Clin. Endocrinol. Metab.,* 34:783–792.
158. Kelch, R. P., Jenner, M. R., Weinstein, R., Kaplan, S. L., and Grumbach, M. M. (1972): Estradiol and testosterone secretion by human, simian, and canine testes, in males with hypogonadism and in male hermaphrodites with the feminizing testes syndrome. *J. Clin. Invest.,* 52:824–830.
159. de Jong, F. H., Hey, A. H., and van der Molen, H. J. (1973): Effect of gonadotrophins on the secretion of oestradiol-17β and testosterone by the rat testis. *J. Endocrinol.,* 57:277–284.

The Testis, edited by H. Burger and D. de Kretser.
Raven Press, New York © 1981.

11

The Influence of Testicular Function on Related Reproductive Organs

M.-C. Orgebin-Crist

*Department of Obstetrics and Gynecology, Vanderbilt University,
Nashville, Tennessee 37232*

The male gonad exerts an early inductive influence on the development of the genital system. At the beginning of this century, Bouin and Ancel (12) postulated that a distinctive cell type in the male gonad produces a male hormone which is responsible for the development of normal male characteristics.

The primary consideration in this chapter is the manner in which the testis influences the differentiation and the growth of the male accessory sex organs. The important influence of the testis and testicular hormones on the external genitalia and phenotypic traits of the male will not be considered.

FETAL PERIOD

Formation of the Male Sex Accessory Organs

Following fusion of the maternal and paternal gametes, the genotypic sex is determined, the Y chromosome being present only in the cells of the male embryo. Male and female embryos pass through a common "indifferent or ambisexual phase" in which the two sexes are morphologically identical.

The indifferent gonad arises as a proliferation of the coelomic epithelium on the surface of the urogenital ridge. The germ cells enter the primitive gonad from an extragonadal source and can be recognized as large round cells distributed among the more elongated and irregularly shaped nongerminal elements. The urogenital ridge comprises also the Wolffian ducts which are situated dorsolaterally in the urogenital ridge. Later they become shifted ventrally and lie ventrolaterally at the summit of the ridge. The Mullerian ducts develop as a thickening of the coelomic epithelium ventral to the Wolffian duct. The epithelial area sinks in forming the Mullerian funnel which then grows caudally as a solid cord, later a duct. At the lower end of the urogenital ridge the Mullerian ducts cross the Wolffian ducts ventrally to meet and fuse in the midline. The fused ducts form the uterovaginal canal which comes in contact with the urogenital sinus causing an elevation of its dorsal wall (the Mullerian tubercle). The Wolffian ducts open in the urogenital sinus on either side of the Mullerian tubercle.

The phase of sexual differentiation follows the ambisexual stage. The mechanisms controlling the initial events in testicular differentiation remain largely unknown. In human fetuses, males can be identified between the 32nd and 65th days (31,39) after fertilization, while females are recognized by their negative features (absence of tunica albuginea and seminiferous cords) and cannot be identified as females before the 65th day or later (32,39). In the rat, the first sign of testicular differentiation occurs on the 13th day by the differentiation of Sertoli cells which enlarge, establish contact with each other, and envelop the germ cells to outline the seminiferous cords (49,50). The process of testicular differentiation begins near the mesonephric tubules, suggesting that they may release an inductive substance. At the same time, a distinct tunica albuginea is formed at the periphery of the gonad. The germ cells continue to divide mitotically within the seminiferous cords and the Sertoli cells form a continuous palisade around the seminiferous cords. At that time the gonocytes lie centrally in the cord. On the 14th day the seminiferous cords are organized in the anterior part of the testis, and differentiation proceeds along an anteroposterior axis. The differentiation of the interstitial tissue parallels the differentiation of the seminiferous cords. The differentiation of the excretory pathway, through which spermatozoa are later transported, begins with the contact of the mesonephric tubules with the rete testis, which in turn contacts the seminiferous cords. Most of the mesonephric tubules which are not incorporated in this new excretory pathway undergo atrophy; a few remain as blind remnants forming the paradidymis and the appendix of the epididymis.

The anterior portion of the Wolffian duct disappears while the middle portion is transformed into the epididymis. The distal portion forms the ductus deferens. The seminal vesicles grow out as a diverticulum of the Wolffian duct and the duct below the diverticulum becomes the common ejaculatory duct. The prostate is derived from the intermediate or pelvic portion of the urogenital sinus which receives the Wolffian and Mullerian ducts in its dorsal wall; it arises as a series of epithelial diverticula which becomes enveloped by mesenchyme. The bulbo-urethral gland (Cowper's gland) develops as a diverticulum of the distal or phallic portion of the urogenital sinus. The Mullerian ducts largely disappear in the male; however, two remnants persist, the appendix of the testis (inconsistent) situated at the anterior pole of the gonad and the utriculus prostaticus derived from the fused terminal portions of the Mullerian ducts at the level of the prostate.

Influence of the Testis on the Development of the Male Genital Tract

Little is known about the mechanisms of early sexual differentiation. From the sequence of events described above, the mesonephric tubules and the early

Sertoli cells may have a preeminent place in this differentiation. The mesenchyme plays a dominant role in regional differentiation (18).

The differentiated testis controls the masculinization of the genital tract and in the absence of testis, even in genetic males, the genital tract develops phenotypically as female. The demonstration of the masculinizing influence of the fetal testis upon the genital system was made by Jost in experiments involving castration of rabbit fetuses before the initiation of sexual differentiation (47,48). The masculinization of the male genital tract comprises several sets of events which are independently controlled: regression of the Mullerian duct, differentiation of the Wolffian duct, and formation of the male sex accessory glands.

Regression of the Mullerian Duct

In male embryos, the onset of Mullerian duct degeneration precedes the regression of Wolffian ducts in the female and degeneration proceeds at a rapid rate. In the rat, at the 14th day of gestation the Mullerian duct is a tube approximately 5 μm in diameter, composed of columnar cells, and surrounded by a ring of undifferentiated mesenchyme. Electron microscopic studies (76) show that at the 15th day of gestation large lysosome-like dense bodies appear in a few columnar cells. Between the 15th day and 16th day, striking changes occur: the number of epithelial cells per cross section is lower (7–10 versus 14–18 2 days earlier), and the cells lose their polarity and organization. Many macrophages are present in the surrounding mesenchyme and among the duct epithelial cells. The mesenchyme condenses to a tight ring around the degenerating duct. By the 17th day, degeneration of the Mullerian duct is complete. An occasional macrophage may be seen in the area, and the mesenchymal cells are dispersed.

The mechanism controlling the rapid regression of Mullerian duct was not understood until Jost's experiments of fetal rabbit castration (5,6). Removal of the gonads on the 19th day resulted in regression of the Wolffian duct but maintenance of the Mullerian ducts in male embryos. Implantation of crystalline testosterone after castration stimulated the Wolffian ducts, but did not induce the regression of the Mullerian ducts. From these experiments, Jost postulated the existence of an anti-Mullerian hormone produced by the fetal testis distinct from the masculinizing hormone responsible for the stimulation of the Wolffian ducts. The specific effect of the fetal testis on Mullerian ducts was clearly demonstrated by Picon in 1969 (69). She showed that rat Mullerian ducts were maintained in explants cultured *in vitro* without gonads, but regressed when explants were co-cultured with fetal testicular tissue. Sensitivity of the Mullerian duct to the testicular hormone is transient and proceeds in the rat craniocaudally from the 14th day to the 16th day.

Introduction of this bioassay for anti-Mullerian activity has permitted rapid advances on the nature of the testicular factor responsible for Mullerian duct regression. As already mentioned, testicular androgens do not induce regression of rat Mullerian ducts *in vitro* (41). Although it has been reported that the Mullerian ducts of birds regress when exposed to testosterone *in vitro* (57,94), a careful study using various concentrations of testosterone showed that the alleged inhibiting effect of testosterone on avian Mullerian ducts was in fact a result of toxicity not observed at lower testosterone concentrations (88).

Interestingly, the factor causing regression of Mullerian ducts is not species-specific. Rat Mullerian ducts regress when co-cultured with fetal testes from humans (42), calves (43), pigs (46), rabbits (70), or even chicks; although in the latter case the reverse was not true, i.e., mammalian tissues (fetal, rat, or calf) did not induce the regression of chick Mullerian ducts (88).

The anti-Mullerian activity of the fetal testis precedes the appearance of Leydig cells, suggesting that these cells are not responsible for it. This was amply confirmed in further experiments where clusters of isolated fetal interstitial cells co-cultured with Mullerian ducts failed to induce their regression (43). From the two main cell populations in the seminiferous cord, the Sertoli cells appear to be the site of production of the anti-Mullerian activity. Human testicular tissues were submitted to radiation and though 3% of germ cells remained, the gonad still possessed a normal anti-Mullerian activity (44). Sertoli cells grown in culture, harvested, and transferred to. organ culture conditions are still able to induce Mullerian duct regression, although to a less extent than cells from whole testis (10).

The presumptive anti-Mullerian substance produced by the fetal Sertoli cells is not of steroidal nature (41), can exert its effect at a distance (24), and is released in the culture medium of fetal testicular explants (45). The substance isolated from such culture media is a protein of relatively high molecular weight, between 200,000 and 320,000 daltons (68).

In summary, in XY embryos a possible secretion of the early mesonephric tubules may be responsible for induction of the seminiferous cords. The fetal Sertoli cells secrete a distinct factor causing the Mullerian ducts to regress, while the Leydig cells secrete androgens which preserve and permit the transformation of the Wolffian duct into the epididymis and ductus deferens.

Differentiation of the Wolffian Ducts and the Urogenital Sinus

Unlike the regression of Mullerian ducts, the differentiation of the Wolffian ducts and the urogenital sinus depends on the presence of testicular steroidal hormones. This has been clearly demonstrated by Jost (47,48), who suppressed the development of male accessory organs in undifferentiated rabbit embryos by surgical castration or administration of antiandrogenic substances such as cyproterone acetate and stimulated it in early female embryos by implantation of testes or testosterone crystals. These *in vivo* experiments were confirmed by Price and co-workers (74,75), who showed that the sexual primordia (Wolffian ducts and cephalic portion of urogenital sinuses) differentiate *in vitro* and form prostatic buds and rudimentary seminal vesicles if cultured in close contact with a fetal testis or testosterone. In the latter system, however, prostatic buds develop spontaneously, although to a lesser extent, in control cultures without androgen. While the role of androgens for growth and maintenance of accessory glands is well established, these observations raised questions about the role of testosterone as an initiator of gland development.

In Wistar rats, prostatic buds appeared in male embryos after 18.5 days of gestation (54). Male urogenital sinuses from 17.5 and 18.5 day fetuses when cultured *in vitro* in control media formed buds which were enhanced in size and number by the addition of testosterone or 5α-dihydrotestosterone to media. Sinuses from 15.5 and 16.5 day embryos did not form buds spontaneously, but responded to either continuous hormone exposure or a short pulse at the initiation of the culture. Sinuses from 14.5 day fetuses did not develop spontaneously nor did they respond to testosterone, but formed prostatic buds after exposure to 5α-dihydrotestosterone (54). The authors concluded that spontaneous prostatic bud formation was owing to exposure to endogenous testosterone prior to explantation. Testes of fetal rats possess the enzymes necessary for converting acetate to testosterone as early as 15.5 days of gestation and contain measurable amounts of testosterone (0.09 ng/mg) (92). The testosterone levels rise to 2.76 ng/ml at 18.5 days of gestation (92). Fetal testis from 15.5 and 18.5 day fetuses grown in close contact with fetal urogenital sinuses or mature prostatic explants induced prostatic bud formation in the former or increased the height of the prostatic epithelium in the latter (54). Testosterone binding protein(s), which in other tissues mediate the action of testosterone, are present in genital tracts of 14.5 to 15 day old fetuses (34).

Considered together, these lines of evidence indicate strongly that the capacity of the fetal testis to synthesize testosterone is acquired early in embryogenesis and that testicular androgens are necessary for the initiation as well as the continued growth of the prostate. The lower affinity of androgen binding protein from reproductive tracts of 14.5 to 15 day rat embryos for 5α-dihydrotestosterone than for testosterone (34) is puzzling, in view of the ability of 5α-dihydrotestosterone (but not testosterone) to induce prostatic bud formation in embryos of identical age (54).

SEXUAL MATURATION PERIOD

The dependence of male sex accessory glands on testicular hormones for growth and differentiation is not restricted to the early fetal period. In the rat, which has been studied most intensively, the rapid growth of the seminal vesicle, prostate, and epididymis parallels the rise in circulating androgen levels and occurs between 35 and 60 days of age in intact but not castrated rats (13,23,35,37,53,62,81,83,87). The same correlation has been observed in other species (17,22,29,60,61,79,82). However, changes do occur in these organs prior to the onset of rapid growth. In the rat and mouse, rapid differentiation of the cells of the seminal vesicle, prostate, epididymis, and vas deferens occurs between 10 and 21 days after birth (19,27,28,55,56). The major changes include proliferation of the endoplasmic reticulum, growth of the Golgi apparatus, appearance in the prostate and seminal vesicle of secretory vacuoles, and stereocilia in the epididymis. How much of this cyto-differentiation is hormonally dependent is unclear in the rat where the prepubertal period is very short. In the rat and the monkey relatively high androgen levels have been recorded at birth (23,80). In the rat a second rise occurs with a maximum on the 20th day prior to the pubertal rise after the 35th day (62), while in the monkey androgen levels remain low until the third year (79,80). The monkey epididymis responds to the late gestation rise in androgens by cyto-differentiation of the epithelium (1). From 130 days of fetal life until parturition, all epithelial cells show marked cellular differentiation: increase in height, development of the Golgi complex and the endoplasmic reticulum, appearance of cilia at the apex of some cells in the ductuli efferentes, and stereocilia in the remaining part of the epididymis. After birth, the epithelial cells of the epididymis regress to an undifferentiated state of low cuboidal epithelium without apical modifications and remain so until puberty. When fetuses are castrated between the 106th and 112th day of gestation, the epididymis does not show any sign of cellular differentiation unless a drug with masculinizing property such as medroxyprogesterone is administered to the pregnant female. Moreover, the regressed epididymal epithelium is able to respond to exogenous androgens at any time during the prepubertal period, even in animals castrated at the 104th day of fetal life and treated with testosterone propionate 6 months after birth (1). These experiments clearly showed that differentiation of epididymal cells is dependent on the testicular androgen output of the fetus or the young.

This does not exclude the possibility that other hormones may have a physiological role in the growth of sex accessory glands acting in synergy with androgens. Rat serum estradiol levels are elevated at birth, thereafter fall, but increase again between the 9th and 19th days to levels higher than those observed later in life (Fig. 1) (23). Prolactin levels are low at birth, but increase between the 20th and 30th days just before the rapid growth of male accessory organs (Fig. 1) (23,25,63). In the lamb where the prepubertal period is longer than in the rat, the rise in prolactin is even more striking (17). Levels of the hormone are basal until the 70th day, then peak sharply concomitantly with the rapid increase of testicular weight and before the rise in accessory gland weights. Receptors for both estrogens and prolactin have been identified in the prostate, seminal vesicle, and epididymis of immature and mature males of several species (2,4,7,8,15,20,21,51,52,90,93), indicating that these hormones could interact with these tissues and have physiological significance in the hormonal regulation of sex accessory glands.

Estrogens have been shown to produce a variety of effects in sex accessory glands, varying from one of enhancement of weight and function to atrophy or the induction of squamous metaplasia (77). These discrepancies may result from a dose-effect relationship, species differences, the type of target organ studied [seminal vesicle being more sensitive than prostate (77)], and within an organ the differential estrogen sensitivity of cellular types. Estrogens appear

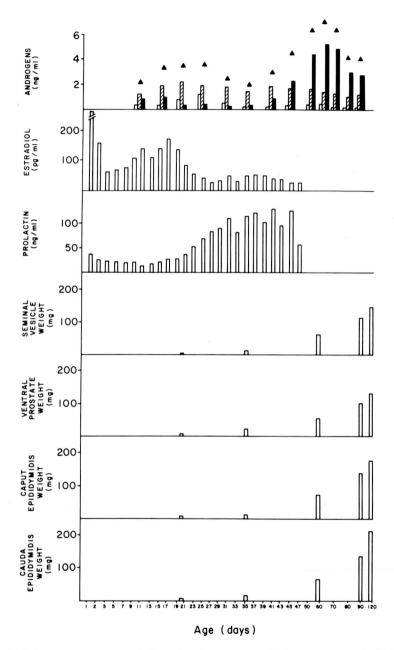

Age (days)

FIG. 1. Androgen:serum concentration of testosterone + dihydrotestosterone (solid bars). 5α-androstane-3α, 17β-diol (stripped bars), and androsterone (open bars) in male rats of various ages. Triangles are the sum of mean concentrations of the three steroids (from ref. 62). Prolactin and estradiol:serum concentration in male rats (from ref. 23). Seminal vesicle, ventral prostate, caput and cauda epididymidis:changes in weight during postnatal maturation in the rat (from ref. 83).

to stimulate, preferentially, growth of fibromuscular tissue (77). This was confirmed in a recent report (8) where separation of the epithelial component from the muscular component of the adult guinea pig seminal vesicle was achieved and where castration produced a much greater regression of the epithelium than the muscle. Estradiol replacement further reduced the epithelium, but caused a significant growth of the fibromuscular component of the gland. The effect of castration and estrogen replacement on prostatic weight parallels the one observed on the weight of the seminal vesicle, but to a lesser extent. Following injection of ^{3}H-estradiol, the highest labeled hormone concentration was recovered from the muscle rather than the epithelial component of the seminal vesicle. The highest amount of specific estrogen binding was also found in the muscle of the seminal vesicle (8). These studies raised the possibility that in addition to a central effect, estrogen may have a physiological role in the hormonal regulation of sex accessory fibromuscular tissues. Whether or not this is of more significance during the prepubertal and pubertal period is not known.

Prolactin has also been implicated in the hormonal regulation of adult male sex accessory glands. Grayhack (33) reported that prostatic atrophy is greater after hypophysectomy than after castration, implying that a pituitary factor is necessary in addition to androgen to maintain the prostate, and in the hypophysectomized castrated adult rat prolactin synergizes with androgen to increase prostatic weight. However, in subsequent studies, the enhancing effect of prolactin was found to be small, and at times at the limit of statistical significance, raising doubt as to the essentiality of prolactin for maintenance of the integrity and function of the sex accessory glands (for review see ref. 95). Recently, Grayhack's observation in the adult rat has been confirmed (84), but, in addition, several reports have clearly demonstrated the role of prolactin in prostatic and seminal vesicular growth in immature rats. Prolactin secreted from a single pituitary graft under the kidney capsule of the 30 day old rat stimulated the sex accessory glands in intact, castrated, castrated-adrenalectomized, or hypophysectomized rats (64). Circulating levels of prolactin were higher than normal, while FSH and LH levels were not changed. Also, prolactin and testosterone in castrated rats had an additive effect. Chronic deficiency of circulating prolactin obtained by repeated injection of an antiserum to prolactin to 3 day old rats for 58 days or by injection of prolactin release inhibitors to 30 day old mice significantly reduces prostatic and seminal vesicular weights (6,38). The effects of prolactin on sex accessory glands are manifold: prolactin augments testicular responsiveness to LH by increasing LH receptor levels in the testis (9,11) and the availability of precursor for the biosynthesis of androgens (5), thereby increasing the secretion of androgenic steroids by the testis (36). Prolactin has also a direct effect on sex accessory glands by increasing the nuclear uptake of 5α-dihydrotestosterone, suggesting that prolactin may increase the number of androgen receptors (3). This could explain the potentiating effect of prolactin on the androgen responsiveness of sex accessory glands and, together with the effect of prolactin on testicular steroidogenesis, points to an important role for prolactin in the stimulation of sex accessory glands before and during sexual maturation.

ADULT PERIOD

The dependence of male sex accessory glands upon testicular hormones does not cease with puberty and continues in the adult. This has long been recognized and numerous recent reviews, which need not be duplicated here, describe various aspects of the regulation of the structure, biochemistry, and function of the male accessory sex organs (59,65,67). Thus, it has been shown that testosterone enters the cells of these organs and becomes transformed into active metabolites, notably 5α-dihydrotestosterone, which after binding to specific cytoplasmic and nuclear receptors control the protein synthetic activity of the cells. Castration or hypophysectomy results in a morphological involution consisting of decreased duct and gland diameter, diminution in epithelial height, reduction in size of the Golgi apparatus and the endoplasmic reticulum. The secretory activity and the biochemical functions of the sex accessory glands are also depressed after castration or hypophysectomy and restored to normal or near normal levels with appropriate androgen therapy.

Circulating androgens are obviously indispensable to normal function, but recent evidence indicates that optimal function may be ensured by different mechanisms. First, depending upon the species, all sex accessory glands may not have the same sensitivity to circulating androgens. It has been reported that a dose of androgens sufficient to restore accessory gland function to normal in castrated rat or monkey maintains the epididymis at only 50% of the intact control levels (78). A further difference in hormone responsiveness between the prostate and the seminal vesicles in the rat has also been reported (85). In the rabbit, this differential sensitivity was not observed and the minimum dose of testosterone propionate necessary to maintain weight and secretory activity of the prostate and seminal vesicle maintained also the weight and secretory activity of the epididymis (40).

Species and organ differences in hormone sensitivity may be related to the existence of mechanisms for local hormonal exchange and control, differences in hormone metabolism, specificity of hormone receptors in the different tissues, and synergy with other hormones.

Androgens are available to all sex accessory glands through the circulatory system; but, in addition, mechanisms exist which enhance the exposure of some organs to higher concentrations of androgens than available to other organs. A counter-current exchange of testosterone has been shown to occur between the closely apposed veins and arteries of the pampiniform plexus in many species, thus increasing arterial testosterone levels. While the cauda epididymidis is supplied by the deferential artery which originates from the hypogastric artery and runs along the vas deferens, the caput epididymidis is vascularized by branches of the internal spermatic artery and is probably subjected to higher androgen levels (30).

Testosterone is also present in high concentration in the luminal fluid entering the epididymis [69 ng/ml testosterone in rabbit rete testis fluid compared to 1.9 ng/ml in peripheral plasma (16)]. The normal exposure of the initial portion of the epididymis to high androgen levels may explain why, after castration and androgen replacement or after ligation of the ductuli efferentes, the biochemical composition and cytological appearance of the epididymis is maintained with the exception of the initial segment of the epididymis (14,26,66).

The possibility that the epididymis exerts a local control on the prostate and seminal vesicles through the excurrent duct system has been suggested (86,89) and seemed to be confirmed when Pierrepoint and co-workers (71) found a significant reduction in the level of androgen-dependent RNA polymerase activity in the ventral prostate after vasectomy. They interpreted this finding as evidence of passage of androgens from the testes along the vas deferens to the prostate. Subsequent experiments suggested that the epididymis alone separated from its gonad could modulate the function of the prostate and seminal vesicle. Thus, the RNA polymerase activity of both glands was significantly increased in castrated rats with an intact androgen-maintained epididymis compared to castrated rats where the epididymis is removed with the testis (73). Further experiments showed that this local influence of the epididymis on the sex accessory glands was not exerted by a direct passage of substance from the lumen of the vas deferens to the prostate and the seminal vesicle, since ligation of the deferential veins produced the same reduction in RNA polymerase activity (72). The anatomical relationship of the deferential vein and the vas deferens is such that it is probably difficult to ligate the vas without some impairment of the blood flow in the deferential veins. It therefore appears that rather than a direct control through the luminal content of the vas (which has a much lower androgen concentration than the rete testis fluid), there is a retrograde flow of the deferential vein draining the cauda epididymidis into the prostatic vein, thus increasing androgen levels in that gland.

In addition to taking account of these local anatomical relationships which may differ in importance between different species, great caution should be exercised in extrapolating findings on the regulation of one sex accessory organ to the others within an animal or for the same organ between different species. For example, circulating testosterone is rapidly metabolized in target organs and metabolites (especially 5α-dihydrotestosterone) appear to be the biologically active androgen for the rat prostate (59,65). The levels of 5α-reductase activity, however, vary considerably between different target organs and between different species. The rabbit prostate, unlike the epididymis, has a very low 5α-reductase activity (58) and 5α-androstane-$3\alpha,17\beta$-diol dipropionate is much more potent than 5α-dihydrotestosterone propionate in promoting secretion of the prostate, but is ineffective in maintaining the function of the epididymis (40). In the dog, 3α-androstanediol is also more potent than 5α-dihydrotestosterone in inducing growth of the prostate (91).

In conclusion, testicular hormones throughout development have an inductive and morphogenetic influence on sex accessory glands. Androgens play a major role in this regulation. Biological activity is very much dependent on the secretion, circulation, and local concentration of testosterone and testosterone metabolites, on the availability of $\Delta 4$, 5α-reductase, and 3α-hydroxysteroid dehydrogenase activity, on the presence and affinity of transport androgen binding protein, on the presence and affinity of cytoplasmic and nuclear androgen receptors in each tissue, and on the possible synergy of androgens with other hormones.

Our understanding of testicular hormone action on male sex accessory glands is far from being complete and calls for a thorough examination of the above parameters in different species before definitive conclusions can be drawn.

ACKNOWLEDGMENT

This review was written in part during the tenure of a Fogarty Senior International Fellowship.

REFERENCES

1. Alexander, N. J. (1972): Prenatal development of the ductus epididymidis in the rhesus monkey. The effects of fetal castration. *Am. J. Anat.,* 135:119.
2. Aragona, C., and Friesen, H. (1975): Specific prolactin binding sites in the prostate and testis of rats. *Endocrinology,* 97:677.
3. Baker, H. W. G., Worgul, T. J., Santen, R. J., Jefferson, L. S., and Bardin, C. W. (1977): Effect of prolactin on nuclear androgens in perfused male accessory sex organs. In: *The Testis in Normal and Infertile Men,* edited by P. Troen and H. R. Nankin. Raven Press, New York.
4. Barkey, R. J., Shani, J., Amit, T., and D. Barzilai (1977): Specific binding of prolactin to seminal vesicle prostate and testicular homogenates of immature, mature and aged rats. *J. Endocrinol.,* 74:163.
5. Bartke, A. (1971): Effects of prolactin and luteinizing hormone on the cholesterol stores in the mouse testis. *J. Endocrinol.,* 49:317.
6. Bartke, A. (1974): Effects of inhibitors of pituitary prolactin release on testicular cholesterol stores, seminal vesicles weight, fertility and lactation in mice. *Biol. Reprod.,* 11:319.
7. Bashirelahi, N., and Armstrong, E. G. (1975): 17β-Estradiol binding by human prostate. In: *Normal and Abnormal Growth of the Prostate,* edited by M. Goland, pp. 632–649. Charles C Thomas, Springfield, Illinois.
8. Belis, J. A., Blume, C. D., and Mawhinney, M. G. (1977): Androgen and estrogen binding in male guinea pig accessory sex organs. *Endocrinology,* 101:726.
9. Bex, F. J., and Bartke, A. (1977): Testicular LH binding in the hamster: Modification by photoperiod and prolactin. *Endocrinology,* 100:1223.
10. Blanchard, M. G., and Josso, N. (1974): Source of the anti-Mullerian hormone synthesized by the fetal testis: Mullerian-inhibiting activity of fetal bovine Sertoli cells in tissue culture. *Pediatr. Res.,* 8:968.
11. Bohnet, H. G., and Friesen, H. G. (1976): Effect of prolactin and growth hormone on prolactin and LH receptors in the dwarf mouse. *J. Reprod. Fert.,* 48:307.
12. Bouin, P., and Ancel, P. (1903): Sur la signification de la glande interstitielle du testicule embryonnaire. *C. R. Soc. Biol.,* 55:1682.
13. Brooks, D. E. (1976): Changes in the composition of the excurrent duct system of the rat testis during postnatal development. *J. Reprod. Fert.,* 46:31.

14. Brooks, D. F. (1977): The androgenic control of the composition of the rat epididymis determined by efferent duct ligation or castration. *J. Reprod. Fert.,* 49:383.
15. Charreau, E. H., Attramadal, A., Torjesen, P. A., Calandra, R., Purvis, K., and Hansson, V. (1977): Androgen stimulation of prolactin receptors in rat prostate. *Mol. Cell. Endocrinol.,* 7:1.
16. Cooper, T. G., Danzo, B. J., DiPietro, D. L., McKenna, T. J., and Orgebin-Crist, M.-C. (1976): Some characteristics of rete testis fluid from rabbits. *Andrologia,* 8:87.
17. Courot, M. (1974): Blood plasma LH, testosterone and prolactin patterns in the male lamb. In: *Sexual Endocrinology of the Perinatal Period.* Colloque INSERM, 32:157.
18. Cunha, G. R. (1973): The role of androgens in the epithelia-mesenchymal interactions involved in prostatic morphogenesis in embryonic mice. *Anat. Rec.,* 175:87.
19. Dahnke, H. G. (1970): Die postnatale Entwicklung des Vesikulardrüsenepithels von Ratten. *Cytobiologie,* 2:445.
20. Danzo, B. J., Eller, B. C., Judy, L. A., Trautman, J. R., and Orgebin-Crist, M.-C. (1975): Estradiol binding in cytosol from epididymidis of immature rabbits. *Mol. Cell. Endocrinol.,* 2:91.
21. Danzo, B. J., Wolfe, M. S., and Curry, J. B. (1977): The presence of an estradiol binding component in cytosol from immature rat epididymides. *Mol. Cell. Endocrinol.,* 6:271.
22. Deane, H. W., and Wurzelmann, S. (1965): Electron microscopic observations on the postnatal differentiation of the seminal vesicle epithelium of the laboratory mouse. *Am. J. Anat.,* 117:91.
23. Döhler, K. D., and Wuttke, W. (1975): Changes with age in levels of serum gonadotropins, prolactin and gonadal steroids in prepubertal male and female rats. *Endocrinology,* 97:898.
24. Donahoe, P. K., Ito, Y., Marfatia, S., and Hendren, W. H. (1976): The production of Mullerian inhibiting substance by the fetal neonatal and adult rat. *Biol. Reprod.,* 15:329.
25. Dowd, A. J., and Bartke, A. (1972): Serum levels of prolactin, LH and FSH and testis cholesterol content in rats from one to ten weeks of age. *Biol. Reprod.,* 7:115.
26. Fawcett, D. W., and Hoffer, A. (1979): Failure of androgen alone to prevent regression of the initial segment of the rat epididymis after castration or efferent duct ligation. *Anat. Rec., Biol. Reprod.,* 20:162–171.
27. Flickinger, C. J. (1969): The pattern of growth of the Golgi complex during the fetal and postnatal development of the rat epididymis. *J. Ultrastruct. Res.,* 27:344.
28. Flickinger, C. J. (1971): Ultrastructural observations on the postnatal development of the rat prostate. *Z. Zellforsch. Mikrosk. Anat.,* 113:157.
29. Frasier, S. D., Gafford, F., and Horton, R. (1969): Plasma androgens in childhood and adolescence. *J. Clin. Endocrinol. Metab.,* 29:1404.
30. Free, M. J. (1977): Blood supply to the testis and its role in local exchange and transport of hormones. In: *The Testis,* Vol. IV, edited by A. D. Johnson and W. R. Gomes, pp. 39–90. Academic Press, New York.
31. Gillman, J. (1948): The development of the gonads in man with a consideration of the role of fetal endocrines and the histogenesis of ovarian tumors. *Carnegie Institute., Washington, D.C. Contributions to Embryology No. 210,* 32:81.
32. Glenister, T. W. (1962): The development of the utricle and of the so-called "middle" or "median" lobes of the human prostate. *J. Anat.,* 96:443.
33. Grayhack, J. T., Bunce, P. L., Kearns, J. W., and Scott, W. W. (1955): Influence of the pituitary on prostatic response to androgen in the rat. *Johns Hopkins Hosp. Bull.,* 96:154.
34. Gupta, D., and Bloch, E. (1976): Testosterone-binding protein in reproductive tracts of fetal rats. *Endocrinology,* 99:389.
35. Gupta, D., Rager, K., Zarzycki, J., and Eichner, M. (1975): Levels of luteinizing hormone, follicle-stimulating hormone, testosterone, dihydrotestosterone in the circulation of sexually maturing intact male rats and after orchidectomy and experimental bilateral cryptorchidism. *J. Endocrinol.,* 66:183.
36. Hafiez, A. A., Lloyd, C. W., and Bartke, A. (1972): The role of prolactin in the regulation of testis function: The effects of prolactin and luteinizing hormone on the plasma levels of testosterone and androstenedione in hypophysectomized rats. *J. Endocrinol.,* 52:327.
37. Hooker, C. W. (1942): Pubertal increase in responsiveness to androgen in the male rat. *Endocrinology,* 30:77.
38. Hostetter, M. W., and Piacsek, B. E. (1977): The effect of prolactin deficiency during sexual maturation in the male rat. *Biol. Reprod.,* 17:574.

39. Jirasek, J. E. (1967): The relationship between the structures of the testis and differentiation of the external genitalia and phenotype in man. *Ciba Foundation Colloquia Endocrinology,* 16:3.

40. Jones, R. (1977): Effect of testosterone, testosterone metabolites and anti-androgens on the function of the male accessory glands in the rabbit and the rat. *J. Endocrinol.,* 74:75.

41. Josso, N. (1971): Effect of testosterone and some of its 17 hydroxylated metabolites on the Mullerian duct of the foetal rat in organ culture. *Eur. J. Clin. Biol. Res.,* 16:694.

42. Josso, N. (1971): Interspecific character of the Mullerian-inhibiting substance: Action of the human fetal testis, ovary and adrenal on the fetal rat Mullerian duct in organ culture. *J. Clin. Endocrinol. Metab.,* 32:404.

43. Josso, N. (1973): In vitro synthesis of Mullerian-inhibiting hormone by seminiferous tubules isolated from the calf testis. *Endocrinology,* 93:829.

44. Josso, N. (1974): Mullerian-inhibiting activity of human fetal testicular tissue deprived of germ cells by in vitro irradiation. *Pediatr. Res.,* 8:755.

45. Josso, N., Forest, M. G., and Picard, J. Y. (1975): Mullerian-inhibiting activity of calf fetal testis. Relationship to testosterone and protein synthesis. *Biol. Reprod.,* 13:163.

46. Josso, N., Picard, J.-Y., and Tran, D. (1977): The anti-Mullerian hormone. Birth defects. In: *Birth Defects,* Vol. XIII. The National Foundation No. 2:59.

47. Jost, A. (1947): Recherches sur la différenciation sexuelle de l'embryon de lapin. III. Rôle des gonades foetales dans la différenciation sexuelle somatique. *Arch. Anat. Microsc. Morphol. Exp.,* 36:271.

48. Jost, A. (1953): Problems of fetal endocrinology: The gonadal and hypophyseal hormones. *Rec. Prog. Horm. Res.,* 8:379.

49. Jost, A. (1972): Données préliminaires sur les stades initiaux de la différenciation du testicule chez le rat. *Arch. Anat. Microsc. Morphol. Exp.,* 61:415.

50. Jost, A., Magre, S., Cressent, M. (1974): Sertoli cells and early testicular differentiation. In: *Male Fertility and Sterility,* edited by R. E. Mancini and L. Martini, pp. 1–11. Academic Press, New York.

51. Jungblut, P. W., Hughes, S. F., Göhrlich, L., Gowers, U., and Wagner, R. K. (1971): Simultaneous occurrence of individual estrogen and androgen receptors in female and male target organs. *Hoppe-Seyler's Z. Physiol. Chem.,* 352:1603.

52. Kledzik, G. S., Marshall, S., Campbell, G. A., Gelato, M., and Meites, J. (1976): Effects of castration, testosterone, estradiol, and prolactin on specific prolactin binding activity in ventral prostate of male rats. *Endocrinology,* 98:373.

53. Knorr, D. W., Vanha-Perttula, T., and Lipsett, M. B. (1970): Structure and function of rat testis through pubescence. *Endocrinology,* 86:1298.

54. Lasnitzki, I., and Mizuno, T. (1977): Induction of the rat prostate gland by androgens in organ culture. *J. Endocrinol.,* 74:47.

55. Leeson, C. R., and Leeson, T. S. (1964): The postnatal development of the ductus epididymis in the rat. *Anat. Anz.,* 114:159.

56. Leeson, T. S., and Leeson, C. R. (1964): An electron microscope study of the postnatal development of the ductus epididymis in the rat. *Anat. Anz.,* 114:168.

57. Lutz-Ostertag, Y. (1974): Nouvelles preuves de l'action de la testosterone sur le développement des canaux de Muller de l'embryon d'oiseau en culture in vitro. *C. R. Acad. Sci. (Paris),* 278:2351.

58. Mainwaring, W. I. P., and Mangan, F. R. (1973): A study of the androgen receptors in a variety of androgen sensitive tissues. *J. Endocrinol.* 59:121.

59. *Male Accessory Sex Organs. Structure and Function in Mammals* (1974), edited by D. Brandes. Academic Press, New York.

60. McKinney, T. D., and Desjardins, C. (1973): Postnatal development of the testis, fighting behavior and fertility in house mice. *Biol. Reprod.,* 9:279.

61. Meusy-Dessolle, N. (1975): Variations quantitatives de la testosterone plasmatique chez le porc mâle de la naissance à l'âge adulte. *C. R. Acad. Sci. (Paris),* 281:1875.

62. Moger, W. H. (1977): Serum 5α-androstane, 3α- 17β-diol, androsterone and testosterone concentrations in the male rat. Influence of age and gonadotropin stimulation. *Endocrinology,* 100:1027.

63. Negro-Vilar, A., Krulich, L., and McCann, S. M. (1973): Changes in serum prolactin and gonadotropins during sexual development of the male rat. *Endocrinology,* 93:660.

64. Negro-Vilar, A., Saad, W. A., and McCann, S. M. (1977): Evidence for a role of prolactin in prostate and seminal vesicle growth in immature male rats. *Endocrinology*, 100:729.
65. *Normal and Abnormal Growth of the Prostate* (1975), edited by M. Goland. Charles C Thomas, Springfield, Illinois.
66. Orgebin-Crist, M.-C. (1973): Maturation of spermatozoa in the rabbit epididymis: Effect of castration and testosterone replacement. *J. Exp. Zool.*, 185:301.
67. Orgebin-Crist, M.-C., Danzo, B. J., and Davies, J. (1975): Endocrine control of the development and maintenance of sperm fertilizing ability in the epididymis. In: *Handbook of Physiology, Endocrinology V*, edited by David W. Hamilton and Roy O. Greep, pp. 319–338. Williams & Wilkins, Baltimore, Md.
68. Picard, J. Y., and Josso, N. (1976): Anti-Mullerian hormone: Estimation of molecular weight by gel filtration. *Biomedicine*, 25:147.
69. Picon, R. (1969): Action du testicule foetal sur le développement in vitro des canaux de Muller chez le rat. *Arch. Anat. Microsc. Morphol. Exp.*, 58:1.
70. Picon, R. (1971): Etude comparée de l'action inhibitrice des testicules de lapin et de rat sur les canaux de Muller de ces deux espèces in vitro. *C. R. Acad. Sci. (D), (Paris)*, 272:98.
71. Pierrepoint, C. G., and Davies, P. (1973): The effect of vasectomy on the activity of prostatic RNA polymerase in rats. *J. Reprod. Fert.*, 35:149.
72. Pierrepoint, C. G., Davies, P., Lewis, M. H., and Moffat, D. B. (1975): Examination of the hypothesis that a direct control system exists for the prostate and seminal vesicles. *J. Reprod. Fert.*, 44:395.
73. Pierrepoint, C. G., Davies, P., and Wilson, D. W. (1974): The role of the epididymis and ductus deferens in the direct and unilateral control of the prostate and seminal vesicles of the rat. *J. Reprod. Fert.*, 41:413.
74. Price, D., and Pannabecker, R. (1956): Organ culture studies of the foetal rat reproductive tracts. *Ciba Foundation Colloquia on Ageing*, 2:3.
75. Price, D., and Pannabecker, R. (1959): Comparative responsiveness of homologous sex ducts and accessory glands of fetal rats in culture. *Arch. Anat. Microsc. Morphol. Exp.*, 48:223.
76. Price, J. M., Donahoe, P. K., Ito, Y., and Hendren, W. H., III (1977): Programmed cell death in the Müllerian duct induced by Müllerian inhibiting substance. *Am. J. Anat.*, 149:353.
77. Price, D., Williams-Ashman, H. G. (1961): The accessory reproductive glands of mammals. In: *Sex and Internal Secretions*, Vol. 1, edited by W. C. Young, pp. 366–448. Williams & Wilkins, Baltimore.
78. Rajalakshmi, M., Arora, R., Bose, T. K., Dinakar, N., Gupta, G., Thampan, T.R.N.V., Prasad, M.R.N., Anand Kumar, T. C., and Mougdal, N. R. (1976): Physiology of the epididymis and induction of functional sterility in the male. *J. Reprod. Fert.*, (Suppl.),24:71.
79. Resko, J. A. (1967): Plasma androgen levels of the rhesus monkey. *Endocrinology*, 81:1203.
80. Resko, J. A. (1970): Androgen secretion by the fetal and neonatal rhesus monkey. *Endocrinology*, 87:680.
81. Resko, J. A., Feder, H. H., and Goy, R. W. (1968): Androgen concentrations in plasma and testis of developing rats. *J. Endocrinol.*, 40:485.
82. Rigaudiere, N., Pelardy, G., Robert, A., and Delost, P. (1976): Changes in the concentrations of testosterone and androstenedione in the plasma and testis of the guinea pig from birth to death. *J. Reprod. Fert.*, 48:291.
83. Setty, B. S., and Jehan, Q. (1977): Functional maturation of the epididymis in the rat. *J. Reprod. Fert.*, 49:317.
84. Slaunwhite, W. R., and Sharma, M. (1977): Effects of hypophysectomy and prolactin replacement therapy on prostatic response to androgen in orchiectomized rats. *Biol. Reprod.*, 17:489.
85. Sufrin, G., and Coffey, D. W. (1974): A comparison of the hormone responsiveness of the prostate and seminal vesicles. *Invest. Urol.*, 11:386.
86. Suzuki, Y., Toshimori, Y., and Mochizuki, K. (1955): Possibility of direct transportation of testicular hormone to some target organs located close to the testicle in the postnatal rats and its physiologic significance. *Endocrinology*, 56:347.
87. Swerdloff, R. S., Walsh, P. C., Jacobs, H. S., and Odell, W. D. (1971): Serum LH and FSH during sexual maturation in the male rat: Effect of castration and cryptorchidism. *Endocrinology*, 88:120.
88. Tran, D., and Josso, N. (1977): Relationship between avian and mammalian anti-Mullerian hormones. *Biol Reprod.*, 16:267.

89. Tuovinen, P. I., and Pohjola, R. (1949): The importance of the epididymis in castration. *Acta Endocrinol.,* 3:1.
90. Van Beurden-Lamers, W. M. O., Brinkmann, A. O., Mulder, E., and van der Molen, H. J. (1974): High-affinity binding of oestradiol-17β by cytosols from testis, interstitial tissue, pituitary, adrenal, liver and accessory sex glands of the male rat. *Biochem. J.,* 140:495.
91. Walsh, P. C., and Wilson, J. D. (1976): The induction of prostatic hypertrophy in the dog with androstanediol. *J. Clin. Invest.,* 57:1093.
92. Warren, D. W., Haltmeyer, G. C., and Eik-Nes, K. B. (1973): Testosterone in the fetal rat testis. *Biol. Reprod.,* 8:560.
93. Witorsch, R. J., and Smith, J. P. (1977): Evidence for androgen-dependent intracellular binding of prolactin in rat ventral prostate gland. *Endocrinology,* 101:929.
94. Wolff, E., Lutz Ostertag, Y., and Haffen, K. (1952): Sur la régression et la nécrose in vitro des canaux de Muller de l'embryon de poulet sous l'action directe des hormones males. *C. R. Soc. Biol., (Paris),* 146:1793.
95. Yamanaka, H., Kirdani, R. J., Saroff, J., Murphy, G. P., and Sandberg, A. A. (1975): Effects of testosterone and prolactin on rat prostatic weight, 5α-reductase and arginase. *Am. J. Physiol.,* 229:1102.

The Testis, edited by H. Burger and D. de Kretser.
Raven Press, New York © 1981.

12

Seasonal Aspects of Testicular Function

G. A. Lincoln

M.R.C. Reproductive Biology Unit,
Edinburgh EH3 9EW, United Kingdom

INTRODUCTION

Seasonal Regression of the Testes

In the majority of mammalian species the testes do not remain uniformly active throughout the year. Instead, there is a period, usually corresponding to the mating season, when the spermatogenic and androgenic functions of the testes are maximally developed, and outside this time regression occurs.

The concept of the testes of the mature animal waxing and waning in activity according to season is strange to those familiar with the reproductive physiology of man or some laboratory and domesticated species (albino rat, mouse, rabbit, guinea pig, cattle, pig) in which a constant state of reproductive activity, once puberty is past, is regarded as the norm. Species such as the golden hamster, ferret, rhesus monkey, sheep, and goat, in which conspicuous seasonal changes in the testes occur, appear to be the exception. Yet when a wider survey of all mammals is conducted this is clearly not the case (9,157). Among wild mammals there are numerous examples in which a seasonal cycle in testicular activity occurs, and in many cases the seasonal regression of the testes renders the males infertile for part of the year (2,37,155,184,190).

When a comparison is made between the different species of mammals it is apparent that seasonal regression of the testes occurs to varying degrees. In the most extreme examples the testes fully regress to a weight less than 10% of the fully active state [e.g., bank vole (155), rock hyrax (122), pipistrelle bat (143).] In other species the regression is less conspicuous and involves about a 50% decrease in size [e.g., wild rabbit, (19), Ile de France ram (134), badger (10)]. The final category is the apparently nonseasonal species in which the regression, if it occurs, is minimal [e.g., brown hare of South Africa (50), hippopotamus (167), African elephant (65)].

As there are examples of all the various degrees of seasonal regression it is

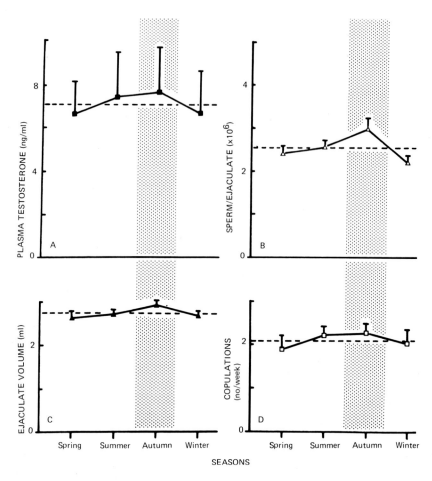

FIG. 1. Seasonal variation ($\overline{m} \pm$ SEM) in various reproductive parameters for normal men living in Europe. **A:** Levels of testosterone in blood plasma based on four samples from 15 people. **B:** Numbers of spermatozoa per ejaculate and **C:** volume of ejaculate after a 2-day period of sexual abstinence based on 83 samples from one man. **D:** Frequency of sexual intercourse based on 960 recordings for 6 men. Note the tendency for all characteristics to be at a maximum in the autumn (stippled). [Data adapted from ref. 169 **(A)** and ref. 97 **(B–D)**].

unsatisfactory to define a species as seasonal or nonseasonal when considering the changes in the reproductive physiology of the male. The important differences between species are not whether or not they are seasonal but in the extent of the seasonal effects. It is probable that even the so-called nonseasonal species show some more subtle changes in testicular activity during a year, a feature borne out in recent studies on a variety of animals [albino rat (89), domesticated rabbit (23), Holstein cattle (6), horse (180)]. Even man is slightly seasonal in his reproductive physiology with a decline in testicular function occurring in the winter and spring, at least amongst European men (97,149,169) (Fig. 1).

Seasonal Puberty

When seasonal regression of the testes occurs to a marked extent, as for example in some of the wild mammals referred to above, both the spermatogenic and androgenic functions of the testes are usually affected. The production of spermatozoa ceases and the testosterone secretion declines to such a low level that the reproductive accessory glands and other androgen dependent tissues become involuted, and the reproductive tract returns to a prepubertal state. Resumption of testicular activity after the quiescent period leads to a reversal of these changes, a sequence of events which is closely comparable to those normally associated with puberty. Males with a pronounced seasonal sexual cycle therefore experience a recurring annual puberty [e.g., red deer (96), fox (81), ferret (126)]. Any growth changes in the size of the testes related to age, occur in addition to the seasonal changes, and even effects of senility on testicular size may be apparent (Fig. 2).

Breeding Seasons

To understand the significance of the seasonal sexual cycle in the male of any species it is necessary to consider the ecology of the animal in its natural environment (13,67,69,117,157). The occurrence of such seasonal changes usually reflects an adaptation to seasonal breeding; the most typical pattern is that full sexual competence in the male is achieved some weeks before receptive females are available and this fertility extends over the full period when successful mating might occur. It is not surprising, therefore, that the most striking examples of seasonal regression of the testes occur in species with the most restricted mating seasons.

The seasonal changes in the testes are dictated by the hypothalamus and anterior pituitary through the secretion of gonadotrophins. Many species have a mechanism which responds to specific cues from the environment, in particular changes in day length and food supply, to regulate hypothalamic activity, and thus time the reproductive changes in the male to the appropriate season (8, 109,133). It is unfortunately outside the scope of this chapter to consider the broad aspects of male seasonality.

The results reviewed here are those dealing with the structural and functional changes in the testes of mammals which occur related to season. The observations on pituitary activity are included since it is the seasonal changes in gonadotrophin secretion which dictate the changes in the testes. Similarly, the variations in the accessory glands and secondary sexual characters, and effects on sexual and aggressive behavior are considered since these are dictated by the testes.

It was over fifty years ago that the French physiologist Courrier produced the first detailed study of the reproductive system of a variety of mammals in which there is a clearly defined sexual cycle (35–37). He investigated the seasonal changes in the testis and accessory glands of several species of bats, the European mole, hedgehog, and marmot, and described the way in which the spermatogenic and androgenic functions of the testes vary, usually in close association, although

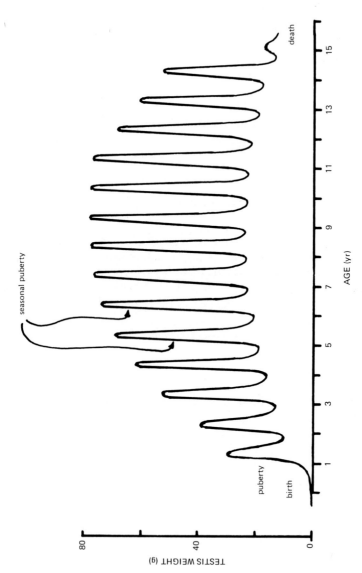

FIG. 2. A summary diagram of the changes which occur in the size of the testes of a red deer stag (*Cervus elaphus*) illustrating the way the seasonal changes in gonad size are superimposed on a longer term change related to age. Each year the testes redevelop and the animal experiences a recurring puberty. (From refs. 95 and 96, and Lincoln, *unpublished observations.*)

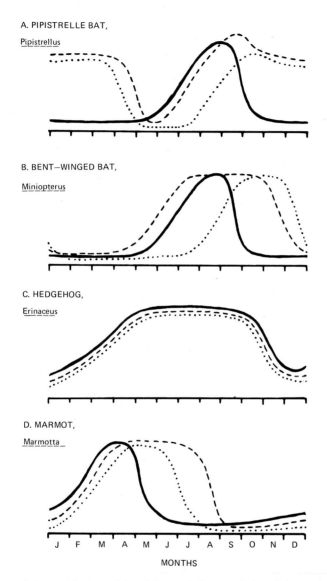

FIG. 3. Seasonal changes in the activity of the seminiferous tubules of the testis (—), Leydig cells of the interstitial tissue of the testis (- -) and accessory sexual glands (. . .) in four species of mammals with a clearly defined annual reproductive cycle. **A:** pipistrelle bat, **B:** bent-winged bat, **C:** hedgehog, **D:** marmot. The assessments of activity are those of Courrier (37) and are only semiquantitative.

not always; in some species of bats the testes can be functionally active at a time when the accessory glands are regressed (Fig. 3). He appreciated that there was a relationship between the histological appearance of the interstitium of the testes, and the activity of the accessory glands.

These deductions were possible only because the activity of the reproductive tract was waxing and waning, and correlations could be drawn between form and function. This is one of the important advantages of studying male reproductive physiology in species in which reproductive function is 'switched off' to a greater or lesser degree for part of the year.

SEASONAL CHANGES IN STRUCTURE OF THE TESTIS

Seminiferous Tubules and Spermatogenesis

The changes in the histological appearance of the seminiferous tubules of the testis throughout the year have been reported for a wide range of mammalian species, mostly selected because the seasonal changes are conspicuous [e.g., bank vole (155), vole (28,29), Indian gerbil (140), red squirrel (41), grey squirrel (3), mole (142), hedgehog (4), pipistrelle bat (143), weasel (72), ferret (2), stoat (62), mink (129), European badger, pine marten, stone marten and polecat (10), mongoose (58), wild rabbit (19), fox (81), masked civet cat (176), grey seal (71), roe deer (163), red deer (95), fallow deer (25), black-tailed deer (186), white-tailed deer (153,191), reindeer (118), blesbok, impala, kudu, springbok (166), red hartebeest and black wildebeest (168), camel (1), rock hyrax (121), green monkey (33), squirrel monkey (42)]. Most of these publications include light microscope photographs of the testicular histology during the active phase of the annual cycle and at the time of regression, along with measurements of the changes in the diameter of the seminiferous tubules.

Seasonal changes in the length of the seminiferous tubules occur in addition to the changes in diameter [Ile de France sheep (75), red deer (74)] and these are correlated with the changes in the bulk of the germinal epithelium. At the time of maximal spermatogenic activity the epithelium consists of germ cells involved in mitosis, and meiosis, and the closely associated Sertoli cells. When seasonal regression occurs the number of germ cells completing spermatogenesis becomes reduced, and this leads to a reduction of the germinal epithelium, so the tubules compensate by shrinking and the basement membrane of the tubules thickens as a consequence (e.g., mink, ref. 129). In some species the seasonal decline in spermatogenesis involves only a slight reduction in the number of cells completing meiosis and thus the reduction in tubule diameter is correspondingly small [e.g., mongoose (58), camel (1), red hartebeest (168)]. In the cases in which the regression is more evident, the reduction in the number of germ cells may be such that no cells fully complete spermatogenesis and the seminiferous tubules are then much reduced in size [e.g., roe deer (163), kudu (166), red deer (95), fox (81)]. For the species which show the most extreme effects of season the process of spermatogenesis virtually ceases so that the germinal epithelium consists of only spermatogonia and Sertoli cells, and in these the tubules become very small [e.g., vole (28), pipistrelle bat (143), mole (142)]. The appearance of the seminiferous tubules during the period of testicular

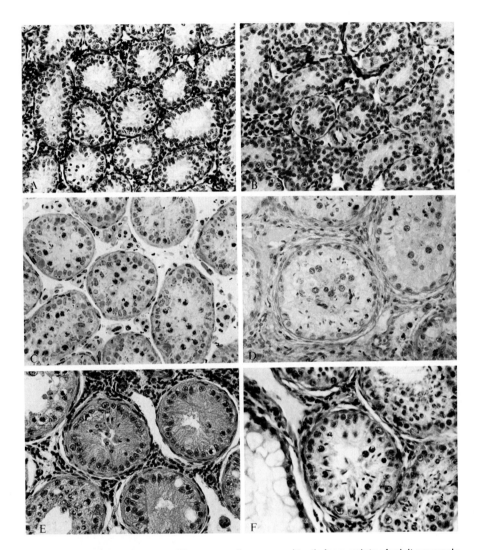

FIG. 4. Histological appearance of the seasonally regressed testis for a variety of adult mammals **A:** vole, *Microtis agrestis* **B:** pipistrelle bat, *Pipistrellus pipistrellus*, **C:** brown hare, *Lepus capensis*, **D:** Soay sheep, *Ovis aries*, **E:** roe deer, *Capreolus capreolus*, **F:** red deer, *Cervus elaphus*. Note the general failure of spermatogenesis; all species with the exception of the Soay sheep fail completely to produce spermatozoa during the period of seasonal quiescence. (Photographs or material supplied by Dr. Anne Grocock—vole, Dr. P. A. Racey—pipistrelle bat, and Professor R. V. Short—roe deer.)

regression is illustrated in Fig. 4 for a number of species in which the seasonal changes are conspicuous.

The seminiferous tubules constitute the bulk of the testicular tissue, and therefore the seasonal changes in the volume of the tubules are closely reflected by

TABLE 1. Seasonal change in the weight of the testes of a variety of wild British mammals

Species	Testis weight (combined)		Size of regressed testes (% of active)	References
	Seasonal maximal (active) (g)	Seasonal minimum (regressed) (g)		
Ungulates				
red deer, Cervus elaphus	151.1(12)[a] Sep–Oct[b]	38.9(8) Apr–June	26	95
fallow deer, Dama dama	133.2(5) Oct	21.0(5) June	16	25
roe deer, Capreolus capreolus	45.0(15) July	6.0(21) Dec	13	20
Canids				
red fox, Vulpes vulpes	13.5(19) Jan	2.3(26) May–Sep	17	82–84
Mustelids				
badger, Meles meles	8.5(16) Feb	4.8(9) Oct	56	10
polecat, Mustela putorius	2.06(22) Mar–May	0.45(2) Nov	22	183
stoat, Mustela erminea	1.01(4) Apr–May	0.16(4) Nov–Dec	16	62
weasel, Mustela nivalis	0.209(104) Mar–May	0.041(8) Nov–Jan	20	72
Lagamorphs				
brown hare, Lepus capensis	19.4(21) Feb–June	4.4(8) Oct–Nov	23	98
mountain hare, Lepus timidus	16.4(16) Feb–Apr	2.2(9) Sep–Nov	13	52
wild rabbit, Oryctolagus cuniculus	3.80(53) Apr	1.40(21) July	37	19
Insectivores				
hedgehog, Erinacius europous	2.95(42) May–June	1.12(4) Oct	38	4
mole, Talpa europaea	1.83(8) Mar	0.22(12) Sep–Dec	12	142
common shrew, Sorex araneus	dies after one season		—	18
nodule bat, Nyctalus noctula	0.520(4) Jul–Aug	0.040(8) Nov–Feb	8	141
pipistrelle bat, Pipistrellus pipistrellus	0.225(3–5) Aug	0.010(3–5) Nov	4	143
Rodents				
red squirrel, Sciurus vulgaris	1.400 Feb–Mar	0.141 Aug–Sep	10	41
brown rat, Rattus norvegicus	no observed change		100?	137
house mouse, Mus musculus	no observed change		100?	93
short-tailed vole, Microtus agrestis	0.550(12) June	0.035(3) Nov	6	195
bank vole, Clethrionomys glareolus	0.682(>50) May	0.024(>25) Nov–Jan	4	155
field mouse, Apodemus sylvaticus	0.882(8)	0.061(14)	7	148
Marine mammals				
grey seal, Halichoerus grypus	166.0(26) Oct–Nov	c 67.5 Apr	41	71
dolphin, Delphinus sp.	Seasonal changes			66

[a] Sample size.
[b] Months when samples collected.

changes in the total size and weight of the testes (e.g., rock hyrax, ref. 122). The seasonal changes in the weight of the testis also reflect the state of spermatogenesis, and this feature is summarized in Table 1 and Fig. 5 for a variety of British mammals. As a general rule when the weight of the testes drops below

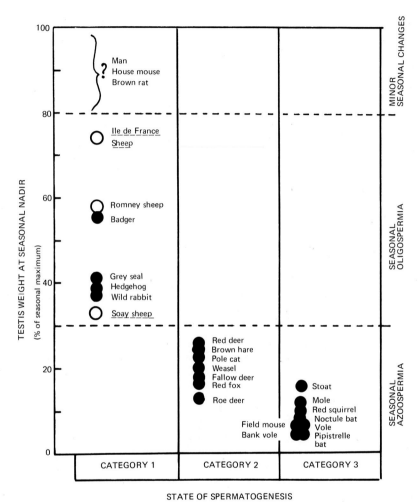

FIG. 5. The relationship between the decline in the weight of the testis (expressed as percent of seasonal maximum) and the state of spermatogenesis at the season of the year when the testes are most regressed, for a variety of wild mammals found in the British Isles. **Category 1:** At least some germ cells complete spermatogenesis although the number may be greatly reduced. **Category 2:** No germ cells complete spermatogenesis although some enter meiosis. **Category 3:** No germ cells complete spermatogenesis or enter meiosis, and the germinal epithelium consists only of spermatozoa and Sertoli cells (data from Table 1). The corresponding values for three breeds of domesticated sheep are shown for comparison: Ile de France (75), Romney (14), Soay (Lincoln, *unpublished observation*).

30% of the seasonal maximum, spermatogenesis is found to be disrupted to the extent that no germ cells complete maturation.

Germ Cells

Quantitative studies on the number of germ cells in the seminiferous tubules at various stages of mitosis and meiosis have been undertaken to establish what happens to the process of spermatogenesis during seasonal regression of the testis. The Ile de France ram has been investigated in most detail (75,130,131,132) and the following changes have been noted in comparing the histology of the seasonally regressed testis (spring) with that of the fully active testis (autumn):

1. The total number of type A spermatogonia is reduced.
2. The efficiency of the mitotic divisions of the spermatogonia is reduced such that fewer primary spermatocytes are formed.
3. The efficiency of the meiotic divisions of the primary spermatocytes is reduced such that fewer spermatids are produced.
4. The number of germ cells completing the final process of spermiogenesis is also reduced.

These changes result in a marked decrease in the number of spermatozoa emanating from the testis. While there are obvious effects of season on the efficiency of spermatogenesis, the duration of the process, and the cell associations within the germinal epithelium are not affected. It is also of interest that even in the fully active testis of the ram the number of germ cells produced is well below the theoretical number expected; thus the efficiency of spermatogenesis is never 100%, and the effect of season is to further decrease the productivity. The 'bottlenecks' in the maturation process at which most cell losses occur, e.g., mitotic divisions of the spermatogonia, are also the stages at which division of the cells fails when the testis is regressed.

The effects of season on the spermatogenic process in the ram are relatively slight compared to the effects seen in some of the wild mammals. Only a few species have been studied in detail, but it appears that during regression, failure of normal mitotic and meiotic divisions contributes to the decline in the number of germ cells completing maturation [hamster (16), vole (60), red deer (74)] (Fig. 6).

In these species the seasonal decline in the efficiency of spermatogenesis is usually paralleled by a decline in the number of spermatogonia. This change may not be true, however, for all forms of spermatogonia. Thus in the studies on the Ile de France sheep and red deer the undifferentiated stem cells (A_0 spermatogonia) have been counted separately from the other spermatogonia which are involved in spermatogenesis (A_1 spermatogonia, refs. 74, 75). In the case of the ram, seasonal regression of testis is accompanied by a decrease in the number of both types of spermatogonia, however, for the red deer the situation is different and in this species the number of A_0 spermatogonia actually

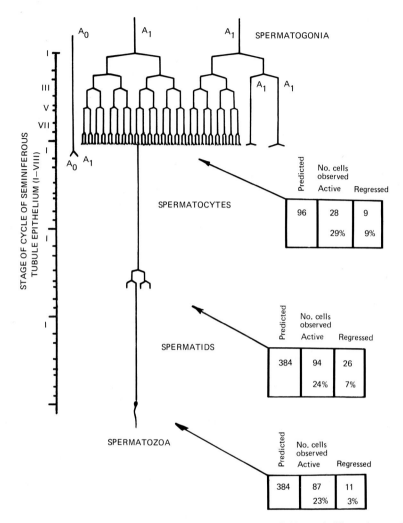

FIG. 6. Theoretical plan of the way in which spermatogonia divide and differentiate to form spermatozoa related to the eight stages of the cycle in the germinal epithelium for the red deer *(Cervus elaphus)*. The figures in the boxes show the number of cells expected to be produced from two A_1 spermatogonia and the number of cells actually counted for the period when the testes are fully developed in the autumn (active) and when the testes are regressing or fully regressed in the spring (regressed). Note at all times less cells are produced than predicted, and in the regressed testes additional losses of germ cells occur during the mitotic divisions of spermatogonia, meiotic divisions of spermatocytes, and during spermiogenesis. When the testes become fully regressed no spermatozoa mature. (From ref. 74.)

increases in the regressed testis (Fig. 7). The significance of this change is not clear but it may be a characteristic feature of very seasonal species that during involution of the testis the undifferentiated spermatogonia become more numerous. The winter spermatogonia described by Courrier (37) in various seasonal

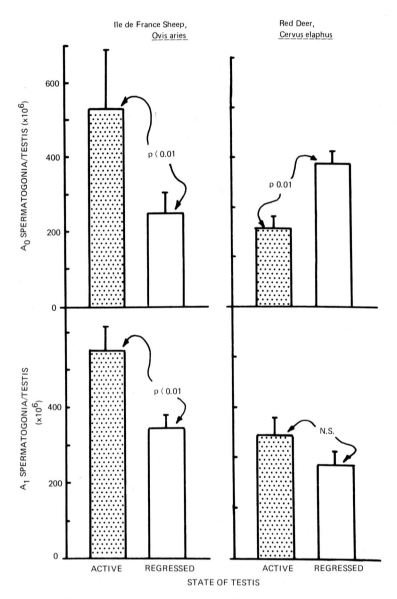

FIG. 7. A comparison of the total number (mean ± SEM) of stem spermatogonia (A_0 and A_1 spermatogonia) in the testis of the Ile de France sheep, *Ovis aries,* and red deer, *Cervus elaphus,* during the season when the testes are fully developed (autumn—stippled) and when regressed (spring—open column). Note the different behavior of the A_0 spermatogonia in the two species related to season. (From refs. 74,75.)

mammals may represent such undifferentiated cells, and these have been described by other workers [ferret (2), weasel (72), vole (28)].

During the season when the testes are regressed and spermatogenesis is disrupted, degenerating germ cells can be seen in the seminiferous tubules. This is especially obvious during the period of regression after full activity when cells of abnormal appearance are more numerous and fragments of disintegrating cells are found in the lumen and in the cytoplasm of the Sertoli cells [e.g., mink (129), grey squirrel (140a)] (Fig. 8). Residual material from the degenerated germ cells may remain in the tubules for many weeks in situations when marked regression of the epithelium occurs (e.g., mole, ref. 5). Abnormalities in the size and Feulgen-staining DNA content of spermatocytes have also been observed (Ile de France Sheep, refs. 48, 75). Amongst the spermatozoa that complete maturation in the regressed testes, abnormalities are common, such as defects in the shape of the head and number and form of the tail [e.g., rock hyrax (120), mole (142)].

Sertoli Cells

The close involvement of the Sertoli cells with the germ cells during spermatogenesis means that seasonal changes occur in these cells in close parallel with the changes in spermatogenesis. The total number of Sertoli cells does not change (e.g., red deer, ref. 74) but the volume of the cytoplasm and size of the nucleus changes in relation to spermatogenic activity.

In the fully active testis the cytoplasm of the Sertoli cells is expanded and surrounds the developing germ cells. The seasonal changes in the fine structure of the cytoplasm have been described for the grey squirrel (140a). In this species, regression of the testes is associated with a change in the shape of the Sertoli cells, there is a decrease in the amount of agranular endoplasmic reticulum which occurs in configurations not seen in the sexually active testes—the association of the agranular reticulum with maturing germ cells is lost and in some situations the reticulum is modified into vacuoles surrounding degenerating spermatids and other cellular debris. There is an increase in the number of inclusions in the cytoplasm apparently derived from degenerating germ cells.

The seasonal changes in the Sertoli cells also include changes in the nucleus which condenses and becomes reduced in size when the testes become regressed. This is especially obvious in the species in which full spermatogenic arrest occurs [e.g., vole (28), pipistrelle bat (143)]. The changes have been quantified for the hamster in which the cross-sectional area of the Sertoli cell nucleus becomes reduced by some 30% at the time of maximum seasonal regression (181) (Fig. 9). When redevelopment of the testes occurs after the seasonal quiescent phase the nucleus and cytoplasm of the Sertoli cell expand. The expansion of the cytoplasm, with associated changes in the size of the seminiferous tubules, is one of the first events noted in the testes at the beginning of the new season [pipistrelle bat (143), mole (142)].

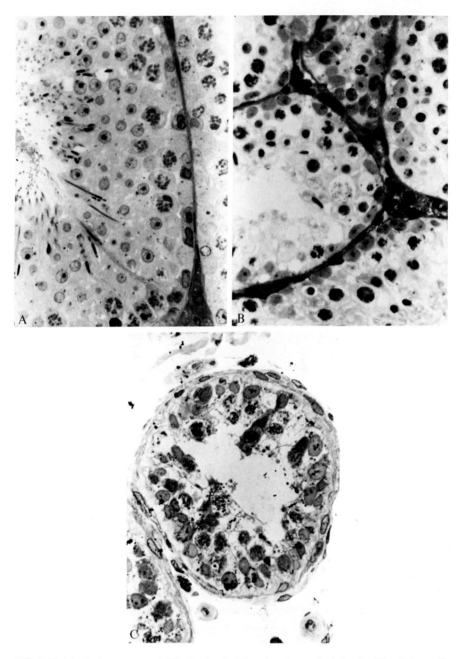

FIG. 8. Histological appearance of the testis of a laboratory housed adult vole, *Microtis agrestis,* **A:** fully sexually active (summer condition)—testis weight 326 mg/pair; **B:** regressed (winter condition)—testis weight 115 mg/pair. Note the decrease in number of germ cells completing maturation during seasonal regression due to the decrease in efficiency of both mitotic and meiotic cell division. In the wild the seasonal regression of the testes occurs to an even greater extent than in captivity. (Data and photographs from Dr. Anne Grocock, Oxford.) **C:** Histological appearance of the testis of a wild adult brown hare, *Lepus capensis,* shot in September at the time of testicular regression following the mating season. A few spermatocytes can be seen nearest the lumen of the seminiferous tubule, but spermatogenesis is markedly disrupted. (Photography from Dr. Anne Grocock, Oxford.)

Intertubular Tissue

The intertubular tissue of the testis undergoes structural changes related to season in many of the species in which the seasonal changes in the seminiferous tubules are conspicuous, regression of the various components of the intertubular tissue occurring often in parallel with regression of the tubules. These changes have been quantified for the red deer, for example, in which a decrease in the volume of Leydig cells, fibroblastic cells, peritubular cells, and blood vessels occur during seasonal regression of the testes (74).

Leydig Cells

The changes in the Leydig cells have been studied at the light microscope level for many species, and a common finding is that the volume of both the nucleus and cytoplasm decreases when the testis regresses during the nonmating season [e.g., woodchuck (146), various bats, mole, and marmot (37), vole (28), hamster (181), roe deer (163), red deer (21,54), mule deer (116)]. The seasonal changes which occur in the ultrastructural appearance of the Leydig cells have been described for several species [e.g., mole (11), myotid bat (63), hamster (189), grey squirrel (140a), rock hyrax (120,127)]. In the case of the rock hyrax, regression of the Leydig cells involves a decrease in the mass of the nucleus and cytoplasm, the agranular endoplasmic reticulum becomes less abundant and more irregular in appearance. There is a decrease in the number of mitochondria, while the number of lipid inclusions increases (120).

The fate of the individual Leydig cells during the seasonal cycle is not established. They appear to develop from undifferentiated cells in the interstitium and subsequently regress again (27), but whether they go through repeated cycles is not clear. It is a common finding that not all the Leydig cells are in a similar stage of development; in the seasonally regressed testis, for example, some Leydig cells may have an expanded nucleus and cytoplasm at a time when the majority of cells are apparently regressed (e.g., mink, ref. 129).

Not all mammals with a seasonal cycle in testicular activity show structural changes in the Leydig cells. In the mole, for example, the ultrastructure of the Leydig cells is not obviously modified during the nonmating season even though dramatic regression of the seminiferous tubules occurs (175).

Blood and Lymph Vessels

The changes in the form of the blood vessels in the testes during seasonal regression and redevelopment of the testes have been described in detail for the red fox (82,86). In this species seasonal regression of the testis results in a reduction in the diameter of the arterioles within the testis which become contorted owing to the shrinkage of the surrounding tissues (Fig. 10). Such changes in the blood vessels probably occur in other seasonal species judging from the

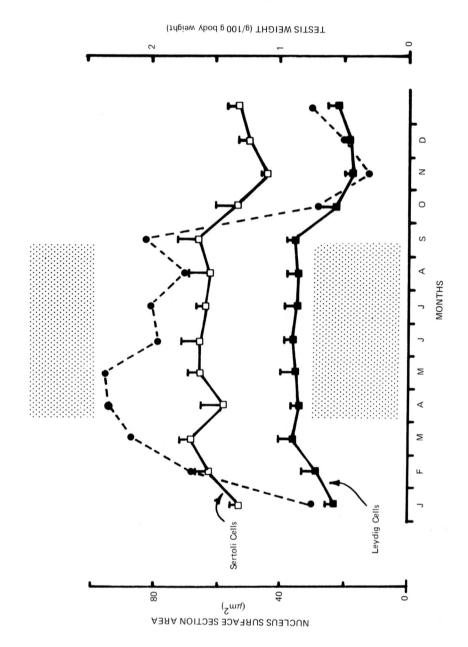

TESTIS WEIGHT (g/100 g body weight)

NUCLEUS SURFACE SECTION AREA (μm^2)

MONTHS

J F M A M J J A S O N D

Sertoli Cells

Leydig Cells

changes in blood flow (ferret and dormouse, ref. 85) and in the macroscopic appearance of the testis (e.g., brown hare, ref. 98). A decrease in the dilation of the lymphatic sinuses has been noted to occur during seasonal regression of the testes of the mole (142), while the reverse change has been reported for a species of Australian native rat, *Rattus fuscipes* in which the lymphatics of the regressed testis are expanded (40).

Tunica Albuginea

The tunica which surrounds the testis accommodates for the seasonal changes in the size of the testes, contracting during the period of regression and expanding during redevelopment. The changes do not occur rapidly so that during the period of regression the testis may be very flaccid, while during development it is relatively turgid (e.g., Soay ram, G. A. Lincoln, *unpublished observation*). Structural changes in the tunica involve alterations in the content of collagen which becomes decreased during regression (fox, ref. 83). In the mole, the tunica is said to be renewed annually (110) but it is not clear whether this is a common feature in all species with a seasonal sexual cycle. During the period of full testicular regression the tunica becomes relatively thickened because of the contraction of the tissue. Animals which have not undergone a previous sexual cycle do not show this characteristic which provides a method of assessing breeding history of animals at this time [vole (28), red squirrel (41), brown hare (106)].

FUNCTIONAL CHANGES OF THE TESTIS

Production of Spermatozoa

The seasonal variation in the number of spermatozoa produced by the testes has been assessed for many species from counts made directly on the testes or from quantitative studies on the spermatozoa present in the epididymis or in the ejaculate [counts made on the testis: vole (60), hamster (16), ram (75), red deer (74); counts made on the epididymides: mole (142), noctule bat (141), mongoose (58), brown hare (98), rock hyrax (121), blesbok, impala, kudu and springbok (166), red hartebeest (168); counts made on the ejaculated semen: domesticated rabbit (23), mink (129), various breeds of domesticated sheep (38,77,92,129,171), goat (164), various breeds of domesticated cattle (6,45,80, 91,162), reindeer (118), rhesus monkey (196)].

FIG. 9. Seasonal variation in the size of the nucleus (surface section area, mean ± SEM) of the Leydig cells and Sertoli cells of the golden hamster, *Mesocricetus auratus,* related to the changes in the total weight of the testes (●---●). The presumed mating season is shown by stippling. Note the decline in the nuclear dimensions at the time of testicular involution in the autumn. (From ref. 181.)

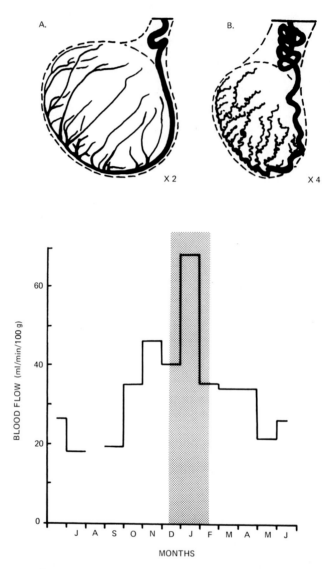

FIG. 10. Macroscopic appearance of the testicular artery and its main branches in the red fox *(Vulpes vulpes)* **A:** January at the time of maximum testicular development (×2) **B:** June at the time of full regression (×4). Note the spiralling appearance of the arterioles which occurs when the testis shrinks in size. The corresponding seasonal changes in the blood flow through the testes of the fox are illustrated below; the mating season is indicated by stippling. (From refs. 82–85.)

In many of the wild species the regression of the testes results in no spermatozoa being produced for several months of the year, and during this period the epididymis becomes devoid of spermatozoa (Fig. 11). In most cases there is a delay of several weeks from the time the production of spermatozoa by the testes ceases, and spermatozoa are lost from the reproductive tract. For those species of bats which indulge in sperm storage during winter hibernation, this period may be 6 months in duration (e.g., pipistrelle bat, ref. 141). When spermatogenesis is resumed after seasonal quiescence there is a delay of several weeks before the caudae epididymides are packed with spermatozoa [e.g., mink (129), red deer (95)].

The structural and biochemical characteristics of the spermatozoa also vary with season in some species. During the period when the testes are regressing or are regressed there is often an increase in the number of immature or abnormal cells emanating from the testes. Structural abnormalities of the acrosome and flagellum occur frequently, and there is an increase in the percentage of dead cells [mole (142), sheep (38,53,92), horse (180), rock hyrax (120), rhesus monkey (196)]. The maturation of the spermatozoa in the epididymis is affected such that more cells retain the cytoplasmic droplet (120). There may be a general decrease in the motility of the spermatozoa during the period of seasonal regression of the testes [mole (142), sheep (38,53,92), blesbok, impala, kudu and springbok (166), horse (180)] and in its fertilizing capacity (cattle, ref. 158). Seasonal changes in the metabolic activity of the spermatozoa include changes in oxygen uptake and fructolysis; the spermatozoa from the seasonally regressed testis use less oxygen and accumulate more lactic acid than normal [sheep (7), cattle (125,165)]. There are seasonal differences also in the enzyme activity of spermatozoa (succinic dehydrogenase activity; cattle spermatozoa, ref. 170) and in their ability to withstand storage at low temperatures (cattle, ref. 158).

Secretion of Testosterone and Related Steroids

The seasonal changes in the endocrine activity of the testis have been documented for many domestic and wild mammals by measurement of testicular content or blood levels of testosterone [testis content of testosterone: pipistrelle and noctule bat (141,143), mole (142), brown hare (98), rock hyrax (122), roe deer (163), red deer (95); blood level of testosterone: mole (142), pipistrelle and noctule bat (141,143), myotid bat (64), hamster (16), stoat (62), red fox (84), rock hyrax (127), sheep (87,100,161), goat (154), roe deer (15), red deer (103), white-tailed deer (114), black-tailed deer (186), reindeer and caribou (187), horse (17,90), Asiatic elephant (78), black bear (115), rhesus monkey (151,152), man (149,169)]. In the few species in which both testicular and blood levels of testosterone have been measured simultaneously, the seasonal changes in both parameters occur in parallel [pipistrelle bat (141), brown hare (98,106)].

The extent to which the testosterone secretion by the testis changes with season varies between species but in some of the more seasonal types the changes are very conspicuous. In the red deer, for example, the testicular content of testosterone may be 3,000 times higher at the peak of activity compared to the nadir (95). The highest recorded levels of testosterone in the blood come from species which are very seasonal in their reproductive activity (64), the record being 134 ng/ml of testosterone in a noctule bat at the peak of the

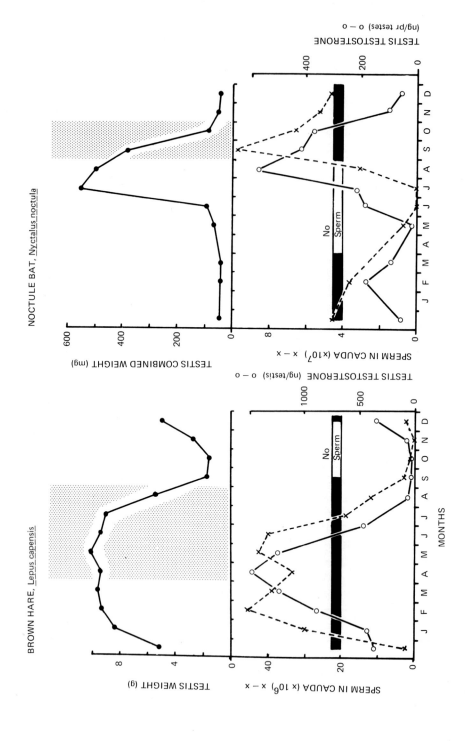

sexual cycle (141). In this species, as in many of the others mentioned above, the blood levels of testosterone become very low or undetectable during the period of testicular regression.

The seasonal changes in the secretion of testosterone occur in parallel with changes in the testicular levels of androstenedione (red deer, ref. 95) and cholesterol (rock hyrax, ref. 120), and the blood levels of dihydrotestosterone [ram (79), rhesus monkey (152)]. In each case testosterone is the major steroid produced by the testes at all seasons.

In Vitro Studies of Steroid Synthesis

Studies involving incubation of testicular tissue with labelled steroid precursors have been performed on a number of species to investigate the way the synthetic activity of the testes changes with season. The most complete study involving separation of testicular tissue into seminiferous tubule and interstitial tissue components, and with careful identification of the products, has been made on the grey squirrel (140a). Testicular tissue from this species taken during the peak of sexual activity will readily synthesize androgens from labelled C_{21} steroid precursors (pregnenolone and progesterone), the synthesis occurring in both testicular compartments. However, the synthesis of androgens is much reduced in testicular tissue taken during seasonal regression of the testes, and at this time a different range of steroid products tends to be produced (Fig. 12). In this situation it appears that the enzyme system necessary for the conversion of pregnenolone to progesterone (3β-hydroxysteroid dehydrogenase-isomerase) is fully active even in the tissue from the regressing testis, yet the enzymes involved in the later stages of biosynthesis are disrupted resulting in the accumulation of progesterone and the synthesis of steroids not produced in significant amounts by the active testis.

Seasonal changes in the synthetic activity of the testis have been described also for the pipistrelle bat, uinta ground squirrel, hamster, and masked civet cat (16,44,141,176). In these species the conversion of pregnenolone or progesterone into androgens is again less efficient when the testes are regressed and at this time the products tend to be androstenedione or progesterone rather than testosterone. These in vitro studies help to illustrate the enzyme capabilities of the testicular tissue, however, they do not necessarily indicate what occurs in vivo at this stage, since the substrates added for incubation are not necessarily freely available in the normal animal. This might explain why the androstenedione concentrations in the testes from culled animals have been found to remain

FIG. 11. Seasonal variation in the weight (●) and content of testosterone (○) of the testis, and the number of spermatozoa (×) in the cauda epididymidis of the brown hare, *Lepus capensis* and noctule bat, *Nyctalus noctula*. The period of the year when the animals are apparently infertile is indicated by a break in the horizontal bar, and the period when most matings occur is shown by stippling. (From refs. 98,141.)

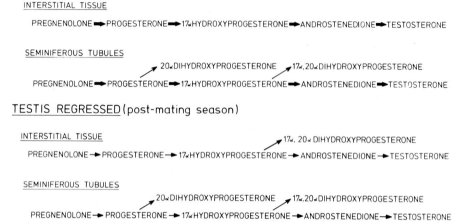

GREY SQUIRREL Scuirus carolinensis

TESTIS FULLY ACTIVE (mating season)

INTERSTITIAL TISSUE

PREGNENOLONE➡PROGESTERONE➡17αHYDROXYPROGESTERONE➡ANDROSTENEDIONE➡TESTOSTERONE

SEMINIFEROUS TUBULES

                     20αDIHYDROXYPROGESTERONE   17α,20αDIHYDROXYPROGESTERONE

PREGNENOLONE➡PROGESTERONE➡17αHYDROXYPROGESTERONE➡ANDROSTENEDIONE➡TESTOSTERONE

TESTIS REGRESSED (post-mating season)

INTERSTITIAL TISSUE   17α, 20α DIHYDROXYPROGESTERONE

PREGNENOLONE→PROGESTERONE→17αHYDROXYPROGESTERONE→ANDROSTENEDIONE→TESTOSTERONE

SEMINIFEROUS TUBULES

                     20αDIHYDROXYPROGESTERONE   17α,20αDIHYDROXYPROGESTERONE

PREGNENOLONE→PROGESTERONE→17αHYDROXYPROGESTERONE→ANDROSTENEDIONE→TESTOSTERONE

FIG. 12. Pathways for androgen biosynthesis in the interstitial tissue and the seminiferous tubules in the testis of the grey squirrel *(Scuirus carolinensis)* during the season of (a) full testicular development and (b) during regression, as indicated by the products formed in the *in vitro* conversion of labelled steroid precursors. The transformation of pregnenolone to testosterone occurs less efficiently during the period of regression, and intermediaries tend to accumulate. (From ref. 140a.)

low during the period when the testes are regressed, and there is no seasonal change in the androstenedione/testosterone ratio (red deer, ref. 95).

Histological Localization of Steroid Synthesis

While there is some evidence that steroid secretion occurs within the seminiferous tubule (140a) the main site of testosterone secretion is the interstitial tissue and in particular the Leydig cells. This is supported by the histochemical localization of cholesterol, lipids, and enzymes associated with steroid synthesis within the cytoplasm of the Leydig cells. Seasonal changes in the intensity of staining reactions for these hormone precursors and enzymes have been observed for several species—the intensity tending to be maximal when the testes are fully active and testosterone secretion is increased [e.g., mole (110), pipistrelle bat (143), mink (129), masked civet cat (176), Virginia deer and sika deer (191), mule deer (116)]. Acid and alkaline phosphatase activity of the Leydig cells also changes with season indicating changes in secretory activity (116,129,191). There is generally a close relationship between the seasonal changes in the structure and histochemistry of the Leydig cells and the secretion of testosterone [myotis bat (63), grey squirrel (140a) rock hyrax (127), red deer (21,95), mule deer (116)] (Fig. 13).

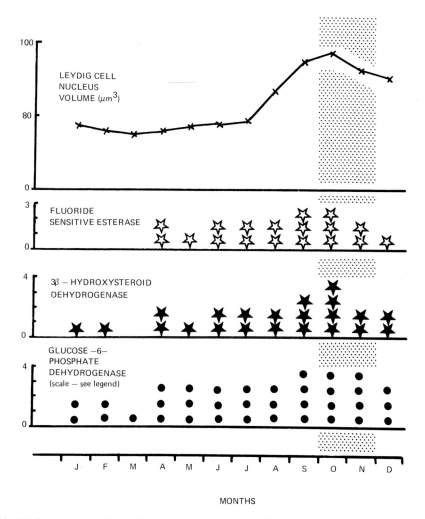

MONTHS

FIG. 13. Seasonal variation in the volume of the nucleus (×) and histochemical reactions of the cytoplasm of the Leydig cells of the mule deer, *Odocoileus hemionus*. The activity of three enzyme systems believed to be involved in steroid biosynthesis (fluoride sensitive esterase, 3β hydroxy-steroid dehydrogenase and glucose-6-phosphate dehydrogenase) was measured semiquantitatively based on the deposition of staining with the reaction product—0 = absent, 1 = trace amount, 2 = small amount, 3 = moderate amount, 4 = large amount. The Leydig cells are apparently least active in spring at the time of full testicular involution and progressively develop over the summer months to reach a peak coinciding with the autumn mating season. (From ref. 116.)

Secretion of ABP and Rete Testis Fluid

The secretion of androgen binding protein (ABP) and fluid by the testis might by expected to change markedly related to season in species in which the Sertoli cells wax and wane in activity. This is borne out in studies on sheep in which both components are at a maximum at the time of full spermatogenic activity when the Sertoli cells are expanded (79; B. Setchell, *personal communication*).

Blood Flow

A seasonal cycle in the blood flow through the testis has been described for a variety of mammals, the maximum rates occurring at the time of maximum testicular size and testosterone secretion [dormouse, ferret, and fox (84,85), sheep (34) (Fig. 10)].

Spermatogenesis in Relation to Testosterone Secretion

The seasonal changes in the exocrine and endocrine functions of the testis usually occur in parallel [e.g., brown hare (98), hedgehog (156), roe deer (163), red deer (95), Soay sheep (100) (Fig. 11)]. An interesting exception to this is provided by the hibernating bats in which testosterone secretion continues, albeit at a reduced rate, for a prolonged period after the production of spermatozoa has ceased (37,143,188). In this situation the spermatozoa remain viable in the reproductive tract for up to 6 months (143). The dissociation of spermatogenesis and androgenesis has also been reported for the golden mole (32). In a few species seasonal changes in the androgenic activity of the testes occur in the absence of obvious changes in spermatogenic activity [e.g., slender loris (145), Australian brushtailed possum (56)]. So far there are no documented examples of the reverse situation in which androgenic activity remains constant but spermatogenesis changes through the year.

PITUITARY CONTROL OF THE TESTIS

Pituitary Content of Gonadotrophins

The role of the anterior pituitary in dictating the seasonal changes in testicular activity has been appreciated for many years. The earliest studies were made with the ferret (73), thirteen-lined ground squirrel (123,184,185), cotton-tailed rabbit (43), and varying hare (111). They illustrated that the levels of the gonadotrophins in the anterior pituitary change during the year, the cycle being closely correlated with the cycle in testicular activity. The period of lowest gonadotrophin levels coincided with the time when the testes were fully regressed. Injections of gonadotrophins stimulated redevelopment of the testis in a way similar to that observed in relation to season, while hypophysectomy induced regression of the testes no more dramatic than that seen in some seasonal species.

Histological evidence for changes in pituitary activity related to the seasonal cycle in testicular activity is available for many species, and the usual finding is that the cells thought to be involved in gonadotrophin secretion increase in size and number during the period of increased testicular activity. Within the cytoplasm the secretory granules become more numerous and enlarged; regression of the cells results in degranulation and return to a chromophobic condition [mole (70), vole (29), ground squirrel (76,113,123), red squirrel (41), cottontailed rabbit (43), red deer (172), rock hyrax (120)]. These changes in the mass of the gonadotrophs is reflected in a change in the total weight of the pituitary gland [noctule bat (141), red squirrel (41), red deer (95)].

Since the early studies on the pituitary content of gonadotrophins a variety of other species have been investigated [vole (30,195), snowshoe hare (39), red deer and roe deer (21), Ile de France sheep (134), rock hyrax (120)]. Some of the more recent studies use specific assays to distinguish LH (luteinizing hormone) and FSH (follicle stimulating hormone) activity and a general finding is that the seasonal changes in the two gonadotrophins occur in parallel [hamster (16), snowshoe hare (39), sheep (135)].

The observations on the variation in LH levels in the pituitary in the deer and sheep are of interest since they show that maximum levels occur not coincident with maximum testicular size but during the phase of redevelopment (21,134). A similar feature occurs in the rock hyrax and the decline in the levels which occurs late in the phase of testicular growth has been attributed to a depletion effect occurring when the release of the gonadotrophins is maximal (122).

Blood Levels of LH and FSH

The advent of sensitive radioimmunoassays has made it possible to investigate the pattern, of secretion of gonadotrophins at different seasons [vole (195), snowshoe hare (39), brown hare (106), Suffolk and Finnish Landrace sheep (87,161), Soay sheep (104), red deer (103)]. The studies on LH have been partly confounded since this gonadotrophin is secreted episodically and thus there can be enormous fluctuations in the values over short periods of time. The most detailed work on the larger species, involving the collection of blood samples at frequent intervals, has illustrated the manner in which the changes in LH secretion occur during the year. The most important change is in the frequency of episodic releases of LH which is maximal at the time of maximal testicular activity and declines outside this period [Suffolk sheep (87), Finnish Landrace and crossbred sheep (159), Soay sheep (99), red deer (103)]. In the most seasonal examples the frequency of episodic releases of LH changes from less than one per day to greater than 10 per day; in these the magnitude of the releases also changes from being maximum during the redevelopment of the testes and decreasing at the time of full testicular activity [Soay sheep (99), red deer (103)] (Fig. 14).

The levels of FSH in the blood do not fluctuate so markedly in the short term compared to those of LH. The changes which occur related to season can be very conspicuous, however, with the increase occurring coincident with the redevelopment of the testes and the maximum levels occurring some weeks before the testes are fully enlarged (Soay sheep, ref. 105) (Fig. 15).

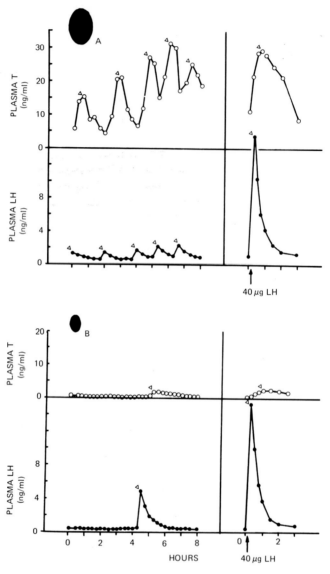

FIG. 14. Short term fluctuations in the level of LH (●) and testosterone (○) in the plasma during an 8-hr period in a Soay ram (A) sampled at the seasonal peak in testicular activity and (B) at the nadir of the sexual cycle. The spontaneous episodic peaks of LH are indicated (◄) along with the corresponding peaks in testosterone. The changes in the levels of LH and testosterone in the plasma following an i.v. injection of 40 μg LH (NIH-LH-S19) are also shown for the two stages of the annual cycle; the testis releases more testosterone in response to LH when the testes are enlarged in the mating season. (From ref. 105.)

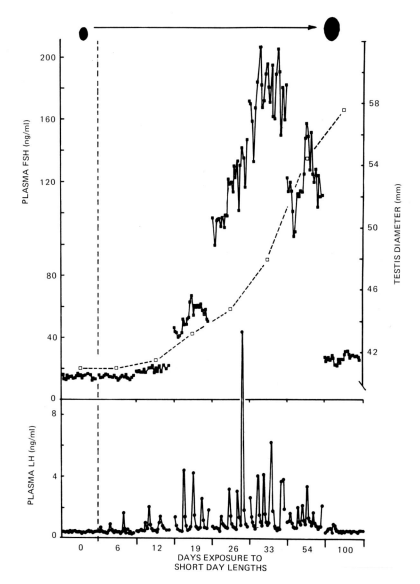

FIG. 15. Changes in the levels of FSH (■) and LH (●) in the plasma in an adult Soay ram in which the seasonal cycle in testicular activity was controlled by an artificial lighting regime: exposure to long-day lengths (16 hr light:8 hr darkness, 16L:8D) for 16 weeks resulted in regression of the testes (Day 0) and the abrupt change to short daylengths (8D:16L) resulted in redevelopment of the testes (□). Blood samples were collected at hourly intervals for 24 hr on the days indicated below. Note the way the levels of LH and FSH decline again once the testes become fully enlarged. (From ref. 104.)

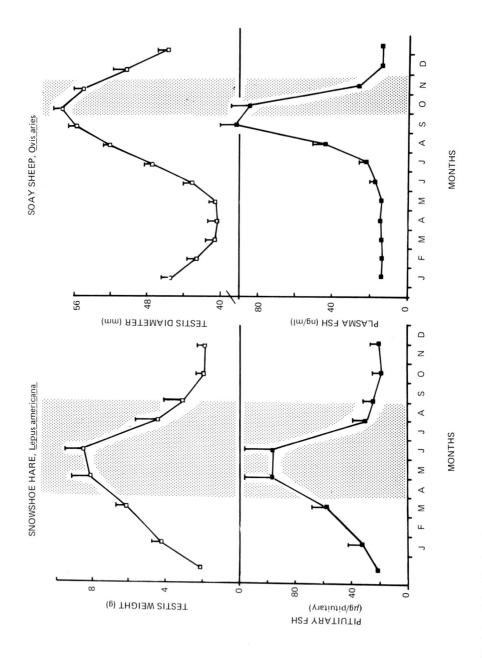

SNOWSHOE HARE, Lepus americana

SOAY SHEEP, Ovis aries

TESTIS WEIGHT (g)

PITUITARY FSH
(μg/pituitary)

TESTIS DIAMETER (mm)

PLASMA FSH (ng/ml)

MONTHS

MONTHS

LH and Testosterone Secretion

The injection of LH stimulates the release of testosterone from the testes, and the changes in the secretion of testosterone which occur during the year in seasonal species appear to be dictated by the pattern of LH secretion [ferret (126), Soay sheep (99)]. From the studies involving serial blood sampling it is apparent that each episodic release of LH stimulates an increase in testosterone secretion, and when there are seasonal changes in LH secretion the levels of testosterone change accordingly (Fig. 14).

Seasonal changes in responsiveness to LH also contribute to the cycle in testosterone secretion. In the Soay ram it has been shown that the release of testosterone to a standardized dose of LH is small and occurs more slowly during the period when the testes are regressed (Fig. 14). The same feature is apparent from the studies on the episodic secretion of LH, from which it is apparent that the peaks of LH are associated with small increases in testosterone during the period of seasonal quiescence, but marked increases in testosterone during the period of maximum testicular activity [Suffolk sheep (87), Soay sheep (99), goat (144), red deer (103)].

FSH and Spermatogenesis

The close correlation between pituitary content or plasma levels of FSH, and the seasonal cycle in the spermatogenic activity of the testes has been commented on above (Figs. 15, 16). In the hamster this close relationship between changes in FSH levels and the efficiency of spermatogenesis has been documented (17) (Fig. 17).

PMSG (pregnant mare serum gonadotrophin) which has principally FSH-like activity, has been used to stimulate testicular growth in the rock hyrax during the period of the year when the testes are regressed, an effect similar to that which occurs related to season (122). The injection of gonadotrophic extracts of pituitaries has had similar effects in other species [ground squirrel (123), varying hare (111)].

Prolactin

Seasonal changes in the levels of prolactin in the blood have been reported for a variety of mammals in which seasonal changes in testicular activity are

---

FIG. 16. Seasonal variation in the weight of the testis (□) and the content of FSH (■) in the pituitary in the snowshoe hare, *Lepus americana,* and the corresponding seasonal changes in diameter of the testis (□) and level of FSH (■) in the plasma in the Soay sheep *(Ovis aries).* Note the way FSH values increase simultaneously with the increase in testicular size following the period of quiescence and the values decline slightly in advance of the decline in the size of the testes. The season when most matings occur is shown by stippling. (From refs. 39,100.)

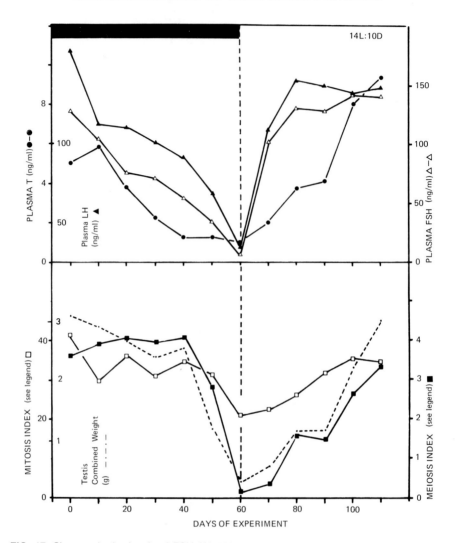

FIG. 17. Changes in the levels of FSH (△), LH (▲) and testosterone (●) in the male golden hamster *(Mesocricetus auratus)* during an experiment in which the animals were exposed to constant darkness (0L:24D) for 60 days and then returned to a normal lighting schedule (14L:10D). The corresponding changes are also shown for the weight of the testis (---) and the efficiency of spermatogonial divisions (□, ratio of leptotene primary spermatocytes: A spermatogonia) and the efficiency of spermatocytic meiotic divisions (■, ratio of round spermatids: leptotene primary spermatocytes). The hormone levels decline during the exposure to darkness and reach relatively low levels before effects on spermatogenesis are apparent, while the hormone levels increase rapidly on exposure to stimulatory lighting and the efficiency of the divisions of germ cells more gradually returns to normal. (From ref. 16.)

also documented. For the ungulates which have been studied the highest prolactin levels generally occur at the time of lowest testicular activity [goat (22), cattle (160), sheep (147)], however, the reverse pattern is apparent for some smaller species [mole (139), hamster (150), brown hare (Lincoln, *unpublished data*)]. The significance of the seasonal changes in prolactin secretion still remains to be established.

ACCESSORY GLANDS, SECONDARY SEXUAL CHARACTERS AND BEHAVIOR

Reproductive Tract and Accessory Glands

The glands of the male reproductive tract which are dependent on androgens for their normal function wax and wane in size and activity during the year in species with a seasonal cycle in testicular activity. When the seasonal regression of the testes is very marked, the reproductive tract may regress to a prepubertal state (Fig. 18).

The changes in the weight of the epididymis and the various accessory glands during the year have been related to the seasonal changes in the testes for a variety of species. The usual pattern is for the accessory glands to become maximally developed at the time when the testes are most expanded or commonly a month or so later (Fig. 19) [mole (142), vole (28), weasel (72), mongoose (58), European badger, pine marten, stone marten, and polecat (10), American badger (195a), brown hare (98), cotton-tailed rabbit (43), fox (81), Virginia deer (190,191), roe deer (163), red deer (95), blesbok, impala, kudu, and springbok (166), black wildebeest and red hartebeest (168), rock hyrax (121)].

Many of the studies referred to above describe the histological changes in the secretory epithelium of the accessory glands with measurements of the changes in the height of the epithelial cells; these attain their maximum dimensions coincident with the time when the glands are of maximum size. The changes in ultrastructure of the secretory cells have also been investigated (mole, refs. 11,174).

The content of fructose or citric acid in the accessory sexual glands (seminal vesicles, prostate, ampullary glands, etc.) provides an index of the secretory activity, and the seasonal changes generally parallel the changes in glandular weight [noctule bat (141), brown hare (98), fox (81), roe deer (163), red deer (95), black wildebeest and red hartebeest (168)]. The seasonal changes in the level of fructose in the semen have been recorded for some domestic species [Merino sheep (53), Awassi, German mutton, Corridale, Border-Leicester and Dorset Horn sheep (7)].

The seasonal changes in the weight and secretory activity of the accessory glands are generally closely correlated with the changes in the activity of the testes and, in particular, the secretion of testosterone. Maximal glandular activity tends to coincide with the time of maximal testosterone secretion and regression

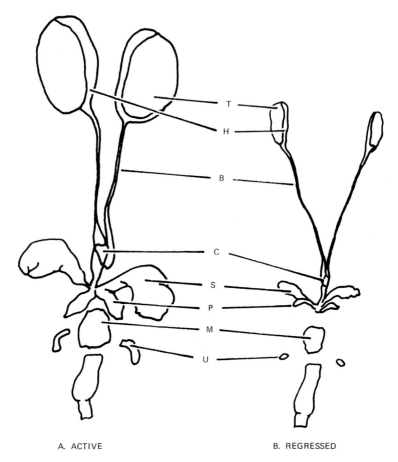

A. ACTIVE   B. REGRESSED

FIG. 18. Outline drawing of the reproductive tract from an adult South African rock hyrax, *Procavia capensis* **A:** at the time of full sexual activity and **B:** during the period of seasonal regression. T: testis; H: head of epididymis, B: body of epididymis, C: sperm store (cauda epididymidis), S: seminal vesicle, P: prostate-type gland, M: urethral muscle, U: bulbo-urethral gland. (Redrawn from ref. 121.)

of the reproductive tract occurs when testosterone secretion declines. At the time of seasonal resurgence of reproductive activity after the quiescent period, the development of the accessory glands usually lags behind the increase in testosterone secretion [roe deer (163), red deer (95) (Fig. 20)]. The cycle in activity of the accessory glands of the hibernating bats is somewhat unusual in that the glands increase in activity relatively slowly after the increase in testosterone levels, while the glands continue to remain enlarged for a prolonged period after testosterone levels have declined [pipistrelle bat (143), noctule bat (141)] (Fig. 20).

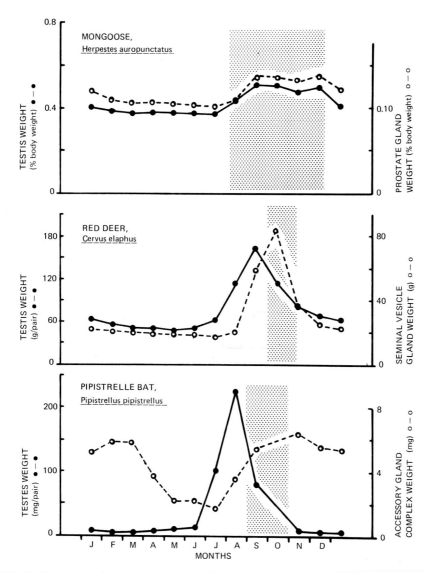

FIG. 19. Seasonal variation in the weight of the testis (●) and the weight of major accessory sexual glands (○) of the adult mongoose, *Herpestes auropunctatus,* red deer, *Cervus elaphus,* and pipistrelle bat, *Pipistrellus pipistrellus.* Note the maintenance of the accessory glands in the species of bat over the winter period during which time the testes regress—a feature related to hibernation and sperm storage. The season when most matings occur is shown by stippling. (From refs. 58,95,141.)

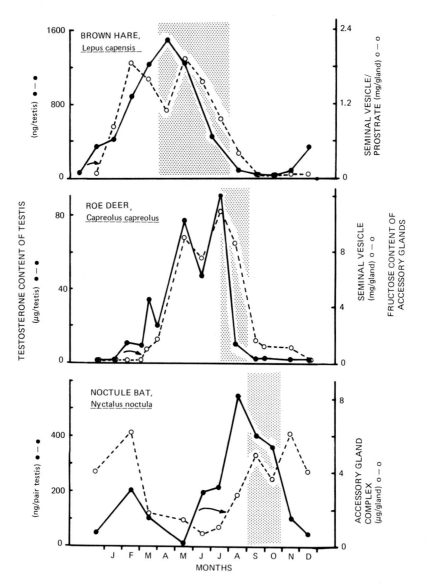

FIG. 20. Seasonal variation in the testosterone content (●) of the testis and the fructose content (○) of the accessory sexual glands for the brown hare, *Lepus capensis*, roe deer, *Capreolus capreolus,* and noctule bat, *Nyctalus noctula*. The changes in the levels of fructose tend to lag behind the changes in testosterone (arrow), a feature especially obvious in the noctule bat. The season when most matings occur is indicated by stippling. (From refs. 98, 141,163.)

Secondary Sexual Characteristics

The seasonal changes in testicular activity are reflected in changes in the male secondary sexual characteristics in some species. This is illustrated especially well amongst the deer, in which the secondary sexual characteristics include the antlers: Virginia deer (190), sika deer (59), red deer (107), and skin glands: musk-pod of musk deer (49a), infra-orbital gland of red deer (95), preputial gland of fallow deer (88), or elaborations of the coat: neck mane of red deer (95), and modifications of the body musculature: neck musculature of red deer (95) (Fig. 21). Each of these features is fully developed for the mating season at the time of maximum testicular development and becomes modified at other times of the year. The annual cycle of casting, growth, and cleaning of the antlers is especially well studied, and the role of testosterone in dictating the changes in the antlers has been demonstrated experimentally [Virginia deer (192), sika deer (59), red deer (107)].

Other examples of male secondary sexual features which change with season related to the activity of the testes include the red skin flush of the rhesus monkey (178), the 'flatted monkey' phenomenon of the green monkey (42), and the soft palate of the camel (26). Many species show seasonal modifications of scent glands: anal gland of wild rabbit and brown hare (124), dorsal gland of rock hyrax (120), sebaceous glands of the goat (112), preputial gland of mole (142), and temporal gland of the Indian elephant (78). In sheep there is a red skin flush which develops seasonally on the exposed skin on the inside of the front and hind legs, and is associated with a sebaceous scent gland which changes in secretory activity during the year (100).

Sexual and Aggressive Behavior

A change in aggressive and sexual behavior is a characteristic feature of many species in which the testes undergo a marked seasonal cycle in activity. Again, the deer provide striking examples in which the so-called rutting behavior develops at the time of peak testicular activity. At this time the males become intensely aggressive towards each other and territoriality appears in some species. They also have increased libido and spend much of the time in pursuit of females [roe deer (20), red deer (107), wapiti (173), fallow deer (24), reindeer (49)].

Beside the studies on deer the seasonal changes in aggressive behavior have been correlated with the cycle in testosterone secretion for such diverse species as the Asiatic elephant (78), brown hare (98), Soay sheep (100), noctule bat (141), and rhesus monkey (152).

Many wild animals lose their normal caution at the time of most intense activity; nocturnal species appear during the day (brown hare, ref. 98), subterranean species sometimes come above ground (mole, ref. 57) and species which normally reside in dense cover can be seen in the open (rabbit, ref. 19). Deaths from accidents reach a peak at this time (mountain hare, ref. 52). In the case

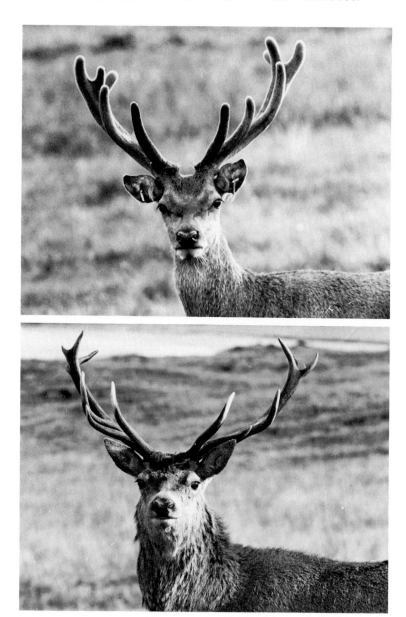

FIG. 21. Photographs of an adult male red deer, *Cervus elaphus,* taken in June **(above)** and November **(below)** showing the changes which occur in the antlers, neck mane and general body coat, and the neck musculature related to season. The animals are sexually quiescent between April and June, redevelopment of the reproductive tract occurs from June to October, and the increase in testosterone secretion results in the seasonal changes in the secondary sexual characteristics.

of the small marsupial rodent, *Antechinus,* the exertions of the rut result in the death of all males (193,194).

Seasonal changes in sexual libido and mating behavior usually occur in parallel with the changes in aggressive behavior (55). Quantitative studies have been made on the sexual behavior of some of the familiar domesticated species, and the usual finding is that the males show a peak in behavior coincident with maximal testicular activity or shortly afterwards; over this time the males usually show greater inclination to mount estrous females. The time from mounting to ejaculation is short and the recovery period following mating is also minimal [sheep (61,92,94,100,108,136,161), goat (46,154,164), cattle (45,91), rhesus mon-

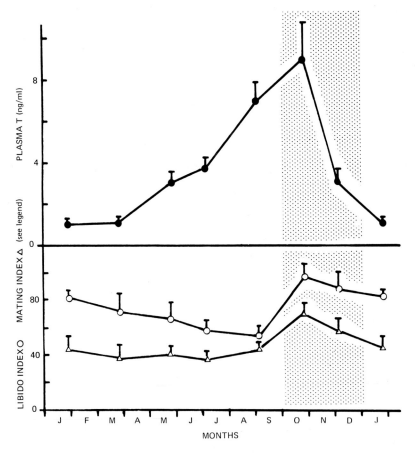

FIG. 22. Seasonal changes (mean ± SEM) in sexual libido (○) and mating behavior (△) of adult Suffolk rams tested with oestrous ewes, and the corresponding changes in the levels of testosterone (●) in the plasma. The values for the two behavioral measures were obtained by scoring various aspects of courtship and mating behavior in rams introduced individually for 20 min to a pen containing 5 ewes induced to show estrus by hormone therapy. (For details see ref. 161.)

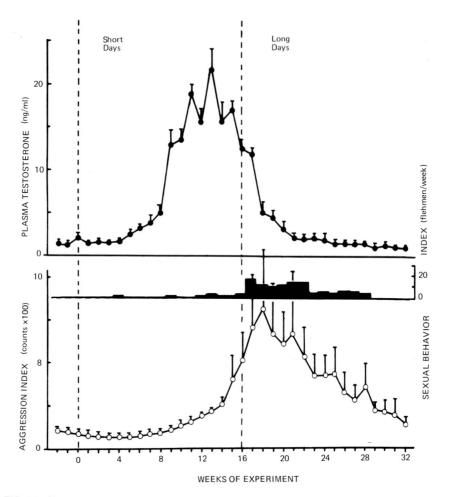

FIG. 23. Changes (mean ± SEM) in the aggressive (○) and sexual behavior (histogram), and the levels of testosterone (●) in the plasma of adult Soay rams induced to show a seasonal cycle in testicular activity by exposure to an artificial lighting regime consisting of 16 week periods of short daylengths (8L:16D) and long daylengths (16L:8D). The animals were penned individually and aggressive behavior was recorded by a mechanical device mounted within each pen; the incidence of flehmen (sexual lip-curl) was used as an index of sexual behavior. Note the long delay between the increase in behavioral activity and the increase in the circulating levels of testosterone. (From ref. 100.)

key (119,152,179)] (Figs. 22 and 23). The role of testosterone in dictating the changes in sexual and aggressive behavior has been demonstrated experimentally for some of the species [sheep (31), red deer (101), rhesus monkey (138)].

CONCLUSIONS

Seasonal changes in daylength, temperature, and food supply are important factors of the environment which dictate the seasonal changes in testicular activ-

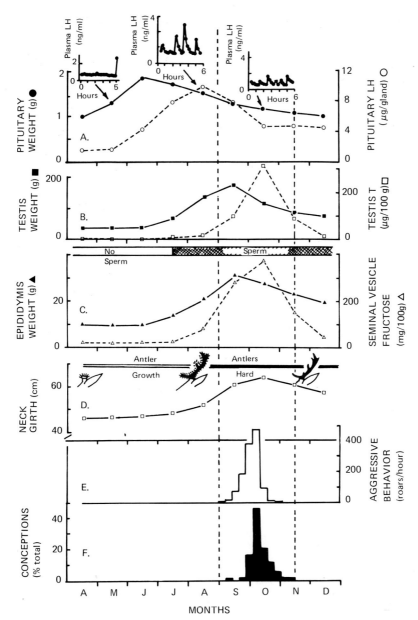

FIG. 24. A composite diagram based on several separate studies summarizing the reproductive changes in the adult red deer stag, *Cervus elaphus,* during part of the year preceding and following the mating season. **A:** Pituitary: weight (●) and LH (○) content of pituitary (from refs. 21,95). Plasma levels of LH are shown above for 3 points in the year (May, August, and October)—samples were collected at 15 min intervals for 6 hr from a single animal (from ref. 103). **B:** Testis: weight (■) and concentration of testosterone (□) in the testes (95). **C:** Accessory glands: weight of epididymides (▲) concentration of fructose in the seminal vesicles (△) and the storage of spermatozoa in the cauda epididymidis (horizontal bar) (95). **D:** Secondary sexual characters: girth of the neck (□) and state of the antlers (95). **E:** Behavior: frequency of roaring in a wild population of deer (from ref. 102). **F:** Conceptions: timing of conceptions amongst female red deer in a wild population (from ref. 102).

ity described in this chapter. It has not been possible to describe the environmental control for the different species, but the general assumption has been that the effects of the environment on the testes are mediated through changes in the secretion of gonadotrophins by the pituitary. The only possible exception to this is where environmental factors directly influence testicular activity. For example, extremes of temperature may directly affect spermatogenesis (177,182).

The general picture is that seasonal regression of the testis results from a decline in pituitary secretion of both LH and FSH, and the differences between species in the extent of regression reflect the degree to which the pituitary becomes 'switched off' for part of the year. In the case of the very seasonal species, complete inactivity of the pituitary occurs and the animals show the symptoms of total hypophysectomy. The decline in gonadotrophin secretion results in regression of the testes and all the associated reproductive functions such that the animal enters a phase of reduced sexual activity. Redevelopment of the reproductive system involves a complete reversal of the changes seen during regression, and a sequence of events occurs at the level of the pituitary, testis, androgen target tissues, and behavior, ultimately resulting in the return of full sexual activity (Fig. 24). The seasonal mammals thus provide a natural experiment in changing pituitary function. Wild mammals as bizarre as the burrowing mole and diminutive short-tailed field mouse may therefore not be totally irrelevant in providing an understanding of male reproductive physiology. In the words of William Harvey in 1653 (68), "It is a wonderful thing to see how great a quantity of geniture both abound in the testicles and much distended seminal vesicles of the very masculine moles and mice, about the time of their coition."

REFERENCES

1. Abdel-Raouf, M., Fateh El-Bab, M. R., and Owaida, M. M. (1975): Studies on reproduction in the camel *(Camelus dromedarius). J. Reprod. Fert.,* 43:109–116.
2. Allanson, M. (1932): The reproductive processes of certain mammals. III. The reproductive cycle of the male ferret. *Proc. R. Soc. Lond. (Biol.),* 110:295–312.
3. Allanson, M. (1933): Changes in the reproductive organs of the male grey squirrel, *Sciurus carolinesis. Philos. Trans. R. Soc. (Biol.),* 222:79–96.
4. Allanson, M. (1934): The reproductive processes of certain mammals. VII. Seasonal variation in the reproductive organs of the male hedgehog. *Philos. Trans. R. Soc. (Biol.),* 223:277–303.
5. Allanson, M. (1963): The reproductive tract of prepubertal and mature moles during the anoestrus. *J. Endocrinol.,* 26:IX–X.
6. Amann, R. P., Almquist, J. O., and Lambiase, J. T. (1966): Seasonal cycles in bull semen characteristics. *J. Anim. Sci.,* 25:916–917.
7. Amir, D., Volcani, R., and Genizi, A. (1965): Seasonal fluctuations in the sexual activity of Awassi, German Mutton, Merino, Corriedale, Border Leicester and Dorset Horn rams. *J. Agric. Sci.,* 64:115–135.
8. Amoroso, E. C., and Marshall, F. H. A. (1960): External factors in sexual periodicity. In: *Marshall's Physiology of Reproduction,* Vol. 1, part 2, edited by A. S. Parkes. Longmans, London.
9. Asdell, S. A. (1964): *Patterns of mammalian reproduction,* 2nd ed. Cornell University Press, Ithaca, New York.

10. Audy, M. C. (1976): Le cycle sexuel saisonnier du male des Mustélidés Europeens. *Gen. Comp. Endocrinol.,* 30:117–127.
11. Aumuller, G., and Greenberg, J. (1976): Seasonal changes in the fine structure of the accessory sex gland in the mole (Talpa europaea). *Cell Tissue Res.,* 175:403–416.
12. Aumuller, G., and Schäfer, A. (1972): Histochemie und Feinstruktur der Zwischenzellen des Maulwurfhodens *(Talpa europaea L.)* während der Abklingphase der Spermatogenese. *Acta Histochem.,* 43:235–253.
13. Baker, J. R. (1938): Evolution of breeding seasons. In: *Evolution Essays on Aspects of Evolutionary Biology,* presented to Professor E. S. Goodrich and G. R. de Beer, p. 350. Clarendon Press, Oxford.
14. Barrell, G. K. (1976). Studies of neuroendocrine mechanisms influencing seasonal variations in semen production and plasma hormone levels in rams. Ph.D. Thesis. Massay University, New Zealand.
15. Barth, V. D., Giménez, T., Hoffmann, B., and Karg, H. (1976): Testosteronkonzentrationen im peripheren Blut beim Rehbock *(Capreolus capreolus).* Z. Jagdwissenschaft, 22:134–148.
16. Berndtson, W. E., and Desjardins, C. (1974): Circulating LH and FSH levels and testicular function in hamster during light deprivation and subsequent photoperiodic stimulation. *Endocrinology,* 95:195–205.
17. Berndtson, W. E., Pickett, B. W., and Nett, T. M. (1974): Reproductive physiology of the stallion. IV. Seasonal changes in the testosterone concentration in peripheral plasma. *J. Reprod. Fert.,* 39:115–118.
18. Brambell, F. W. R. (1935): Reproduction in the common shrew *(Sorex araneus). Philos. Trans. R. Soc.,* 225B:1–62.
19. Brambell, F. W. R. (1944): The reproduction of the wild rabbit, *Oryctolagus cuniculus. Proc. Zool. Soc. (Lond),* 114:1–45.
20. Bramley, P. S. (1970). Territoriality and reproductive behaviour of roe deer. *J. Reprod. Fert.,* Suppl. 11:43–70.
21. Bruggemann, J., Adam, A., and Karg, H. (1965): ICSH-bestimmungen in hypophysen von rehböcken *(Capreolus capreolus)* und hirschen *(Cervus elaphus)* unter berücksichtigung des saisoneinflusses. *Acta Endocrinol.,* 48:569–580.
22. Buttle, H. L. (1974): Seasonal variation of prolactin in plasma of male goats. *J. Reprod. Fert.,* 37:95–99.
23. Carson, W. S., and Amann, R. P. (1972): The male rabbit. VI. Effects of ejaculation and season on testicular size and function. *J. Anim. Sci.,* 34:302–309.
24. Chaplin, R. A., and White, R. W. (1970): The sexual cycle and associated behaviour patterns in the fallow deer. *Deer,* 2:561.
25. Chaplin, R. E., and White, R. W. G. (1972): The influence of age and season on the activity of the testes and epididymides of the fallow deer, *Dama dama. J. Reprod. Fert.,* 30:361–369.
26. Charnot, Y. (1963): Synchronisation of growth of the palatal expansion and the testis during the sexual cycle in the dromedary. *Bull. Soc. Sci. Nat. Maroc.,* 43:49–54.
27. Christensen, A. K. (1975): Leydig cells. In: *Handbook of Physiology,* Vol. V., Male Reproductive System, edited by D. W. Hamilton and R. O. Greep, pp. 57–94. American Physiological Society, Washington, D.C.
28. Clarke, J. R., and Forsyth, I. A. (1964*a*): Seasonal changes in the gonads and accessory reproductive organs of the vole *(Microtus agrestis). Gen. Comp. Endocrinol.,* 4:233–242.
29. Clarke, J. R., and Forsyth, I. A. (1964*b*): Seasonal changes in the adenohypophysis of the vole *(Microtus agrestis). Gen. Comp. Endocrinol.,* 4:243–252.
30. Clarke, J. R., and Greig, F. (1971): Seasonal changes in the adenohypophysis of the bank vole, *Clethrionomys glareoulus. J. Reprod. Fert.,* 25:310–311.
31. Clegg, M. T., Beamer, W., and Bermant, G. (1969): Copulatory behaviour of the ram, *Ovis aries.* III. Effects of pre- and postpubertal castration and androgen replacement therapy. *Anim. Behav.,* 17:712–717.
32. Conaway, C. H. (1959): The reproductive cycle of the eastern mole. *J. Mammal,* 40:180–194.
33. Conaway, C. H., and Sade, D. S. (1969): Annual testis cycle of the green monkey *(Cercopithecus aethiops)* on St Kitts, West Indies. *J. Mammal,* 50:833–835.
34. Courot, M., and Joffre, M. (1976): Testicular capillary blood flow in the impuberal lamb and ram during the breeding and non-breeding seasons. *Ann. Biol. Anim. Biochem. Biophys.,* 16:171.

35. Courrier, R. (1923a): Sur la cycle de la glande interstitielle et l'évolution des caractéres sexuels secondaires chez les mammifères a spermatogénèse periodique. *C. R. Soc. Biol.,* 89:1311–1313.
36. Courrier, R. (1923b): Cycle annuel de la glande interstitielle du testicule chez les cheiroptères. Coexistence du repos seminal et de l'activité génitale. *C. R. Soc. Biol.,* 88:1163–1166.
37. Courrier, R. (1927): Étude sur le eterminisme des caractères sexuels secondaires chez quelques mammifères à activité testiculaire périodique. *Arch. Biol. (Paris),* 37:173–334.
38. Cupps, P. T., McGowan, B., Rahlmann, D. F., Reddon, A. R., and Weir, W. C. (1960): Seasonal changes in the semen of rams. *J. Anim. Sci.,* 19:208–213.
39. Davis G. J., and Meyer, R. K. (1973): Seasonal variation in LH and FSH of bilaterally castrated Snowshoe hares. *Gen. Comp. Endocrinol.,* 20:61–68.
40. De Kretser, D. M., Bremner, W. J., Burger, H. G., Hudson, B., Irby, D. C., Kerr, J. B., and Less V. W. K. (1977): The interaction between the hypothalamo-hypophyseal system and the testis in mammalian species. In: *Reproduction and Evolution,* edited by J. H. Calaby, and C. H. Tyndale-Biscoe, pp. 111–120. Australian Academy of Science.
41. DeLost, P. (1966): Reproduction et cycles endocrines de l'ecurcuil *(Sciurus vulgaris) Arch. Sci. Physiol.,* 20:425–457.
42. Dumond, F. V., and Hutchinson, T. C. (1967): Squirrel monkey reproduction: the 'flatted' male phenomenon and seasonal spermatogenesis. *Science,* 158:1067–1070.
43. Elder, W. H., and Finerty, J. C. (1943): Gonadotrophic activity of the pituitary gland in relation to the seasonal sexual cycle of the cotton-tail rabbit, *Sylvilagus floridanus mearnsi. Anat. Rec.,* 85:1–16.
44. Ellis, L. C., and Balph, D. F. (1976): Age and seasonal differences in the synthesis and metabolism of testosterone by testicular tissue and pinal HIOMT activity of uinta ground squirrels. *Spermophilus armalus. Gen. Comp. Endocrinol.,* 28:42–55.
45. Elsawaf, S., Badaway, A, and Elwishy, A. (1971): Seasonal variation in sexual desire and semen characteristics of buffalo bulls. *Z. Tierzücht Zucht Biol.* 88:222–230.
46. Elwishy, A., Elsawaf, S, and Elmikkawi, F. (1971): Monthly and seasonal variation in sexual activity of male Damascus goats. *Indian J. Anim. Sci.,* 41:562–569.
47. Erb, R. E., Andrews, F. N., and Hilton, J. H. (1942): Seasonal variation in semen quality of the dairy bull. *J. Dairy Sci.,* 25:815.
48. Esnault, C., Fautréz, F., and Ortavant, R. (1964): The development of the level of Feulgen-DNA material of the germ cells of rams submitted to different photoperiods. *Proc. 5th Int. Congr. Anim. Reprod. Artif. Insem.* Trento. 2:419.
49. Espmark, Y. (1964): Rutting behaviour in reindeer, *Rangifer tarandus* L. *Anim. Behav.,* 12:420–426.
49a. Flerov, K. K. (1952): Musk deer and deer. *Fauna of USSR, Mammals,* 1(2):123–131. The Academy of Sciences of the USSR, Moscow.
50. Flux, J. E. C. (1969): Current work on the reproduction of the African hare, *Lepus capensis,* in Kenya. *J. Reprod. Fert.,* Suppl. 6:225–235.
52. Flux, J. E. C. (1970): Life history of the mountain hare *(Lepus timidus scoticus)* in north east Scotland. *J. Zool. (Lond),* 161:75–123.
53. Fowler, D. G. (1965): Semen quality 2. The effects of seasonal changes in day length on semen quality. *Aust. J. Exp. Agric. Anim. Husb.,* 5:247–251.
54. Frankenberger, Z. (1954): Interstitial cells in the deer *(Cervus elephus* L). *Cesk. Morfol.,* 2:36.
55. Frazer, A. (1968): *Reproductive Behaviour in Ungulates.* Academic Press, London.
56. Gilmore, D. P. (1969): Seasonal reproductive periodicity in the male Australian brush-tailed possum (Trichosurus vulpecula) *J. Zool. (Lond),* 157:75–98.
57. Godfrey, G., and Crowcroft, P. (1960): *Life of the Mole, Talpa europaea.* Museum Press, London.
58. Gorman, M. L. (1976): Seasonal changes in the reproductive pattern of feral *Herpestes auropunctatus* (Carnivora: Viverridae) in the Fijian Islands. *J. Zool. (Lond),* 178:237–246.
59. Gross, R. J. (1963): The deciduous nature of deer antlers. In: *Mechanisms of Hard Tissue Destruction,* publication No. 75, pp. 339–369. American Association for the Advancement of Science, Washington, D.C.
60. Grocock, C. A., and Clarke, J. R. (1975): Spermatogenesis in mature and regressed testes of the vole, *Microtus agrestis. J. Reprod. Fert.,* 43:461–470.
61. Grubb, P., and Jewell, P. A. (1973): The rut and occurrence of estrus in the Soay sheep on St. Hilda. *J. Reprod. Fert.,* Suppl. 19:491–502.

62. Gulamhusein A. P., and Tam, W. H., (1974): Reproduction in the male stoat, *Mustela erminea. J. Reprod. Fert.,* 41:303–312.
63. Gustafson, A. W. (1975): Observations on the hydroxysteroid dehydrogenase and lipid histochemistry and ultrastructure of the Leydig cells in adult *Myotis l. lucifugus* during the annual reproductive cycle. *Anat. Rec.,* 181:366–367.
64. Gustafson, A. W., and Shemesh, M. (1976): Changes in plasma testosterone levels during the annual reproductive cycle of the hibernating bat, *Myotis lucifugus lucifugus* with a survey of plasma testosterone levels in adult male vertebrates. *Biol. Reprod.,* 15:9–24.
65. Hanks, J. (1977): Comparative aspects of reproduction in the male hyrax and elephant. In: *Reproduction and Evolution,* edited by J. H. Calaby and C. H. Tyndale-Biscoe, pp. 155–164. Australian Academy of Science.
66. Harrison, R. J., and Ridgway, S. H. (1971): Gonadal activity in some bottlenose dolphins *Turiops truncatus J. Zool.,* 165:355–366.
67. Hart, J. S. (1964): Geography and season: mammals and birds. In: *Handbook of Physiology, Adaptations to the Environment,* edited by D. B. Dill. American Physiological Society, Washington, D.C.
68. Harvey, W. (1653): *Anatomical Exercitations Concerning the Generation of Living Creatures: To Which are Added Particular Discourses, of Births and of Conceptions, etc.* J. Young for O. Pulleyn, London.
69. Heape, W. (1901): The sexual season of mammals and the relation of the pro-oestrum to menstruation. *J. Microsc. Sci.,* 44:1–70.
70. Herlant, M. (1959): L'hypophyse de la Taupe au cours de la phase d'activité sexuelle. *C.R. Acad. Sci. (Paris),* 248:1033–1036.
71. Hewer, H. R. (1964): The determination of age, sexual maturity longevity and a life table in the grey seal. *Halichoerus grypus. Proc. Zool. Soc. (Lond),* 142:593–624.
72. Hill, M. (1939): The reproductive cycle of the male weasel *Mustela nivalis. Proc. Zool. Soc., (Lond) (B)* 109:481–512.
73. Hill, M., and Parkes, A. S. (1933): Studies on the hypophysectomised feret IV. Comparison of the reproductive organs during anestrous and after hypophysectomy. *Proc. R. Soc. (B.),* 113:530–536.
74. Hochereau-De Reviers, M. T., and Lincoln, G. A. (1978): Seasonal variation in the testicular histology of the red deer stag *(Cervus elaphus). J. Reprod. Fert.,* 54:209–213.
75. Houchereau-De Reviers, M. T., Loir, M., and Pelletier, J. (1976): Seasonal variation in the response of the testis and LH levels to hemicastration of adult rams. *J. Reprod. Fert.,* 46:203–209.
76. Hoffman, R. A., and Zarrow, M. X. (1955): Changes in the cytology of the pituitary gland of *Citellus* as demonstrated by the periodic acid-Schiff reaction. *Anat. Rec.,* 122:476–477.
77. Islam, A. B. M. M., and Land, R. B. (1977): Seasonal variation in testis diameter and sperm output of rams of breeds of different prolificacy. *Anim. Prod.,* 25:311–317.
78. Jainudeen, M. R., Katongole, C. B., and Short, R. V. (1972): Plasma testosterone levels in relation to musth and sexual activity in the male Asiatic elephant, *Elaphas maximus. J. Reprod. Fert.,* 29:99–103.
79. Jegou, B., Terqui, M., Gardier, D. H., Dacheux, J. L., and Courot, M. (1976): Variations saisonnieres de la proteine de liaison des androgenes dans les secretions exocrines du testicule de belier. *Ann. Endocrinol.* 37:489–490.
80. Jochle, W. (1972): Seasonal fluctuations of reproductive functions in zebu cattle. *Int. J. Biometeorol.* 16:131–144.
81. Joffre, M. (1976): Puberté et cycle génital saisonnier du renard mâle *(Vulpes vulpes). Ann. Biol. Anim. Biochem. Biophys.,* 16: 503–520.
82. Joffre, M. (1977a): Circulation testiculaire chez le renard roux (*Vulpes vulpes* L) adulte. *J. Physiol. (Paris),* 73:155–176.
83. Joffre, M. (1977b): La capsule testiculaire du renard roux (*Vulpes vulpes* L): relation avec l'activité testiculaire pendant la periode prépubere et au cours du cycle saisonnier. *Ann. Biol Anim. Biochem. Biophys.,* 17:695–712.
84. Joffre, M. (1977c): Relationship between testicular blood flow, testosterone secretion and spermatogenic activity in young and adult wild red foxes *(Vulpes vulpes). J. Reprod. Fert.,* 51:35–40.

85. Joffre, J., and Joffre, M. (1973): Seasonal changes in the testicular blood flow of seasonally breeding mammals: dormouse *(Glis glis)* ferret *(Mustela furo)* and fox *(Vulpes vulpes). J. Reprod. Fert.,* 34:227–233.

86. Joffre, M., and Kormano, M. (1975): An angiographic study of the fox testis in various stages of sexual activity. *Anat. Rec.,* 183:599–601.

87. Katongole, C., Naftolin, F., and Short, R. V. (1974): Seasonal variation in blood luteinizing hormone and testosterone levels in rams. *J. Endocrinol.,* 60:101–106.

88. Kennaugh, J. H., Chapman, D. I., and Chapman, N. G. (1977): Seasonal changes in the prepuce of adult Fallow deer *(Dama dama)* and its probable function as a scent organ. *J. Zool. (Lond),* 183:301–310.

89. Kinson, G., and Liu, C. (1973): Further evidence of inherent testicular rhythms in the laboratory rat. *J. Endocrinol.,* 56:337–338.

90. Kirkpatrick, J. F., Wiesner, L., Kenney, R. M., Ganjam, V. K., and Turner, J. W. (1977): Seasonal variation in plasma androgens and testosterone in the North American wild horse. *J. Endocrinol.,* 72:237–238.

91. Kushwahaws, R., Mukhergee, D., and Bhattacharya, P. (1955): Seasonal variation in reaction time and semen quality of buffalo bulls. *Indian J. Vet. Sci.,* 25:317.

92. Land, R. B (1970): The mating behaviour and semen characteristics of Finnish landrace and Scottish blackface rams. *Anim. Prod.,* 12:551–560.

93. Laurie, E. M. O. (1946): The reproduction of the house-mouse *Mus musculus* living in different environments. *Proc. R. Soc.,* 133B:248–281.

94. Lees, J. (1965): Seasonal variation in the breeding activity of rams. *Nature (Lond),* 207:221–222.

95. Lincoln, G. A. (1971*a*): The seasonal reproductive changes in the red deer stag *(Cervus elaphus). J. Zool. (Lond),* 163:105–123.

96. Lincoln, G. A. (1971*b*): Puberty in a seasonally breeding male, the red deer stag *(Cervus elaphus L). J. Reprod. Fert.,* 25:41–54.

97. Lincoln, G. A. (1973): Cyclical and seasonal changes in human testicular activity. *J. Reprod. Fert.,* 33:365.

98. Lincoln, G. A. (1974): Reproduction and 'March madness' in the brown hare, *Lepus europaeus. J. Zool. (Lond),* 174:1–14.

99. Lincoln, G. A. (1976): Seasonal variation in the episodic secretion of LH and testosterone in the ram. *J. Endocrinol.,* 69:213–226.

100. Lincoln, G. A., and Davidson, W. (1977): The relationship between sexual and aggressive behaviour, and pituitary and testicular activity during the seasonal sexual cycle of rams, and the influence of photoperiod. *J. Reprod. Fert.,* 49:267–276.

101. Lincoln, G. A., Guinness, F., and Short, R. V. (1972): The way in which testosterone controls the social and sexual behaviour of the red deer stag *(Cervus elaphus). Horm. Behav.,* 3:375–396.

102. Lincoln, G. A., and Guinness, F. (1973): The sexual significance of the rut in red deer. *J. Reprod. Fert.,* Suppl. 19:475–489.

103. Lincoln, G. A., and Kay, R. N. B. (1978): Effects of season on the secretion of luteinizing hormone and testosterone in intact and castrated red deer stags *(Cervus elaphus). J. Reprod. Fert.,* 55:75–80.

104. Lincoln, G. A., and Peet, M. J. (1977): Photoperiodic control of gonadotrophin secretion in the ram: A detailed study of the temporal changes in plasma levels of follicle-stimulating hormone, luteinizing hormone and testosterone following an abrupt switch from long to short days. *J. Endocrinol.,* 74:355–367.

105. Lincoln, G. A., Peet, M. J., and Cunningham, R. A. (1977): Seasonal and circadian changes in the episodic release of follicle stimulating hormone, luteinizing hormone and testosterone in rams exposed to artificial photoperiods. *J. Endocrinol.,* 72:337–349.

106. Lincoln, G. A., and Mackinnon, P. C. B. (1976): A study of seasonally delayed puberty in the male hare, *Lepus europaeus. J. Reprod. Fert.,* 46:123–128.

107. Lincoln, G. A., Youngson, R. W., and Short, R. V. (1970): Social and sexual behaviour of the red deer stag. *J. Reprod. Fert.,* Suppl. 11:71–103.

108. Lindsay, D., and Ellsmore, J. (1968): The effect of breed, season and competition on mating behaviour of rams. *Aust. J. Exp. Agric. Anim. Husb.,* 8:649–652.

109. Lodge, J. R., and Salisbury, G. W. (1970): Seasonal variation and male reproductive efficiency. In: *The Testis*, Vol. III, edited by A. D. Johnson, W. R. Gomes, and N. L. Vandemark. Academic Press, London.
110. Lofts, B. (1960): Cyclical changes in the distribution of the testis lipids of a seasonal mammal *(Talpa europaea). Q. J. Microsc. Sci.*, 101:199–205.
111. Lyman, C. P. (1943): Control of coat colour in the varying hare, *Lepus americanus. Bull. Mus. Comp. Zool. (Harvard)*, 93:393–461.
112. Macewan Jenkinson, D., Blackburn, D., and Proudfoot, R. (1967): Seasonal changes in the skin glands of the goat. *Br. Vet. J.*, 123:541–549.
113. McKeever, S. (1963): Seasonal changes in body weight, reproductive organs, pituitary, adrenal glands, thyroid gland and spleen of the Belding ground squirrel, *Citellus beldingi. Am. J. Anat.*, 113:153–167.
114. McMillin, J. M., Seal, U. S., Keenlyne, K. D., Erickson, A. W., and Jones, J. E. (1974): Annual testosterone rhythm in the adult white-tailed deer *(Odocoileus virginianus borealis). Endocrinology*, 94:1034–1040.
115. McMillin, J. M., Seal, U. S., Rogers, L., and Erickson, A. W. (1976): Annual testosterone rhythm in the black bear *(Ursus americanus). Biol. Reprod.*, 15:163–167.
116. Markwald, R. R., Davis, R. W., and Kainer, R. A. (1971): Histological and histochemical periodicity of cervine Leydig cells in relation to antler growth. *Gen. Comp. Endocrinol.*, 16:268–280.
117. Marshall, F. H. A. (1942): Exteroceptor factors in sexual periodicity. *Biol. Rev.*, 17:69–89.
118. Meschaks, P., and Nordkvist, M. (1962): On the sexual cycle in the reindeer male. *Acta Vet. Scand.*, 3:151–162.
119. Michael, R. P., Zumpe, D., Plant, T. M., and Evans, R. G. (1975): Annual changes in the sexual potency of captive male rhesus monkeys. *J. Reprod. Fert.*, 45:169–172.
120. Millar, R. P. (1972): Reproduction in the rock hyrax *(Procavia capensis)* with special reference to seasonal sexual activity in the male. Ph.D. Thesis, University of Liverpool.
121. Millar, R. P., and Glover, T. D. (1970): Seasonal changes in the reproductive tract of the male rock hyrax, *Procavia capensis. J. Reprod. Fert.*, 23:497–499.
122. Millar, R. P., and Glover, T. D. (1973): Regulation of seasonal sexual activity in an ascrotal mammal, the rock hyrax, *Procavia capensis. J. Reprod. Fert.*, Suppl. 19:203–220.
123. Moore, C. R., Simmons, G. F., Wells, L. J., Zalesky, M., and Nelson, W. O. (1934): On the control of reproductive activity in an annual breeding mammal *(Citellus tridecemlineatus). Anat. Rec.*, 60:279–289.
124. Mykytowycz, R. (1966): Observations on odiferous and other glands in the Australian wild rabbit, *Oryctolagus cuniculus,* and the hare *Lepus europaeus. The anal gland. CSIRO Wild. Res.*, 11:11.
125. Nakabayashi, N. T., and Salisbury, G. W. (1959): Factors influencing the metabolic activity of bovine spermatozoa. V. Season. *J. Dairy Sci.*, 42:1806–1814.
126. Neal, J., Murphy, B. D., Moger, W. H., and Oliphant, L. W. (1977): Reproduction in the male ferret: gonadal activity during the annual cycle; recrudescence and maturation. *Biol. Reprod.*, 17:380–385.
127. Neaves, W. B. (1973): Changes in testicular Leydig cells and in plasma testosterone levels among seasonally breeding rock hyrax. *Biol. Reprod.*, 8:451–466.
128. Newsome, A. E. (1973): Cellular degeneration in the testis of red kangaroos during hot weather and drought in central Australia. *J. Reprod. Fert.*, Suppl. 19:191–201.
129. Onstad, O. (1967): Studies on postnatal testicular changes, semen quality and anomalies of the reproductive organs in the mink. *Acta Endocrinol.* Suppl., 117:29–55.
130. Ortavant, R. (1956): Action de la durée d'eclairement sur les processus spermatogénétiques chez le Bélier. *C. R. Soc. Biol. (Paris)*, 150:471–474.
131. Ortavant, R. (1958): Le cycle spermatogénétique chez le bélier. Thèse de Doctoral D'état Es-sciences Naturelles, pp. 1–127. Université de Paris.
132. Ortavant, R., Courot, M., and Hochereau-De-Reviers, M. T. (1969): Spermatogenesis and morphology of the spermatozoon. In: *Reproduction in Domestic Animals,* 2nd ed., edited by H. H. Cole and P. T. Cupps, pp. 251–276. Academic Press, London.
133. Ortavant, R., Mauleon, P., and Thibault, C. (1964): Photoperiodic control of gonadal and hypophyseal activity in domestic mammals. *Ann. N.Y. Acad. Sci.*, 177:157–192.

134. Pelletier, J. (1971): Influence du photopériodisme et des androgènes sur la synthese et la libération de LH chez le bélier. Thèse de Doctoral D'état Es-sciences Naturelles, pp. 1–243. Université de Paris.

135. Pelletier, J., and Ortavant, R. (1964): Influence de la durée d'éclairement sur le contenu hypophysaire en hormones gonadotropes FSH et ICSH chez le bélier. *Ann. Biol. Anim. Biochem. Biophys.,* 4:17–26.

136. Pepelko, W. E., and Clegg, M. T. (1965): Influence of season of the year upon patterns of sexual behaviour in male sheep. *J. Anim. Sci.,* 24:633–637.

137. Perry, J. S. (1945): The reproduction of the wild brown rat, *Rattus norvegicus. Proc. Zool. Soc. (Lond),* 115:19–46.

138. Phoenix, C., Slob, A., and Goy, R. (1973): Effects of castration and replacement therapy on sexual behaviour of adult male rhesus monkeys. *J. Comp. Physiol. Psychol.,* 84:472–481.

139. Pieters, A., and Herlant, M. (1972): Modification saisonnières des cellules à prolactine dans l'antehypophyse de la Taupe male. *C. R. Acad. Sci. (Paris),* 274:3002–3006.

140. Prasad, M. R. N. (1956): Reproductive cycle of the male Indian gerbil, *Tatera indica cuvierii, Waterhouse. Acta Zool. Stockh.,* 37:87–122.

140a. Pudney, J., and Lacy, D. (1977): Correlation between ultrastructure and biochemical changes in the testis of the American grey squirrel, *Sciurus carolinensis,* during the reproductive cycle. *J. Reprod. Fert.,* 49:5–16.

141. Racey, P. A. (1974): The reproductive cycle in male noctule bats, *Nyctalus noctula. J. Reprod. Fert.,* 41:169–182.

142. Racey, P. A. (1978): Seasonal changes in testosterone levels and androgen-dependent organs in male moles *(Talpa europaea). J. Reprod. Fert.,* 52:195–200.

143. Racey, P. A., and Tam, W. H. (1974): The reproductive cycle in the male pipistrelle bat, *Pipistrellus pipistrellus. J. Zool. (Lond),* 172:101–122.

144. Racey, P. A., Rowe, P. H., and Chesworh, J. M. (1975): Changes in the LH and testosterone system of the male goat during the breeding season. *J. Endocrinol.,* 65:8P–9P.

145. Ramakrishna, P. A., and Prasad, M. R. N. (1967): Changes in the male reproductive organs of *Loris tardigradus lydekkerianus. Folia Primatol.,* 5:176–189.

146. Rasmussen, A. T. (1918): Cyclic changes in the interstitial cells of the ovary and testis in the woodchuck *(Marmota monax). Endocrinology,* 2:353.

147. Ravault, J. P. (1976): Prolactin in the ram: seasonal variation in the concentration of blood plasma from birth to three years old. *Acta Endocrinol. (Kbh),* 83:720–725.

148. Raynaud, A. (1950): Variations saisonnieres des organes genitaux des mulots *(Apodemus sylvaticus)* de sexe male. Donnees pondérales et histologiques. *C. R. Soc. Biol.,* 144:941–945.

149. Reinberg, A., Lagoguey, M., Chauffournier, J-M, and Cesselin, F. (1975): Circannual and circadian rhythms in plasma testosterone in five healthy young Parisian males. *Acta Endocrinol. (Kbh),* 80:732–743.

150. Reiter, R. J. (1975): Exogenous and endogenous control of the annual reproductive cycle in the male golden hamster: participation of the pineal gland. *J. Exp. Zool.,* 191:111–126.

151. Resko, J. A. (1967): Plasma androgen levels of the rhesus monkey: effects of age and season. *Endocrinology,* 81:1203–1212.

152. Robinson, J. A., Scheffler, G., Eisele, S. G., and Goy, R. W. (1975): Effects of age and season on sexual behaviour and plasma testosterone and dihydrotestosterone concentration of laboratory-housed male rhesus monkeys *(Macaca mulatta). Biol. Reprod.,* 13:203–210.

153. Robinson, R. M., Thomas, J. W., and Marburger, R. G. (1965): The reproductive cycle of male white-tailed deer in central Texas. *J. Wildl. Manag.,* 29:53–59.

154. Rouger, Y. (1974): Étude des interactions de l'environment et des hormones sexuelles dans la regulation du comportement sexuel des bovidae. Thèse de Doctoral D'état Es-sciences Naturelles, Université de Rennes, France.

155. Rowlands, I. W. (1936): Reproduction of the bank vole *(Evolonys (Clethrionomys) glareolus).* II. Seasonal changes in the reproductive organs of the male. *Philos. Trans. R. Soc. Lond. (Biol),* 226:99–120.

156. Saboureau, M., and Peyre, A. (1970): Le décalage des activités endocrine et spermatogénétique du testicule au cours du réveil printanier chez le Hérisson mâle. *C. R. Soc. Biol. (Paris),* 164:2364–2367.

157. Sadleir, R. M. F. S. (1969): *The Ecology of Reproduction in Wild and Domestic Mammals.* Methuen, London.

158. Salisbury, G. W. (1967): Aging phenomena in spermatozoa. III. Effect of season and storage at −79°C to −88°C on fertility and prenatal losses. *J. Dairy Sci.,* 50:1683–1689.
159. Sanford, L. M., Winter, J. S. D., Palmer, W. M., and Howlands, B. E. (1974): The profile of LH and testosterone secretion in the ram. *Endocrinology,* 95:627–631.
160. Schams, D., and Reinhardt, V. (1974): Influence of season on plasma prolactin levels in cattle from birth to maturity. *Horm. Res.,* 5:217–226.
161. Schanbacher, B. D., and Lunstra, D. D. (1976): Seasonal changes in sexual activity and serum levels of LH and testosterone in Finnish Landrace and Suffolk rams. *J. Anim. Sci.,* 43:644–650.
162. Sen Gupta, B. P., Misra, M. S., and Roy, A. (1963): Climatic environment and reproductive behaviour of buffaloes. I. Effect of different seasons on various seminal attributes. *Indian J. Diary Sci.,* 16:150–160.
163. Short, R. V., and Mann, T. (1966): The sexual cycle of a seasonally breeding mammal, the roebuck, *Capreolus capreolus. J. Reprod. Fert.,* 12:337–351.
164. Shukla, D., and Bhattacharya, P. (1953): Seasonal variation in reaction time and semen quality in goats. *Indian J. Vet. Sci.,* 22:179–190.
165. Sinha, R. C., Sen Gupta, B. P., and Roy, A. (1966): Climatic environment and reproductive behaviour of buffaloes. IV. Comparative study of oxygen uptake and aerobic fructolysis by Murrah *(B. bubalis)* and Hariana *(B. indicus)* spermatozoa during different seasons. *Indian J. Diary Sci.,* 19:18–25.
166. Skinner, J. D. (1971): The effect of season on spermatogenesis in some ungulates. *J. Reprod. Fert.,* Suppl. 13:29–37.
167. Skinner, J. D., Scorer, J. A., and Millar, R. P. (1975): Observations on the reproductive physiological status of mature herd bulls, bachelor bulls and young bulls in the hippopotamus, *Hippopotamus amphibius amphibius* L. *Gen. Comp. Endocrinol.,* 26:92–95.
168. Skinner, J. D., Van Zyl, J. H. M., and Van Heerden, J. A. H. (1973): The effect of season on reproduction in the black wildebeest and red hartebeest in South Africa. *J. Reprod. Fert.,* Suppl. 19:101–110.
169. Smals, N. H., Kloppenborg, P. W. C., and Benraad, T. J. (1976): Annual cycle in plasma testosterone levels in man. *J. Clin. Endocrinol. Metab.,* 42:979–982.
170. Smith, J. T., Mayer, D. T., and Merilan, C. P. (1957): Seasonal variation in the succinic dehydrogenase activity of bovine spermatozoa. *J. Dairy Sci.,* 40:516–520.
171. Smyth, P., and Gordon, I. (1967): Seasonal and breed variations in the semen characteristics of rams in Ireland. *Irish Vet. J.,* 21:222–225.
172. Stosic, N., and Pantic, V. (1966): Cyclic changes in deer pituitary. *Jugoslav. Physiol. Pharmacol. Acta,* 2:231–237.
173. Struhsaker, T. T. (1967): Behaviour of elk *(Cervus canadensis)* during the rut. *Z. Tierpsychol.,* 24:80–114.
174. Suzuki, F., and Racey, P. A. (1976): Fine structural changes in the epididymal epithelium of mole *(Talpa europaea)* throughout the year. *J. Reprod. Fert.,* 47:47–54.
175. Suzuki, F., and Racey P. A. (1978): The organization of testicular interstitial tissue and changes in the fine structure of the Leydig cells of European moles, *Talpa europaea* throughout the year. *J. Reprod. Fert.,* 52:189–194.
176. Tsui, H. W., Tam, W. H., Lofts, B., and Phillips, J. G. (1974): The annual testicular cycle and androgen production *in vitro* in the masked civet cat, *Paguma larvata. J. Reprod. Fert.,* 36:283–293.
177. Van Demark, N. L., and Free, M. J. (1970): Temperature effects. In: *The Testis,* Vol. 3, edited by A. D. Johnson, W. R. Gomes, and N. L. Vandemark, pp. 233–313. Academic Press, London.
178. Vandenbergh, J. G. (1965): Hormonal basis of sex skin in male rhesus monkeys. *Gen. Comp. Endocrinol.,* 5:31–34.
179. Vandenbergh, J. G., and Vessey, S. (1968): Seasonal breeding of free-ranging rhesus monkeys and related ecological factors. *J. Reprod. Fert.,* 15:71–79.
180. Van Der Holst, W. (1975): A study of the morphology of stallion semen during the breeding and non-breeding seasons. *J. Reprod. Fert.,* Suppl. 23:87–89.
181. Vendrely, E., Guerillot, C., and Lage Da, C. (1972): Variations saisonnières des cellules de Sertoli et de Leydig dans le testicule de hamster dore. Étude caryometrique. *C. R. Acad. Sci. (Paris),* 275:1143–1146.

182. Waites, G. M. H., and Ortavant, R. (1968): Effets précoces d'une breve élévation de la température testiculaire sur la spermatogenèse du bélier. *Ann. Biol. Anim. Biochem. Biophys.,* 8:323–331.
183. Watson, K. C. (1976): The reproductive cycle in the male polecat, *Putorius putorius* in Britain. *J. Zool. (Lond),* 180:498–503.
184. Wells, L. J. (1935): Seasonal sexual rhythm and its experimental modification in the male of the thirteen-lined ground squirrel, *Citellus tridecemlineatus. Anat. Rec.,* 62:409–447.
185. Wells, L. J. (1938): Gonadotrophic potency of the hypophysis of a male rodent with annual rut. *Endocrinology,* 22:588–594.
186. West, N. O., and Nordan, H. C. (1976): Hormonal regulation of reproduction and the antler cycle in male Columbian black-tailed deer *(Odocoileus sp).* Part 1, Seasonal changes in the histology of the reproductive organs, serum testosterone, sperm production and the antler cycle. *Can. J. Zool.,* 54:1617–1636.
187. Whitehead, P. E., and McEwan, E. H. (1973): Seasonal variation in the plasma testosterone concentration of reindeer and caribou. *Can. J. Zool.,* 51:651–658.
188. Wimsatt, W. A. (1960): Some problems of reproduction in relation to hibernation in bats. *Bull. Mus. Comp. Zool. Harvard,* 124:249–263.
189. Wing, T-Y, and Lin, H.-S. (1977): The fine structure of testicular interstitial cells in the adult golden hamster with special reference to seasonal changes. *Cell Tissue Res.,* 183:385–393.
190. Wislocki, G. B. (1943): *Studies on growth of deer antlers.* 2. Seasonal changes in the male reproductive tract of the Virginia deer *(Odocoileus virginianus borealis)* with a discussion of the factors controlling the antler-gonad periodicity. Essays in Biology in honour of H. M. Evans, p. 631. University of California Press.
191. Wislocki, G. B. (1949): Seasonal changes in the testes, epididymides and seminal vesicles of deer investigated by histochemical methods. *Endocrinology,* 44:167–189.
192. Wislocki, G. B., Aub, J. C., and Waldo, C. M. (1947): The effects of gonadectomy and the administration of testosterone proprionate on the growth of antlers in male and female deer. *Endocrinology,* 40:202–224.
193. Wood, D. H. (1970): An ecological study of *Antechinus stuartii (Marsupialia)* in a Southeast Queensland rain forest. *Aust. J. Zool.,* 18:185–207.
194. Wooley, P. (1966): Reproduction in *Antecinus sp* and other Dasyurid marsupials. *Symp. Zool. Soc. (Lond),* 15:281–294.
195. Worth, R. W., Charlton, H. M., and Mackinnon, P. C. B. (1973): Field and laboratory studies on the control of luteinizing hormone secretion and gonadal activity in the vole, *Microtus agrestis. J. Reprod. Fert.,* Suppl. 19:89–99.
195a. Wright, P. L. (1969): The reproductive cycle of the male American badger, *Taxidea taxus. J. Reprod. Fert.,* Suppl. 6:435–445.
196. Zamboni, L., Conaway, C. H., and Van Pelt, L. (1974): Seasonal changes in production of semen in free-ranging rhesus monkeys. *Biol. Reprod.,* 11:251–267.

The Testis, edited by H. Burger and D. de Kretser.
Raven Press, New York © 1981.

13

Clinical Evaluation and Management of Testicular Disorders Before Puberty

Pierre C. Sizonenko, Anne-Marie Schindler, and Antoine Cuendet

*Endocrinology Unit and Pediatric Surgery Unit, Department of Pediatrics and Genetics,
1211 Geneva 4, Switzerland*

As presented in this volume, the testis plays a very important part in sexual differentiation during fetal life and in the development of the reproductive functions at puberty. It has also been shown that the testicular endocrine secretion might be of importance in infancy. Later, the testis is quiescent and although it does not play an important role before puberty, clinical evaluation and management of prepubertal testicular disorders are important for a boy's future. After describing the pattern of change in testicular size before puberty, three important pathological conditions met before puberty will be discussed: testicular tumors threatening life, precocious puberty leading to possible adult short stature, and cryptorchidism, in which condition the fertility of the male may be seriously affected.

TESTICULAR VOLUME

An accurate evaluation of testicular volume is frequently needed by clinicians dealing with testicular disorders. Leydig cell function can be assessed clinically by observation of the secondary sex characteristics and determination of plasma and/or urinary testosterone. Some estimate of tubular function can be achieved before puberty by the measurement of testicular volume. This measurement, combined with the clinical ratings of Tanner (112), is of particular value at the very beginning of pubertal development when an increase of testicular volume only is observed. Little has been published on standards for testicular volume.

Prader (90) has introduced an orchidometer made of ellipsoids of different volumes, from 1 to 25 ml. In relation to chronological age (126), the first major increase of testicular volume was between 11.5 to 12 years (2.1 ml $\pm$ 0.8 to 4 ml $\pm$ 2.7). In another study in which the product of mean testicular length and width was used as an index of testicular volume (25), the increase of testicular size also occurred between 11.5 and 12 years (Fig. 1).

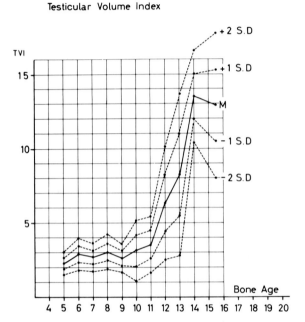

FIG. 1. Testicular volume index (TVI) in relation to bone age. (From ref. 25.)

Our own longitudinal study of testicular volume for boys from 7 to 16 years of age has confirmed that boys who have started their pubertal development have a testicular volume index above 4. This is usually observed at a median age of 11.5 years. However, the beginning of the increase in testicular size can be observed from 9.5 to 14 years. This range must be taken into consideration when the diagnosis of precocious puberty or delayed puberty is to be made.

TESTICULAR TUMORS

Although testicular tumors are rare before puberty, and are of little relevance to the endocrinologist, as secreting tumors of the testis are exceptional, new endocrine aspects of testicular tumors have been described recently and are useful to clinicians (59). Both benign and malignant tumors of the testis are less common in children than in adults. Only about 2 to 5% of testicular tumors occur in childhood (32). Sixty-five percent of these tumors are derived from germinal cells (7, 124). They are predominantly limited to infancy and adolescence.

Several classifications have been proposed for these tumors. The most widely accepted is presented in Table 1 and is derived from the classification of Mostofi (85), slightly modified by the World Health Organization (11). Because the differential diagnosis includes a tumor of the adnexae, and because the symptom-

TABLE 1. *Classification of tumors of the testis during childhood*[a]

Germ-cell tumors (65–70%)

  Tumors showing one histological pattern
    Embryonal carcinoma (25–40%)
    Teratoma (17–27%)
      a. mature
      b. immature
    Seminoma (2.5%)
    Choriocarcinoma (rare)
      a. infantile
      b. adult
      c. polyembryoma
    Teratocarcinoma (21%)
    Teratoma + embryonal carcinoma
    Others (7.3%)
      Epidermal cyst
      Retinal anlage tumor

Non-germ-cell tumors (31–35%)

  Tumors of gonadal stroma
    Leydig-cell tumors (10–27%)
    Sertoli-cell tumors (5–15%)
    Tumors of primitive gonadal stroma (9.5%)
  Tumors with germ-cell and gonadal stroma
    Gonadoblastoma (12%)
  Tumors of the adnexae
    Benign
      Adenomatoid tumor
      Adenoma
      Soft tissue tumors
    Malignant
      Carcinoma
      Sarcomas (paratesticular rhabdomyosarcoma)
  Metastatic tumors
    Malignant lymphoma (20%)
    Leukemia
    Neuroblastoma
    Others

[a] From refs. 1,7,11,14,32,42,59,85,124.

atology is very similar, tumors of the "adnexae," i.e., vas deferens, epididymis, etc., have also been presented in Table 1 and will be discussed later. In 90%, the reason for presentation and the main clinical finding is a painless swelling in the scrotum which grows progressively, but slowly (11). Other methods of presentation are less frequently observed: pain alone, a mass and pain suggesting acute epididymo-orchitis, trauma, metastases, firmness of testis, accidental finding (14). Often, the scrotal swelling is owing not only to the testicular mass but to the presence of a cystic hydrocele. Transillumination of the scrotum is helpful for differentiation. Twenty-five to sixty percent of testicular tumors are associated with hydrocele (1,11,14,42,85). The dangers of diagnostic puncture

TABLE 2. *Nontumoral lesions of the testis and of paratesticular tissues*

Lesions of the testis
    Contusion
    Hematoma
    Torsion
    Orchitis
    Epididymo-orchitis

Lesions of paratesticular tissues
    Hematocele
    Hydrocele
    Torsion of the testis
    Appendix
    Spermatocele
    Epidermoid cyst

of the hydrocele, or of needle biopsy must be stressed in all scrotal swellings in infancy. A good prognosis depends largely on the early diagnosis of malignant testicular tumors. The differential diagnosis includes nontumoral lesions of the testis or of paratesticular tissues as listed in Table 2. Transillumination must be attempted, as failure to transilluminate a painless scrotal mass must always lead to the suspicion of a testicular neoplasm which needs prompt treatment.

Staging of malignant tumors has been described by several authors and recently modified (14). Because of the characteristic features of some tumors, details concerning age of occurrence, therapy, and prognosis will be given in relation to the type of tumor.

Embryonal Carcinoma of Infancy

Embryonal carcinoma of infancy (or yolk-sac tumor, adenocarcinoma, or orchioblastoma) forms a network of undifferentiated embryonal tubular structures. However, the current concept does not accord with derivation from the undifferentiated testicular tubule. It is thought, by some, to belong to the germ-cell tumors and to derive from extra embryonal yolk-sac, or by others, to represent a teratoma (23). Almost all tumors are present in the first 4 years of life with a peak at 1 to 2 years. Treatment is orchiectomy, associated with chemotherapy, and abdominal radiotherapy (62,100). In adults, retroperitoneal lymphadenectomy has been recommended. In children, this surgical approach remains controversial. *Teratomas* represent about 30% of germ-cell testicular tumors in children. Contrary to their malignant behavior in adulthood, teratomas during childhood are more frequently benign. From review of the literature, there was only one proven case in which metastases may have occurred in the total series of 109 cases studied (23,29). The tumor appears in the first 5 years of life and usually enlarges and largely replaces the testis. The usual microscopic pattern is a wide variety of tissues derived from all three germ layers. Glial and retinal tissues are not uncommon. Mesodermal structures include muscle, cartilage, and bone. Numerous mitoses may be observed but areas resembling embryonal carcinoma are very rarely present. The mode of presentation, investigations, and diagnosis are similar to those described for embryonal carcinoma. As teratomas are benign tumors, the treatment is orchiectomy. Teratomas in adolescent boys may behave like adult teratomas, and if malignancy is found on histology of a teratoma from a postpubertal boy, additional treatment such as lymphadenectomy, radiotherapy, and/or chemotherapy should be considered.

Seminoma

Seminoma is one of the rarest tumors of the testis in childhood. Most of the tumors appear in pubescent boys 12 to 16 years of age. Several reviews have attempted to show a relationship of such tumors with undescended and dysgenetic testes (36). Three to 7% of tumors are associated with cryptorchid testes. From series published (36,40), it can be stated that an undescended testis is more susceptible to malignant degeneration, although tumors can arise in the contralateral testis (normally descended). This strongly suggests that dysgenetic tissue may be present in the testis and may account for the development of tumor. From observations of undescended and/or dysgenetic gonads, it is suggested that the malignancy may be related to the chromosome constitution of the gonad (107). It is recognized that bringing down an undescended testis surgically does not decrease the chance that a malignant tumor will develop in it but, at least, the testis is more accessible to observation and palpation (59). Currently reported observations suggest that surgery performed at an early age (before or at 4–5 years of age) diminishes the incidence of tumoral degeneration as compared to subjects operated at a later age (3). Para-aortic lymph nodes are often involved. Treatment is very comparable to the embryonal carcinoma involving retroperitoneal lymphadenectomy (although this point remains controversial in the case of seminoma), radiotherapy (seminoma and its metastases are very sensitive to radiation) following orchiectomy, and chemotherapy (although again this latter therapy has not been proved to improve survival) (59).

Because *Leydig cell adenomas* present with endocrine symptomatology, they will be discussed in the paragraph devoted to precocious puberty (50)

Sertoli-Cell Tumor

Sertoli-cell tumor, often called gonocytoma, gonadoblastoma, granulosa theca cell tumor, gonadal "stromal" tumor, is very rare during childhood, the incidence being around 1 to 12% (42). It originates from the stromal cell and is in fact mostly found in patients with dysgenetic testes, and in the testicular feminization syndrome. Sexual ambiguity is present and is beyond the scope of this chapter. A painless testicular swelling is the commonest presentation. Some endocrine symptoms may be present such as gynecomastia. Radical orchiectomy is the usual therapeutic approach (59).

For completeness, paratesticular rhabdomyosarcoma and retinal anlage tumor should be mentioned. Paratesticular rhabdomyosarcoma may be difficult to distinguish from a predominantly sarcomatous element arising in a malignant teratoma. It occurs more frequently in adolescents and may invade the testis. Because the tumor may expand and give metastases quickly, an early pathological diagnosis is necessary. Treatment will include radical orchiectomy, retroperitoneal lymphadenectomy, radiotherapy, and chemotherapy (59). Retinal anlage tumor is rare and should be diagnosed by histological appearance. Simple orchiectomy is the treatment of choice. Testes may be the site of lymphoma, lymphosarcoma, Hodgkin's disease, neuroblastoma, and leukemia. The latter condition is the most frequent cause of bilateral enlargement of the testes by metastases.

Biologic tumor markers like α-fetoprotein (α-FP) and human chorionic gonadotropin (hCG) have been extremely helpful in detecting recurrence, staging, and monitoring of testicular cancer (19,22,54). Sensitive and specific radioimmunoassays have been developed for hCG and for α-FP which are capable of measuring minute amounts of these markers in the serum. When these two serum markers are utilized together, they are the best serologic and cellular markers available. They may also be very useful in the understanding of the cell origin of the tumors by using immunohistochemical methods to localize hCG and α-FP and to correlate the serum levels of hCG and α-FP with the various types of germ cell tumors present. Based on these findings an immunohistologic classification of germ-cell tumors has been proposed (Fig. 2). Pure semi-

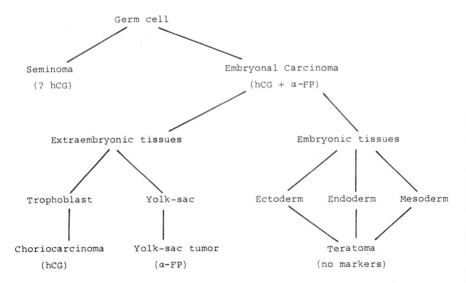

FIG. 2. Cell origin of α-fetoprotein (α-FP) and human chorionic gonadotropin and the possible biological markers secreted by testicular tumors. (From ref. 54.)

noma and teratoma derived from embryonic tissues do not produce biological markers. Embryonal carcinoma containing extraembryonic tissues is capable of secreting α-FP and hCG. More differentiated than embryonal carcinoma, choriocarcinoma can secrete hCG, whereas tumors coming from the yolk-sac will produce α-FP. Discrepancies between these markers and the histological diagnosis may often be based upon the fact that syncytiotrophoblastic giant cells which may synthesize hCG are associated with pure seminoma, embryonal carcinoma, or yolk-sac tumor. Also the discordance between α-FP and hCG could be explained on the basis of the findings that the cells producing hCG and α-FP are different.

Because germ-cell tumors may produce abnormal amounts of α-FP and human chorionic gonadotropin, or its β-subunit, it is important to follow the plasma levels of these markers (19,22). Notwithstanding the discrepancies between these two biological markers, clearly both should be measured in order to follow remission and make an early diagnosis of relapse. In children there have been higher percentages of positive secretion of α-FP than in adults (19). When a nonseminomatous germ-cell tumor is confined to the scrotum, the markers may or may not be elevated. In addition, α-FP is not usually elevated in seminomas (72,89); as already discussed, elevated levels of hCG have occasionally been reported in patients said to have pure seminoma (31,54,68,72). These markers are extremely sensitive postoperative indicators of metastatic disease. Elevated levels in postorchiectomy and prelymphadenectomy patients are good indicators of metastases to the retroperitoneal lymph nodes. They are very useful in monitoring radio- and chemotherapy (54,72).

PRECOCIOUS PUBERTY

Precocious pubertal development can be defined as the appearance of secondary sexual characteristics before the age of 9 years in boys. From Tanner's data, the first signs of puberty appeared between 9.5 and 13.5 years (112). In our own longitudinal study, they also occurred at 9.5 years and affected 50% of the boys at 11 years, 9 months. Ninety-five percent of the boys had some signs of pubertal development by 14 years.

Two types of precocious puberty should be defined: true precocious puberty (or isosexual precocity) in which there is a precocious, always isosexual, activation of the hypothalamic-pituitary-gonadal axis, and pseudo-precocious puberty, which results from an adrenal, gonadal, or extragonadal tumor. In the latter, the precocious pubertal development can be either isosexual or heterosexual, i.e., in the boy with virilization (isosexual) or with feminization (heterosexual). In addition, precocious puberty can be complete or incomplete.

True Precocious Puberty

True precocious puberty is related to an early triggering mechanism which activates the hypothalamic-pituitary-gonadal axis. It is often called the cerebral

TABLE 3. *Etiology of isosexual precocious puberty in boys*

Complete or cerebral (true isosexual precocity)

1. Idiopathic
   A. Familial
   B. Sporadic (rare in the male)
2. Neurogenic
   A. Tumoral lesion of the posterior hypothalamus (pinealoma, hamartoma)
   B. Other lesions
      neurofibromatosis
      hydrocephalus
      encephalitis
      meningitis
      McCune-Albright's syndrome

Incomplete pseudo-precocious puberty

1. Isosexual
   A. Gonadotropin-producing tumors
      testicular tumors (chorioepitheliomas, teratomas)
      hepatoblastoma
      chorioepitheliomas of other regions
   B. Hormonal overlap syndrome (primary hypothyroidism with sexual precocity and galactor-
      rhea)
   C. Adrenal lesions
      congenital adrenal hyperplasia
      Cushing's syndrome: hyperplasia, tumor
      adrenal adenoma or carcinoma
   D. Testicular tumors (Leydig cell tumor)
   E. Exogenous androgens
   F. Premature adrenarche
2. Heterosexual
   A. Feminizing adrenal tumors (rare)
   B. Exogenous estrogens

form of precocious puberty, although the lesions may be so small as to be undetectable by our present means of investigation.

Because cerebral forms of true precocious puberty are very heterogenous, it is advantageous to separate them into two groups: idiopathic, which are much more frequent in girls than in boys (30,58,108,113,120,121), and neurogenic, which can be owing to cerebral tumors (Table 3). For the whole group, precocious puberty is much more frequent in girls than in boys (4:1 to 7–8:1) as is true for the idiopathic forms (4:1). On the contrary, neurogenic causes are more frequent in boys than in girls (2:1) (17). From the literature, it can be stated that in boys 55% of cases of true precocious puberty are of idiopathic origin and 44% can be attributed to a neurogenic origin: among all these boys, 22% are tumoral, i.e., 50% of all the neurogenic forms (16).

Among idiopathic forms, some cases are sporadic, others familial, the latter occurring predominantly in males. Transmission is supposed to be as a sex-linked autosomal dominant, with either variable or complete penetrance (38). Some cases of idiopathic precocious puberty have been said to be associated with abnormalities of the electroencephalogram (79) which should suggest the existence of very small cerebral organic lesions responsible for the EEG and the pubertal changes.

Among the neurogenic forms of true precocious puberty, expanding lesions in the region of the posterior hypothalamus have been found more frequently in boys than in girls (8,12,16). Pineal gland lesions have been reported more frequently (pinealoma or ectopic pinealoma, teratoma, hamartoma). Tumors that cause precocious puberty are those which involve the pineal region (13, 24,66,99). They produce pathological lesions of the hypothalamus. Clinical symptoms such as diabetes insipidus, polyphagia, and obesity often occur. Astrocytomas or craniopharyngiomas rarely cause precocious puberty. Other central nervous system lesions can induce precocious puberty: neurofibromatosis, hydrocephalus, meningitis, encephalitis. McCune-Albright's syndrome is rarely observed in boys. This syndrome should probably be placed in the neurogenic category as it is postulated that precocious puberty is owing to the hypersecretion of hypothalamic-releasing hormone (48,77). In the case of hypothalamic hamartoma, luteinizing hormone-releasing factor has been found present by immunofluorescence (60). As in all forms of true sexual precocity, premature isosexual development is followed by accelerated physical development with tallness and advanced bone age. In boys, both testes enlarge with growth of the penis; the appearance of pubic or axillary hair follows much later. The very sudden appearance of secondary sex characteristics leads to the suspicion of a rapidly growing tumor of the brain or the gonads, or of an ectopic gonadotropin-producing tumor. Early in development, increased height and accelerated skeletal growth are observed (Fig. 3). The increased height and the considerably advanced bone age lead to premature closure of the epiphyses and, so, to a cessation of growth at an early age with consequent short adult stature.

An organic cerebral lesion should always be suspected when both testes are enlarged. Examination of the fundi and visual fields and performance of an EEG are important clinically. X-rays of the skull and of the sella turcica, pneumoencephalography, and computerized axial tomography should be done to try to localize the tumor or the abnormality. In some cases, idiopathic precocious puberty is diagnosed. In very rare cases, the precocious puberty appears only temporarily.

Laboratory findings are of great help although none of them is completely conclusive. Basal plasma and urine gonadotropins have often been found to be elevated compared to values obtained in normal boys at the same age and are generally in the range of values observed at a similar stage of puberty. Sleep-associated release of luteinizing hormone (LH) has been observed in boys with idiopathic and tumoral precocious puberty (18). Testosterone levels are usually higher than normal for chronological age and correspond with the size of the testes and the stage of pubertal development. During stimulation with luteinizing hormone-releasing hormone (LHRH), increased gonadotropin responses have been observed in the few males studied, with a mature pattern of gonadotropin release, corresponding to the clinical stage of puberty (55,56).

In tumoral cases, it is clear that therapy is initially directed to the tumor using neurosurgery, radiotherapy, or chemotherapy. In the case of idiopathic or nontumoral origin, treatment of precocious puberty has been based on the use of antigonadotropic drugs, such as medroxyprogesterone, or more recently in Europe, cyproterone acetate. Before 1974, many articles in the literature reported the arrest of penile growth or sexual hair development (33,34,71,96,105) with medroxyprogesterone (100–300 mg of depot-medroxyprogesterone every 2 weeks or 20–40 mg/day orally). Excretion of sex steriods and gonadotropins in the urine decreased. However, in most cases, the volume of the testes did not decrease greatly, although spermatogenesis was suppressed. The effects of medroxyprogesterone on growth and on advancement of bone age have generally been poor and remain controversial. The eventual adult short stature characteristic of patients with sexual precocity is not prevented. Undesirable side-effects have also been observed. Medroxyprogesterone acetate has slight glucocorticoid activity which can partially suppress ACTH secretion and adrenal cortical function, and can cause signs of Cushing's disease (81,95,101). Cyproterone acetate also has an antigonadotropic action and reduces the LH response to LHRH stimulation (64,86). The extent of clinical improvement of patients with true isosexual precocity treated with cyproterone acetate (150 mg/m²/day) has been very controversial. Clinical signs of puberty have regressed in most instances but the advancement of bone age and growth (Fig. 3) was not significantly affected by therapy (119). These were diminished in other studies, however (15,63,92), suggesting an improvement of the final predicted height. It has also been observed that cyproterone acetate has an anti-ACTH action and the possibility of induced

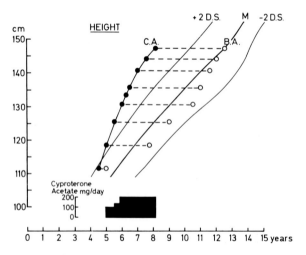

FIG. 3. Effect of therapy (cyproterone acetate) on growth of a boy aged 4 years 6 months with idiopathic precocious puberty. C.A. (*closed circle:* height with chronological age) B.A. = corresponding bone ages *(open circles).*

adrenal glucocorticoid deficiency should be considered (43). Plasma cortisol levels can be low. Clinically, some treated children complain of asthenia, particularly after gymnastics. Replacement with hydrocortisone or cortisone acetate might be helpful in the cases of severe asthenia. The final outcome of such anitgonadotropic therapy has not been well studied in the male. Whether fertility is affected during adulthood remains to be determined.

Pseudo-Precocious Puberty

Pseudo-precocious puberty is usually characterized by incomplete sexual maturation. Two types can be defined (Table 3), isosexual and heterosexual. The former can be owing to tumors producing gonadotropins or to excessive androgen production by the testis or the adrenal in boys. The latter is owing to feminizing hormones secreted by tumors in the male infant.

Gonadotropin-producing tumors are always malignant. They are usually either chorioepitheliomas or teratomas derived from the trophoblast, or nontrophoblastic ectopic neoplasms of the liver which have been observed only in boys (52,94). These tumors produce either genuine hCG or compounds with LH activity, or β-subunits. Chorioepitheliomas and teratomas originate from the gonads, from the pineal, or the mediastinum. Metastases occur early, in particular to the lung (11,31,51). As the result of the secretion of hCG or LH-like compounds, activation of the Leydig cells occurs with an increase in testosterone secretion.

Another condition is the association of genuine precocious puberty with untreated primary hypothyroidism. It is believed that the increased production of TSH overlaps with the production of other tropic glycoprotein hormones like FSH and LH. Prolactin is also secreted in excessive amounts accounting for the galactorrhea often met. In several children with severe untreated hypothyroidism, expansion of the sella turcica was observed as a result of the reactive enlargement of the hypophysis (39,74,123). If thyroid hormone replacement is instituted, the symptoms of precocious puberty disappear. Abnormal adrenal secretions are frequently the cause of pseudo-precocious puberty. Congenital adrenal hyperplasia (or adrenogenital syndrome) is the most common cause. In boys, this condition might be difficult to recognize as there are no heterosexual symptoms as in girls. Macrogenitosomia praecox, presence of pubic hair with small testes, and pigmentation of the scrotum are clinical signs generally found. However, in some untreated cases, testicular enlargement can occur owing to the presence of large hyperplastic adrenal remnants in the testis (91). Gonadotropin determinations show low levels with high levels of adrenal androgens such as dehydroepiandrosterone and its sulfate (69,93,109). Determinations of urinary pregnanetriol excretion, plasma 17-hydroxy-progesterone, 11-deoxycorticosterone and ACTH levels are necessary. The high levels of the adrenal steroids are decreased following cortisone suppression. Another adrenal cause of pseudo-precocious puberty is Cushing's syndrome. In this condition, signs of precocious puberty are associated with symptoms owing to excessive glucocorticoid se-

TABLE 4. *Sexual precocity in boys*

Testes	Pathological	Gonadotropins	Testosterone
Both large	True sexual precocity		
	idiopathic	slightly elevated	moderately elevated
	CNS lesions	slightly elevated	moderately elevated
	Pseudo-precocious puberty		
	gonadotropin-producing tumor	high	moderately elevated
	hormonal overlapping (hypothyroidism)	slightly elevated	moderately elevated
	congenital adrenal hyperplasia (testicular remnants)	low	adrenal androgens elevated
One large	Benign scrotal tumor (Leydig cell tumor)	low	elevated
	Malignant scrotal tumor (Chorioepithelioma)	high	moderately elevated
Both small	Congenital adrenal hyperplasia	low	adrenal androgens elevated
	Exogenous administration of androgens	low	high or very low
	Premature adrenarche	normal	adrenal androgens slightly elevated

cretion. Adrenal tumors such as adenomas or carcinomas secreting only androgens are rare but can be observed (121). Similarly, feminizing adrenal tumors, such as estrogen-producing carcinomas or adenomas are extremely rare (84). Secreting testicular tumors (Leydig cell tumors) are rare, as already mentioned. The tumors vary in size and are usually well separated from the rest of the testicular tissue. They have a firmer consistency than the testis and are usually unilateral and benign. Hormone production is often increased: high levels of plasma testosterone (and 17-ketosteroids) with low levels of gonadotropins (117). In some cases, other androgenic steroids can be increased such as Δ^4-androstenedione (98,117). After surgical removal of the Leydig cell tumor, arrest or regression of clinical symptoms occurs in most cases. In some, advanced bone age has led to tall stature and, in these patients, puberty can progress further. This is observed if the bone age is greater than 12 years. Pituitary production of gonadotropins which was suppressed by the excessive androgens produced by the tumor, increases as pubertal maturation of the hypothalamic-pituitary-testicular axis occurs.

Finally, because of the rare conditions which can be observed in sexual precocity in boys, their features have been summarized (Table 4). When both testes are small, it is always important to rule out the exogenous administration of androgens. If human gonadotropin is given, both testes are enlarged.

Among the incomplete forms of isosexual pseudo-precocious puberty, premature adrenarche is often observed in the boy. This condition represents the early appearance of pubic and often axillary hair between 7 and 10 years of age. It represents an early and excessive maturation of the androgenic zone of the adrenal cortex. Testes are small, as well as the penis. Bone age is slightly advanced and may be associated with tall stature. Adrenal androgens such as dehydroepiandrosterone and its sulfate are moderately elevated for age (109). Congenital adrenal hyperplasia should be ruled out. No treatment is required and normal puberty occurs.

CRYPTORCHIDISM

Undescended testis is a common and difficult problem in pediatric practice. There has been a great deal of controversy over the physiopathology and the management of this condition. Undescended testes can be classified as totally undescended, incompletely descended, or ectopic. The condition can be unilateral or bilateral. The incompletely descended testis is found somewhere along the normal route of descent, in the abdomen, in the inguinal canal, or beyond the inguinal ring. The undescended testis is often associated with a patent processus vaginalis. Conversely, the ectopic testis, which is usually not associated with a hernial sac, is located outside the normal route of descent: in the superficial inguinal area, between the external oblique aponevrosis and the fascia of Scarpia lateral to the superficial ring. Ectopic testes can also be found in the pubic, perineal, and femoral positions.

A cryptorchid or an ectopic testis should be defined as a testis which is permanently located outside the scrotum and which cannot be brought completely into the scrotum by manual traction. As soon as the traction is discontinued, the testis is back to its previous location. Therefore, the condition has to be carefully distinguished from the retractile testis which may be present within the inguinal canal. Contraction of the cremasteric muscle causes elevation of the testis. Careful and repeated examination with warm hands is often necessary before the retractile testis can be palpated. In this case, spontaneous descent usually occurs and testicular function is not impaired.

The incidence of cryptorchidism is said to be between 0.4 to 2% after the first year of age. Before 1 year of age, a higher incidence of cryptorchidism has been observed, in particular in premature newborns (106). The physiopathology of failure of descent of the testis is poorly understood. There is considerable heterogeneity in cryptorchidism. In some instances, mechanical and intrinsic abnormalities of the testis are present. In other instances, endocrine abnormalities have been suspected. Chromosome abnormalities have been looked for in such undescended testes (10,114). No abnormal pattern was observed except for the finding of some XXY subjects. In some families, more than one male is affected (67). It is evident, however, that there is not a simple mendelian mode of inheritance of this condition which is multifactoral. Cryptorchidism may be associated with many congenital syndromes: Beckwith's syndrome, Cornelia de Lange syndrome, Fanconi syndrome, Leopard syndrome, Noonan syndrome, prune-belly syndrome, Silver Russell syndrome. Abnormalities of the epididymis (3.6%), ductus deferens (7.8%), shortness of spermatic vessels (8.3%) are observed with undescended testis (45,114). Inguinal hernia is very frequent. Its incidence varies from author to author (28,114). The consequences of these findings are that undescended testes can be classified into two groups: the first with some mechanical obstacle to normal descent, the second with no mechanical obstacle, in which an abnormal testis or an endocrine cause could explain the nondescent.

Many studies concerning the endocrine functions of the hypothalamic-pituitary-testicular axis and the testicular secretions have been performed. In bilateral cryptorchidism, conflicting results have been obtained. No differences in the testosterone response to hCG were noted by several investigators between normal and cryptorchid boys (27), or between unilateral and bilateral cryptorchid boys at the same stage of puberty (110). Other groups have observed decreased testosterone responses to hCG both in bilateral and/or unilateral cryptorchidism (26,41,116). The hCG stimulation test also gives information in cases of bilateral cryptorchidism in which no testis can be palpated. The absence of response of testosterone is in favor of anorchia (6,27,44,109,125). It is then thought that surgical search for testicular tissue is not necessary. Surgery may be indicated for implantation of prosthetic testes. On the contrary, if the testosterone response is present, bilateral surgical search and bringing down of the testis is necessary in order not to leave the abdominal testes *in situ*. It has also been suggested that bilateral cryptorchidism could be caused by hypogonadotropic hypogonad-

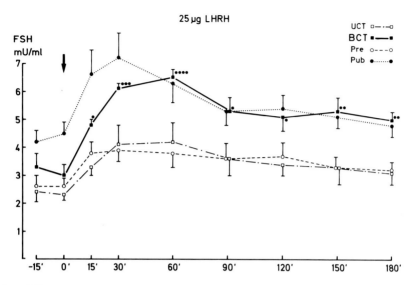

FIG. 4. FSH response to LHRH (25 μg) in prepubertal boys with unilateral cryptorchid testes (UCT), bilateral cryptorchid testes (BCT), and in normal prepubertal (pre) and pubertal (pub: stage P_2) boys. Significance: $*p < 0.05$; $**p < 0.01$; $***p < 0.005$; $****p < 0.001$. (From ref. 111.)

ism (103). Reduced or normal LH response to LHRH was observed by some groups in uni- and bilateral prepubertal cryptorchidism (41). Conversely, in bilateral cryptorchidism with low counts of spermatogonia on testicular biopsies (111), FSH responses to LHRH were increased before puberty (Fig. 4). LH responses were similar to normal (Fig. 5). These findings suggest that a selective increase of FSH in response to LHRH is owing to the presence of an active negative feedback mechanism between inhibin (20,70) produced by the seminifer-ous tubule and the prepubertal pituitary. Increased basal levels of FSH have been observed in pubertal boys with bilateral cryptorchidism or unilateral cryp-torchidism with or without compensatory testicular hypertrophy (5,73,76,115).

Because of the different responses obtained with endocrine stimulation, hetero-geneity of the cryptorchid syndrome has been proposed (9). It is clear that in some cases hypogonadotropic hypogonadism can be observed (103), in particular in specific syndromes like the Prader-Willi syndrome. Other authors have sug-gested that an early defect or a delay of LH secretion during fetal life might be responsible for the cryptorchidism (57). This theory is also sustained by electron microscopic findings demonstrating structural abnormalities of Leydig cells in cryptorchid babies suggesting again a possible defect in LH secretion (47).

This has not yet been proven for it has been postulated that only hCG might be necessary during fetal life (61). Cryptorchidism is also observed in defects of testosterone metabolism although these defects induce sexual ambiguity and

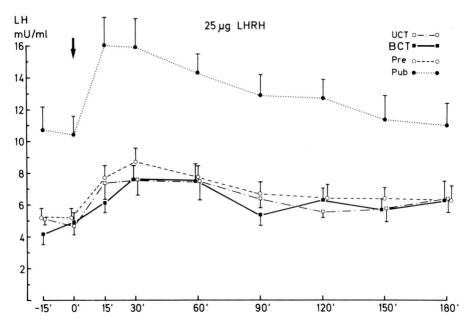

FIG. 5. LH responses to LHRH (25 μg) in prepubertal boys with unilateral cryptorchid testis (UCT), bilateral cryptorchid testes (BCT), and in normal prepubertal (pre) and pubertal (pub: stage P_2) boys. (From ref. 111.)

are therefore beyond the scope of this chapter. The possible neoplastic transformation of intra-abdominal testes has already been discussed (see above), and will not be further developed (40).

The undescended testis is usually smaller than the normally descended testis in unilateral cryptorchidism (Fig. 6). Although individual values are not plotted in the figure, we have not found any case of compensatory testicular hypertrophy of the normal side (73). Most of the work on cryptorchidism has been based on the histological lesions observed in the testis which has been undescended for several years. The diameter of the seminiferous tubules has been found to be reduced compared to normal values for age (83,97). Interstitial fibrosis has also been observed, but the main lesion observed even before puberty has been the reduced number of spermatogonia found in the tubules of the undescended testis (35,37,80,82,83,102,104). These findings were derived from testicular biopsies taken during surgery (Fig. 7). The incidence of these lesions varies from 30% to 100% in the undescended testis. Using refined methods of counting the numbers of spermatogonia per 50 tubules (80,82), it has been shown by some authors that the number of spermatogonia decreases with age in the undescended testis, and that the number remains normal before 3 years of age (37,83). These findings have led to the conclusion that early surgery should be performed in cryptorchid boys. This point will be discussed later. Many authors have

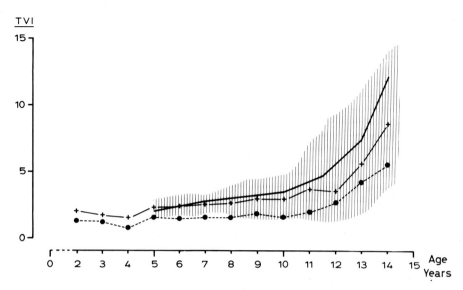

FIG. 6. Mean testicular volume index (TVI) of undescended testes *(closed circles)* and of normally descended testes *(crosses)* in relation to age in 205 boys with undescended testes. Hatched area: normal TVI.

also found histological lesions in up to 20% of the normally descended testis in unilateral cryptorchidism (Fig. 7).

For many years, medical treatment of cryptorchidism by the administration of hCG has been advocated. Because of the great heterogeneity of this syndrome and of the presence of mechanical factors preventing the normal descent of the testis, it is very difficult to compare the findings in the literature concerning the positive results of this therapy. In our own experience, the number of cases which could be treated with hCG administration is very small compared to the number of cryptorchid boys seen (5%). The only indication is when a testis remains high in the scrotum and cannot be brought fully intrascrotally. In this case, successful therapy has been observed in more than 50% of the cases treated with hCG, 5,000 U/m² twice a week during 2 weeks. More recently, the treatment of cryptorchidism with intranasal synthetic LHRH has been advocated in both uni- and bilateral cryptorchidism with apparently some positive results (53).

If the medical treatment is successful, with descent of the testis into the scrotum 7 to 10 days after the last injection, a yearly follow-up examination is advised. In case the testis cannot be brought down at a following examination, surgery should be advised.

Early surgery (before the age of 3 years) has been suggested (37,51,83,102) compared to previous recommendations between 10 to 11 years (51), or more recently between 5 and 7 years of age (49,75). There is, however, no real evidence

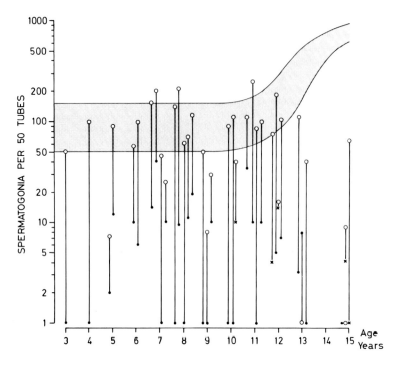

FIG. 7. Number of spermatogonia *(logarithmic scale)* in relation to age in cryptorchid *(full dot)*, ectopic testes *(crosses)* and in contralateral normally descended testes *(open circles)*. The shaded area represents the normal range. (From ref. 104.)

that surgery before 3 years of age does improve fertility rate. One should be aware that surgery is much more difficult at younger ages and only skilled surgeons should perform it. The chance of secondary hypoplasia of the surgically descended testis is high at this young age and should not be underestimated. We recommend that surgery should be performed between 5 and 7 years of age if the medical treatment, if indicated, has failed.

The reduced number of spermatogonia found before puberty raises the question of testicular function in adulthood, particularly in bilateral cryptorchidism in which the number of spermatogonia is reduced on both sides. Previous studies have shown that sterility is very frequent, the incidence varying from one author to another: 50 to 70% in bilateral cryptorchidism (4,21,51,78,118,122). In unilateral cryptorchidism, the rate of fertility is slightly lower than in the normal male population. It is clear that azoospermia and severe oligospermia are seen mainly in bilateral cryptorchidism; moderate oligospermia or normospermia are observed in unilateral cryptorchidism. If the data on semen analysis from the different published series are combined, it can be stated that 70% of patients with unilateral cryptorchidism treated surgically in the 6 or so years before puberty are likely to have normal semen analyses, while only 25% of bilaterally

TABLE 5. *Iterative biopsies in the 37 contralateral normally descended testes at puberty in unilateral cryptorchidism*

Stages of lesions	A[a]	B[b]	C[c]
Cryptorchid testis	12	10	0
Ectopic testis	10	3	0
Testicular agenesis	1	1	0
Total	23	14	0

In all the surgically descended testes, severe lesions were observed (stage B and C).
[a] Stage A: no lesion of spermatogenetic maturation.
[b] Stage B: moderate lesions consisting of (a) incomplete spermatogenetic maturation; (b) spermatogenesis with hypocellularity; and (c) peritubular sclerosis.
[c] Stage C: complete arrest of spermatogenesis.

cryptorchid patients so treated have normal semen analyses (2). Among 205 prepubertal children (representing 356 biopsies) we have been able to follow, we have found low numbers of spermatogonia in 90% of undescended testes and lesions in the normally descended testis in 30% of unilateral cryptorchid cases (Fig. 7). In 37 cases, we were able to biopsy both sides again at puberty in order to evaluate the pubertal maturation of the testis. In order to analyze the lesions, three histological stages were defined according to the spermatogenetic maturation. With this classification, it can be seen (Table 5) that in 23 contralateral normally descended testes, stage A (i.e., normal spermatogenesis) was achieved. All the surgically descended testes showed severe lesions and were classified in stages B and C. It is clear from this study that normal pubertal maturation fails to occur in the surgically treated cryptorchid testis. In one-third of the normally descended testes, moderate lesions could still be observed. However, in 5 cases, there was an increase of the number of spermatogonia with puberty. In 5 other cases, no increase was observed (Fig. 8). The outcome of cryptorchidism still remains to be defined.

PREPUBERTAL TESTIS AND CHEMOTHERAPY

Although the prepubertal testis is not fully active, it has been shown recently that chemotherapy may induce nonreversible lesions, as may radiotherapy. Treatment of the nephrotic syndrome in prepubertal boys with cytotoxic or immunosuppressive drugs, such as cyclophosphamide, azathioprine, or chlorambucil, has induced oligo- or aspermia and abnormalities of testicular histology as observed in the same patients during adulthood (46,65,87,88).

ACKNOWLEDGMENTS

Some of the studies presented in the paper were supported by Grant No. 3.747.76 of the Swiss National Science Foundation. Our thanks are expressed to Mrs. M. Pasche and Mr. D. Furrer for their secretarial and drawing assistance.

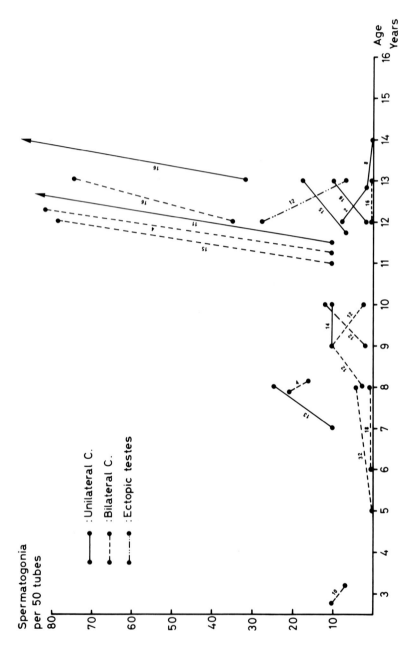

FIG. 8. Evolution of the number of spermatogonia (per 50 tubules) in repeated biopsies after surgery (number of months after surgery indicated along the individual curves) in 18 boys with unilateral or bilateral cryptorchidism (C.) or ectopic testes, in relation to age. (From ref. 104.)

REFERENCES

1. Abell, M. R., and Holtz, E. (1963): Testicular neoplasms in infants and in children. I. Tumors of germ cell origin. *Cancer,* 16:965–981.
2. Albescu, J. Z., Bergada, C., and Cullen, M. (1971): Male fertility in patients treated for cryptorchidism before puberty. *Fertil. Steril.,* 22:829–833.
3. Altman, B. L., and Malament, M. (1967): Carcinoma of the testis following orchidopexy. *J. Urol.,* 97:498–504.
4. Atkinson, P. M. (1975): A follow up study of surgically treated cryptorchid patients. *J. Pediatr. Surg.,* 10:115–119.
5. Atkinson, P. M., Epstein, M. T., and Rippon, A. E. (1975): Plasma gonadotropins in surgically treated cryptorchid patients. *J. Pediatr. Surg.,* 10:27–33.
6. Aynsley-Green, A., Zachmann, M., Illig, R., Rampini, S., and Prader, A. (1976): Congenital bilateral anorchia in childhood: A clinical, endocrine and therapeutic evaluation of twenty-one cases. *Clin. Endocrinol.,* 5:381–391.
7. Bachmann, K. D., and Grawert, H. von (1972): Tumoren des Hodens im Kindesalter: Bericht über 545 Fälle. *Monatsschr. Kinderheilkd.,* 120:40–46.
8. Barnes, N. D., Cloutier, M. D., and Hayles, A. B. (1974): The central nervous system and precocious puberty. In: *"The Control of the Onset of Puberty,"* edited by M. M. Grumbach, G. D. Grave, and F. E. Mayer, pp. 211–228. Wiley, New York.
9. Battin, J., and Colle, M. (1977): Hétérogénéité du syndrome "cryptorchidie." *Arch. Fr. Pediatr.,* 34:595–603.
10. Bergada, C., Farias, N. E., Romero de Behar, M., and Cullen, M. (1969): Abnormal sex chromatin pattern in cryptorchidism, girls with short stature and other endocrine patients. *Helv. Paediatr. Acta,* 24:372–377.
11. Bergami, F., Caione, P., and Rivosecchi, M. (1977): Testicular tumors in infancy and childhood. *Z. Kinderchir.,* 20:57–70.
12. Bierich, J. R. (1975): Sexual precocity. *Clin. Endocrinol. Metab.,* 4:107–142.
13. Bing, J. F., Globus, J. H., and Simon, H. (1938): Pubertas praecox: A survey of the reported case and verified anatomical findings. *J. Mt. Sinaï Hosp.,* 4:935–965.
14. Borski, A. A. (1973): Diagnosis, staging and natural history of testicular tumors. *Cancer,* 32:1202–1205.
15. Bossi, E., Zurbrügg, R. P., and Joss, E. E. (1973): Improvement of adult height prognosis in precocious puberty by cyproterone acetate. *Acta Paediatr. Scand.,* 62:405–412.
16. Bovier-Lapierre, M. (1972): Aspects particuliers des pubertés précoces neurogènes. *Pédiatrie,* 27:611–622.
17. Bovier-Lapierre, M., Sempé, M., and David, M. (1972): Aspects étiologiques cliniques et biologiques des pubertés précoces d'origine centrale. *Pédiatrie,* 27:587–609.
18. Boyar, R. M., Finkelstein, J. W., David, R., Roffwarg, H., Kapen, S., Weitzman, E. D., and Hellman, L. (1973): Twenty-four hour patterns of plasma luteinizing hormone and follicle-stimulating hormone in sexual precocity. *N. Engl. J. Med.,* 289:282–286.
19. Bracken, R. B., Johnson, D. E., and Samuels, M. L. (1975): Alpha-foetoprotein determinations in germ cell tumors of testis. *Urology,* 6:382–384.
20. Bramble, F. J., Houghton, A. L., Eccles, S. S., Murray, M. A. F., and Jacobs, H. S. (1975): Specific control of the follicle-stimulating hormone in the male: Postulated site of action of inhibin. *Clin. Endocrinol.,* 4:443–449.
21. Bramble, F. J., Houghton, A. L., Eccles, S. S., O'Shea, A., and Jacobs, H. S. (1974): Reproductive and endocrine function after surgical treatment of bilateral cryptorchidism. *Lancet,* 2:311–314.
22. Braunstein, G. D., McIntire, K. R., and Waldmann, T. A. (1973): Discordance of human chorionic gonadotropin and alpha-foetoprotein in testicular teratocarcinomas. *Cancer,* 31:1065–1068.
23. Brown, N. J. (1976): Yolk-Sac tumour (orchioblastoma) and other testicular tumours of childhood. In: *Pathology of the Testis,* edited by R. C. B. Pugh, pp. 356–370. Blackwell Scientific Publications, London.
24. Bruton, O. C., Martz, D. C., and Gerard, E. S. (1961): Precocious puberty due to secreting chorioepithelioma (teratoma) of the brain. *J. Pediatr.,* 59:719–725.
25. Burr, I. M., Sizonenko, P. C., Kaplan, S. L., and Grumbach, M. M. (1970): Hormonal changes

in puberty. I. Correlation of serum luteinizing hormone and FSH with stages of puberty, testicular size, and bone age in normal boys. *Pediatr. Res.,* 4:25–35.

26. Cacciari, E., Cicognani, A., Pirazzoli, P., Zappula, F., Tassoni, P., Bernardi, F., and Salardi, S. (1976): Hypophyso-gonadal function in the cryptorchid child: Differences between unilateral and bilateral cryptorchids. *Acta Endocrinol.,* 83:182–189.

27. Cacciari, E., Cicognani, A., Tassoni, P., Flamigi, P., Bolelli, F., Pirazzoli, P., and Salardi, S. (1974): Plasma testosterone and estradiol concentration in prepubertal boys with cryptorchidism before and after dexamethasone and after human chorionic gonadotropin administration. *Helv. Paediatr. Acta,* 29:27–34.

28. Canlorbe, P., Borniche, P., Bader, J. C., Vassal, J., Toublanc, J. C., and Job, J. C. (1974): La cryptorchidie. *Arch. Fr. Pediatr.,* 31:145–156.

29. Carney, J. A., Kelalis, P. P., and Lynn, H. B. (1973): Bilateral teratoma of the testis in an infant. *J. Pediatr. Surg.,* 8:49–54.

30. Cloutier, M. D., and Hayles, A. B. (1970): Precocious puberty. *Adv. Pediatr.,* 17:125–138.

31. Cochran, J. S., Walsh, P. C., Porter, J. C., Nicholson, T. C., Madden, J. D., and Peters, P. C. (1975): The endocrinology of human chorionic gonadotropin-secreting tumors: New methods in diagnosis. *J. Urol.,* 114:549–555.

32. Collins, D. H., and Pugh, R. C. B. (1964): Classification and frequency of testicular tumors. *Br. J. Urol.,* (Suppl.) 36:1–11.

33. Collip, P. J., Kaplan, S. A., Boyle, D. C., Plachte, F., and Kogut, M. D. (1964): Constitutional isosexual precocious puberty. Effects of medroxyprogesterone acetate therapy. *Am. J. Dis. Child.,* 108:399–405.

34. David, M., Bovier-Lapierre, M., and Sempé, M. (1972): Le traitement des pubertés précoces par l'acétate de medroxyprogesterone. *Pédiatrie,* 27:623–645.

35. Dougall, A. J., Maclean, N., and Wilkinson, A. W. (1974): Histology of the maldescended testis at operation. *Lancet,* 1:771–774.

36. Dow, J. A., Oteen, N. C., and Mostofi, F. K. (1967): Testicular tumors following orchidopexy. *South. Med. J.,* 60:193–195.

37. Farrington, G. H. (1969): Histologic observations in cryptorchidism: the congenital germinal-cell deficiency of the undescended testis. *J. Pediatr. Surg.,* 4:606–613.

38. Ferrier, R. P., Shepard, T. H., and Smith, E. H. (1961): Growth disturbances and values for hormone excretion in various forms of precocious sexual development. *Pediatrics,* 28:258–275.

39. Franks, R. C., and Stempfel, R. S. (1963): Juvenile hypothyroidism and precocious testicular maturation. *J. Clin. Endocrinol.,* 23:805–810.

40. Gehring, G. G. Rodriguez, F. R., and Woodhead, D. M. (1974): Malignant degeneration of cryptorchid testes following orchiectomy. *J. Urol.,* 112:354–356.

41. Gendrel, D., Roger, M. Chaussain, J. L., Canlorbe, P., and Job, J. C. (1977): Correlation of pituitary and testicular responses to stimulation tests in cryptorchid children. *Acta Endocrinol.,* 86:641–650.

42. Giebink, G. S., and Ruymann, F. B. (1974): Testicular tumors in childhood. *Am. J. Dis. Child.,* 127:433–438.

43. Girard, J., and Baumann, J. B. (1977): Corticotropin-releasing hormone-adreno-corticotropin suppression by an antiandrogenic drug (cyproterone acetate). A therapeutic possibility for congenital adrenal hyperplasia. In: *Congenital Adrenal Hyperplasia,* edited by P. A. Lee, L. P. Plotnick, A. A. Kowarski, and C. J. Migeon, pp. 217–230. University Park Press, Baltimore.

44. Grant, D. B., Laurance, B. M., Atherden, S. M., and Ryness, J. (1976): HCG stimulation test in children with abnormal sexual development. *Arch. Dis. Child.,* 51:596–601.

45. Gross, R. E., and Jewett, T. C. Jr. (1956): Surgical experiences from 1,222 operations for undescended testis. *JAMA,* 160:634–641.

46. Guesry, P., Lenoir, G., and Broyer, M. (1977): Actions à long terme des immunosuppresseurs sur la fonction de reproduction. *Arch. Fr. Pediatr.,* 34:792–798.

47. Hadziselimovic, F., Herzog, B., and Seguchi, H. (1975): Surgical correction of cryptorchidism at 2 years: Electron miscroscopic and morphometric investigations. *J. Pediatr. Surg.,* 10:19–26.

48. Hall, R., and Warrick, C. (1972): Hypersecretion of hypothalamic releasing hormones: A possible explanation of the endocrine manifestations of polyostotic fibrous dysplasia (Albright's syndrome). *Lancet,* 1:1313–1316.

49. Hinman, F., Jr. (1955): The implications of testicular cytology in the treatment of cryptorchidism. *Am. J. Surg.,* 90:381–386.
50. Holtz, F., and Abell, M. R. (1963): Testicular neoplasms in infants and in children. II. Tumors of non-germ cell origin. *Cancer,* 16:982–986.
51. Hösli, P. O. (1971): Zum Kryptorchismus: welcher ist der optimale Zeitpunkt der Behandlung? *Schweiz. Med. Wochenschr.,* 101:1090–1096.
52. Hung, W., Blizzard, R. M., Migeon, C. J., Camacho, A. M., and Nyhan, W. L. (1963): Precocious puberty in a boy with hepatoma and circulating gonadotropin. *J. Pediatr.,* 63:895–903.
53. Illig, R., Exner, G. U., Kollmann, F., Kellerer, K., Borkenstein, M., Lungmayr, L., Kuber, W., and Prader, A. (1977): Treatment of cryptorchidism by intranasal synthetic luteinizing—hormone releasing hormone. *Lancet,* 2:518–520.
54. Javadpour, N. (1978): Biologic tumor markers in management of testicular and bladder cancer. *Urology,* XII:177–183.
55. Jenner, M. R., Kelch, R. P., Kaplan, S. L., and Grumbach, M. M. (1972): Hormonal changes in puberty. IV: plasma estradiol, LH and FSH in prepubertal children, pubertal females, and in precocious puberty, premature thelarche, hypogonadism and in a child with a feminizing ovarian tumor. *J. Clin. Endocrinol. Metab.,* 34:521–530.
56. Job, J. C., Garnier, P. E., Chaussain, J. L., and Canlorbe, P. (1973): Effect of synthetic luteinizing hormone—releasing hormone (LHRH) on the release of gonadotropins in hypophyso-gonadal disorders of children and adolescents. III. Precocious puberty and premature thelarche. *Biomed. Exp.,* 19:77–81.
57. Job, J. C., Gendrel, D., Safar, A., Roger, M., and Chaussain, J. L. (1977): Pituitary LH and FSH and testosterone secretion in infants with undescended testes. *Acta Endocrinol.,* 85:644–649.
58. Jolly, H. (1955): *Sexual Precocity, American Lectures in Endocrinology,* No. 200. Charles C Thomas, Springfield, Illinois.
59. Jones, P. G., and Campbell, P. E. (1976): Tumors of the testis and breast. In: *Tumors of Infancy and Childhood,* Chapter 25, pp. 869–897. Blackwell Scientific Publications, London.
60. Judge, D. M., Kulin, H. E., Page, R., Santen, R., and Trapukdi, S. (1977): Hypothalamic hamartoma. A source of luteinizing hormone—releasing factor in precocious puberty. *N. Engl. J. Med.,* 296:7–10.
61. Kaplan, S. L., Grumbach, M. M., and Aubert, M. L. (1976): The ontogenesis of pituitary hormones and hypothalamic factors in the human fetus: Maturation of the central nervous system regulation of the anterior pituitary function. *Rec. Prog. Horm. Res.,* 32:161–234.
62. Karamehmedovic, O., Woodtli, W., and Plüss, H. J. (1975): Testicular tumors in childhood. *J. Pediatr. Surg.,* 10:109–114.
63. Kauli, R., Pertzelan, A., Prager-Lewin, R., Grünebaum, M., and Laron, Z. (1976): Cyproterone acetate in treatment of precocious puberty. *Arch. Dis. Child.,* 51:202–208.
64. Kauli, R., Prager-Lewin, R., Keret, R., and Laron, Z. (1975): The LH response to LH-releasing hormone in children with true isosexual precocious puberty treated with cyproterone acetate. *Clin. Endocrinol.,* 4:305–311.
65. Kirkland, R. T., Bongiovanni, A. M., Cornfeld, D., McCormick, J. B., Parks, J. S., and Tenore, A. (1976): Gonadotropin responses to luteinizing releasing factor in boys treated with cyclophosphamide for nephrotic syndrome. *J. Pediatr.,* 89:941–944.
66. Kitay, J. I. (1954): Pineal lesions and precocious puberty, a review. *J. Clin. Endocrinol.,* 14:622–625.
67. Klein, D., Ferrier, P., and Ammann, F. (1963): La génétique de l'ectopie testiculaire. *Pathol. Biol.,* 11:1214–1221.
68. Kohn, J., Orr, A. H., McElwain, T. J., Bentall, M., and Peckham, M. J. (1976): Serum alpha-foetoprotein in patients with testicular tumors. *Lancet,* ii:433–436.
69. Korth-Schutz, S., Levine, L. S., and New, M. I. (1976): Dehydroepiandrosterone sulfate (DS) levels, a rapid test for abnormal adrenal androgen secretion. *J. Clin. Endocrinol. Metab.,* 42:1005–1013.
70. de Kretser, D. M., Burger, H. G., and Hudson, B. (1974): The relationship between germinal cells and serum FSH levels in males with infertility. *J. Clin. Endocrinol. Metab.,* 38:787–793.

71. Kupperman, H. S., and Epstein, J. A. (1962): Medroxyprogesterone acetate in the treatment of constitutional sexual precocity. *J. Clin. Endocrinol.,* 22:456–458.
72. Lange, P. H., McIntire, K. R., Waldmann, T. A., Hakala, T. R., and Fraley, E. E. (1976): Serum alpha-foetoprotein and human chorionic gonadotropin in the diagnosis and management of non-seminatous germ-cell testicular cancer. *N. Engl. J. Med.,* 295:1237–1240.
73. Laron, Z., Dickerman, Z., Prager-Lewin, R., Keret, R., and Halabe, E. (1975): Plasma LH and FSH response to LRH in boys with compensatory testicular hypertrophy. *J. Clin. Endocrinol. Metab.,* 40:977–981.
74. Laron, Z., Karp, M., and Dolberg, L. (1970): Juvenile hypothyroidism with testicular enlargement. *Acta Paediatr. Scand.,* 59:317–322.
75. Lattimer, J. K., Smith, A. M., Dougherty, L. J., and Beck, L. (1974): The optimum time to operate for cryptorchidism. *Pediatrics,* 53:96–99.
76. Lee, P. A., Hoffmann, W. H., White, J. J., Rainer, M. E., Engel, M. E., and Blizzard, R. M. (1974): Serum gonadotropins in cryptorchidism. An indicator of functional testes. *Am J. Dis. Child.,* 127:530–532.
77. Lightner, E. S., Penny, R., and Frasier, S. D. (1975): Growth hormone excess and sexual precocity in polyostotic fibrous dysplasia (McCune-Albright's syndrome): Evidence for abnormal hypothalamic function. *J. Pediatr.,* 87:922–927.
78. Lipschultz, L. I., Camino-Torres, R., Greenspan, P. S., and Snyder, P. J. (1976): Testicular function after orchidopexy for unilaterally undescended testes. *N. Engl. J. Med.,* 295:15–18.
79. Liu, N., Grumbach, M. M., De Napoli, R. A., and Morishima, A. (1965): Prevalence of electroencephalographic abnormalities in idiopathic precocious puberty and premature pubarche. *J. Clin. Endocrinol.,* 25:1296–1308.
80. Mancini, R. A., Rosenberg, E., Cullen, M., Lavieri, J. C., Villar, O., Bergada, C., and Andrada, J. A. (1965): Cryptorchid and scrotal human testes. I. Cytological, cytochemical and quantitative studies. *J. Clin. Endocrinol. Metab.,* 25:927–942.
81. Mathews, J. H., Abrams, C. A. L., and Morishima, A. (1970): Pituitary-adrenal function in ten patients receiving medroxyprogesterone acetate for true precocious puberty. *J. Clin. Endocrinol. Metab.,* 30:653–658.
82. Mengel, W., Heinz, H. A., Sippe, W. G., and Hecker, W. C. (1974): Studies on cryptorchidism: A comparison of histological findings in the germinative epithelium before and after the second year of life. *J. Pediatr. Surg.,* 9:445–450.
83. Meyer, J. M., Goldschmidt, P. A., Sauvage, P., and Buck, P. (1977): Étude histologique et histométrique du testicule ectopique en fonction de l'âge, Incidences thérapeutiques. *Ann. Chir. Infant.,* 18:371–378.
84. Mosier, H. D., and Goodwin, W. E. (1961): Feminizing adrenal adenoma in a seven-year-old boy. *Pediatrics,* 27:1016–1021.
85. Mostofi, F. K. (1974): International histological classification of tumors. A report by the Executive Committee of the International Council of Societies of Pathology. *Cancer,* 33:1480–1483.
86. Neumann, F. (1977): Pharmacology and potential use of cyproterone acetate. *Horm. Metab. Res.,* 9:1–13.
87. Pennisi, A. J., Grushkin, C. M., and Lieberman, E. (1975): Gonadal function in children with nephrosis treated with cyclophosphamide. *Am. J. Dis. Child.,* 129:315–318.
88. Penso, J., Lippe, B., Ehrlich, R. and Smith, F. G. (1974): Testicular function in prepubertal and pubertal male patients treated with cyclophosphamide for nephrotic syndrome. *J. Pediatr.,* 84:831–836.
89. Perlin, E., Engeler, J. E., Edson, M., Karp, D., McIntire, R., and Waldmann, T. A. (1976): The value of serial measurement of both human chorionic gonadotropin and alpha-foetoprotein for monitoring germinal cell tumors. *Cancer,* 37:215–219.
90. Prader, A. (1975): Delayed adolescence. *Clin. Endocrinol. Metab.,* 4:143–155.
91. Radfar, N., Kolins, J., and Bartter, F. C. (1977): Evidence for cortisol secretion by testicular masses in congenital adrenal hyperplasia. In: *Congenital Adrenal Hyperplasia,* edited by P. A. Lee, L. P. Plotnick, A. A. Kowarski, and C. J. Migeon, pp. 331–338. University Park Press, Baltimore.
92. Rager, K., Huenges, R., Gupta, D., and Bierich, J. R. (1973): The treatment of precocious puberty with cyproterone acetate. *Acta Endocrinol.,* 74:399–408.
93. Reiter, E. O., Fuldauer, U. G., and Root, A. W. (1977): Secretion of the adrenal androgen,

dehydroepiandrosterone sulfate, during normal infancy, childhood, and adolescence, in sick infants, and in children with endocrinologic abnormalities. *J. Pediatr.,* 90:766–770.

94. Reeves, R. S., Tesluk, H., and Harrison, C. E. (1959): Precocious puberty associated with hepatoma. *J. Clin. Endocrinol.,* 19:1651–1660.

95. Richman, R. A., Underwood, L. E., French, F. S., and Van Wyk, J. J. (1971): Adverse effects of large doses of medroxyprogesterone (MPA) in idiopathic isosexual precocity. *J. Pediatr.,* 79:963–971.

96. Rivarola, M. A., Camacho, A. M., and Migeon, C. J. (1968): Effect of treatment with medroxyprogesterone acetate (Provera) on testicular function. *J. Clin. Endocrinol.,* 28:679–684.

97. Robinson, J. N., and Engle, E. T. (1954): Some observations on cryptorchid testes. *J. Urol.,* 71:726–734.

98. Root, A., Steinberger, E., Smith, K., Steinberger, A., Russ, D., Somers, L., and Rosenfeld, R. (1972): Isosexual pseudoprecocity in a 6-year old boy with testicular interstitial cell adenoma. *J. Pediatr.,* 80:264–268.

99. Russell, D. S., Rubinstein, L. J., and Lumsden, C. E. (1963): Pineal neoplasm. In: *Pathology of Tumors of the Nervous System,* pp. 173–183. Edward Arnold, London.

100. Sabio, H., Burgert, E. O., Jr., Farrow, G. M., and Kelalis, P. P. (1974): Embryonal carcinoma of the testis in childhood. *Cancer* 34:2118–2121.

101. Sadeghi-Nejad, A., Kaplan, S. L., and Grumbach, M. M. (1971): The effect of medroxyprogesterone acetate on adrenocortical function in children with precocious puberty. *J. Pediatr.,* 78:616–624.

102. Salle, B., Hedinger, C., and Nicole, R. (1968): Significance of testicular biopsies in cryptorchidism in children. *Acta Endocrinol.,* 58:67–76.

103. Santen, R. J., and Paulsen, C. A. (1973): Hypogonadotropic eunuchoidism. II. Gonadal responsiveness to exogenous gonadotropins. *J. Clin. Endocrinol. Metab.,* 36:55–63.

104. Schindler, A. M., Cuendet, A., Paunier, L., and Sizonenko, P. C. (1974): Etude bilatérale et évolutive de l'histologie des testicules cryptorchides et ectopiques. *Helv. Paediatr. Acta,* (Suppl.) 32:17–18 (Abstract).

105. Schoen, E. J. (1966): Treatment of idiopathic precocious puberty in boys. *J. Clin. Endocrinol. Metab.,* 26:363–370.

106. Scorer, C. G. (1964): Descent of the testis. *Arch. Dis. Child.,* 39:605–609.

107. Scully, R. E. (1970): Gonadoblastoma: A review of 74 cases. *Cancer,* 25:1340–1356.

108. Sigurjonsdottir, T. S., and Hayles, A. B. (1968): Precocious puberty. Report of 96 cases. *Am. J. Dis. Child.,* 115:309–321.

109. Sizonenko, P. C. (1975): Endocrine laboratory findings in pubertal disturbances. *Clin. Endocrinol. Metab.,* 4:173–206.

110. Sizonenko, P. C., Cuendet, A., and Paunier, L. (1973): FSH. I. Evidence for its mediating role on testosterone secretion in cryptorchidism. *J. Clin. Endocrinol. Metab.,* 37:68–73.

111. Sizonenko, P. C., Schindler, A. M., Paunier, L., and Cuendet, A. (1978): FSH. III. Evidence for a possible prepubertal regulation of its secretion by the seminiferous tubules in cryptorchid boys. *J. Clin. Endocrinol. Metab.,* 46:301–308.

112. Tanner, J. M. (1975): Growth and endocrinology of the adolescent. In: *Endocrine and Genetic Diseases of Childhood and Adolescence,* 2nd ed., edited by L. I. Gardner, pp. 14–64. Saunders, Philadelphia.

113. Thamdrup, E. (1961): *Precocious Sexual Development. A Clinical Study of 100 Children.* Charles C Thomas, Springfield, Illinois.

114. Waaler, P. E. (1976): Clinical and cytogenetic studies in undescended testes. *Acta Paediatr. Scand.,* 65:553–558.

115. Waaler, P. E. (1976): Endocrinological studies in undescended testes. *Acta Paediatr. Scand.,* 65:559–564.

116. Walsh, P. C., Curry, N., Mills, R. C., and Siiteri, P. K. (1976): Plasma androgen response to hCG stimulation in prepubertal boys with hypospadias and cryptorchidism. *J. Clin. Endocrinol. Metab.,* 42:52–59.

117. Wegienka, L. C., and Kolb, F. O. (1967): Hormonal studies of a benign interstitial cell tumor of the testis producing androstenedione and testosterone. *Acta Endocrinol.,* 56:481–489.

118. Werder, E. A., Illig, R., Torresani, T., Zachmann, M., Baumann, P., Ott, F., and Prader, A. (1976): Gonadal function in young adults after surgical treatment of cryptorchidism. *Br. Med. J.,* 2:1357–1359.

119. Werder, E. A., Mürset, G., Zachmann, M., Brook, G. D., and Prader, A. (1974): Treatment of precocious puberty with cyproterone acetate. *Pediatr. Res.,* 8:248–256.
120. van der Werff ten Bosch, J. J. (1975): Isosexual precocity. In: *Endocrine and Genetic Diseases of Childhood and Adolescence,* 2nd ed., edited by L. I. Gardner, pp. 619–639. Saunders, Philadelphia.
121. Wilkins, L. (1965): *The Diagnosis and Treatment of Endocrine Disorders in Childhood and Adolescence,* 3rd ed., Charles C Thomas, Springfield, Illinois.
122. Woodhead, D. M., Pohl, D. R., and Johnson, D. E. (1973): Fertility of patients with solitary testes. *J. Urol.,* 109:66–67.
123. van Wyk, J. J., and Grumbach, M. M. (1960): Syndrome of precocious menstruation and galactorrhea in juvenile hypothyroidism. *J. Pediatr.,* 57:416–435.
124. Young, P. G., Mount, B. M., Foote, F. W., Jr., and Whitmore, W. F., Jr. (1970): Embryonal adenocarcinoma in the prepubertal testis. A clinico-pathologic study of 18 cases. *Cancer,* 26:1065–1075.
125. Zachmann, M. (1972): Evaluation of testicular endocrine function before and in puberty. *Acta Endocrinol.,* (Suppl.) 164:1–94.
126. Zachmann, M., Prader, A., Kind, H. P., Häfliger, H., and Budliger, H. (1974): Testicular volume during adolescence. Cross-sectional and longitudinal studies. *Helv. Paediatr. Acta,* 29:61–72.

The Testis, edited by H. Burger and D. de Kretser.
Raven Press, New York © 1981.

14

Hypogonadotropic Hypogonadism and Delayed Puberty

Richard J. Santen and Howard E. Kulin

*Departments of Medicine and Pediatrics, Division of Endocrinology, The Milton S. Hershey
Medical Center, The Pennsylvania State University, College of Medicine,
Hershey, Pennsylvania 17033*

Clinical evaluation of patients with delayed adolescence requires a thorough understanding of the normal anatomic and endocrine changes which occur prior to and during puberty. These principles can then be applied in the utilization of static and dynamic endocrine tests for diagnosis. In this chapter, we shall first review the physiology of normal puberty and then discuss the clinical disorders resulting from a derangement of this process.

ANATOMIC AND PHYSIOLOGIC CHANGES ASSOCIATED WITH PUBERTY

Anatomic

Between the ages of 1 and 9 the male external genitalia gradually enlarge, but these changes are small and proportionate to somatic growth. Penis length increases from 3 to 5 cm (Fig. 1). Testicular size is stable until age 6 and then gradually increases between the ages of 6 and 9.

Puberty is typified by an increase in growth rate and the appearance of striking somatic differences between boys and girls. The onset of these changes actually antedates the appearance of secondary sex characteristics by a few years. Thus, if bodily changes are considered, sexual maturation may be a longer process than ascribed to the period of visible changes in genital development. The acceleration in growth of body constituents during puberty is most impressively reflected by increments in height and weight. The adolescent growth spurt begins approximately 1 year before the development of secondary sex characteristics. Peak height velocity is attained 2 years after the appearance of notable testicular enlargement. Other parameters of somatic growth, including lean body mass and muscle mass, also increase at this time. Total body water, which is reflective

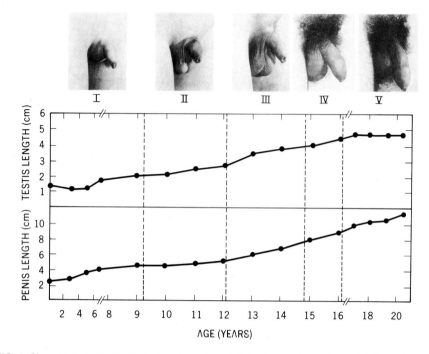

FIG. 1. Changes in penis and testis length and genital development prior to and during puberty. The stages of genital development are depicted in the photographs and are classified as **I–V** according to Tanner. (From ref. 10.)

of lean body mass, increases significantly in boys beginning at age 9½ years. Muscle mass doubles between the ages of 10 and 17; the skeletal mass doubles between the ages of 12 and 16.

The first readily detectable genital change during puberty in boys is an increase in rate of testicular growth. Significantly stimulated testes (a length of approximately 2.5 cm) can be noted at a mean age of 11.6 years, with a normal range (±2.5 standard deviations) which extends from ages 9 through 13. Pubertal maturation is delayed if the testes are smaller than 2.5 cm by age 14. Marshall and Tanner (24) developed rating scales describing the pubic hair and genital changes; the latter are shown in Fig. 1. Pubic hair of males can be rated as follows:

Stage 1: Prepubertal, no true pubic hair

Stage 2: Sparse growth of long, slightly pigmented hair

Stage 3: Hair becomes darker, coarser, and more curled and begins to spread over the pubic symphysis

Stage 4: Hair is adult in character but not in distribution; no spread to medial surface of thighs

Stage 5: Adult

TABLE 1. *Pattern of pubertal changes in a British population*

Pubertal event	Mean age at onset	
	Boys[a]	Girls[b]
Breast development		11.2
Testicular enlargement	11.6	
Pubic hair development	13.4	11.7
Peak height velocity	14.1	12.1
Menarche		13.5
Adult pubic hair configuration	15.2	14.4
Adult type breast		15.3

[a] From ref. 24.
[b] From ref. 23a.

Marked variation may occur in the pattern of pubertal development regarding both onset and duration of pubic hair and genital stages. For instance, a boy with midpubertal genital development may have no pubic hair or nearly adult amounts and still fall within the range of normal. Despite this variability, knowledge of the mean time of onset and duration of various pubertal stages will provide the physician with a reliable index of suspicion regarding abnormalities of sexual maturation. Skeletal age varies less than chronologic age for most pubertal events and remains as an excellent predictor of pubertal onset.

The very first signs of pubertal development in boys, i.e., enlargement of testicular size, occurs approximately 6 months later than the first change in girls, which usually is breast development. Thus, the time of onset of the pubertal process may be similar for boys and girls, even though the development of secondary sex characteristics may progress at a different rate. Pubic hair, for instance, appears approximately 1½ years later in boys than in girls, and peak height velocity is reached approximately 2 years later in boys than in girls (Table 1). In both sexes it takes approximately 4½ years from the first appearance of secondary sex characteristics until adult configuration is attained.

Endocrine

Although the secretory products of the hypothalamic-pituitary-gonadal axis are the primary modulators of the somatic changes which appear during puberty, other hormones do play a role. In particular, somatotropin appears to be necessary in order to realize the full growth-promoting effects of the gonadal steroids. Growth hormone deficient boys will exhibit a growth spurt when exposed to testosterone, but to a lesser degree than in the presence of somatotropin. While changes in growth hormone production with age have been described, the adolescent growth spurt appears to be independent of these variations.

Change in the adrenal production of weakly androgenic substances, as represented by an increase in urinary 17-ketosteroid (17-KS) production, is a well-

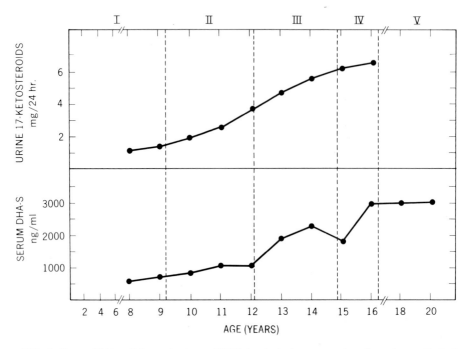

FIG. 2. Serum DHA-sulfate and urinary 17-KS levels in boys as a function of age. Dotted horizontal lines divide figures into five stages of development, as shown in Fig. 1. (From ref. 13.)

known pubertal event. The primary circulating adrenal androgen is dehydro-epiandrosterone (DHA) and its sulfate (DHAS) (Fig. 2). These hormones have now been assayed in childhood and during the course of puberty (13,35). The precise cause of the rise in adrenal androgens remains unknown and is apparently not ACTH or gonadotropin mediated. The significant somatic changes (e.g., increments in lean body mass and height acceleration) which precede by a year or more the appearance of secondary sex characteristics could be a result of adrenal steroids or a subliminal increase in the production of gonadal hormones.

Gonadal Function

Although the testis increases significantly in size in the several years prior to the onset of puberty, testosterone levels appear to remain constant at less than 20 to 30 ng/100 ml, in boys and girls, for the duration of childhood. Once testosterone levels begin to rise in boys, they do so relatively rapidly (15). Many androgen-mediated changes, such as the pubertal growth spurt, occur in the presence of relatively low testosterone levels. There is great variability between pubic hair development and plasma testosterone; even with advanced

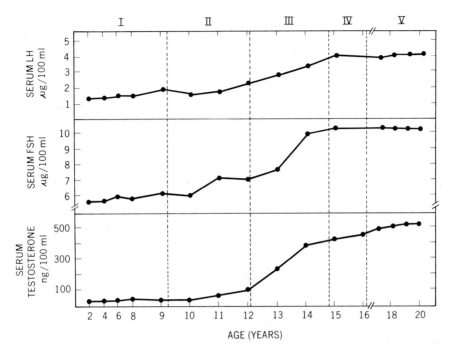

FIG. 3. Serum testosterone, LH, and FSH in boys as a function of age. Dotted horizontal lines divide figure into five stages of development, as shown in Fig. 1. (From ref. 10.)

stages of pubic hair development, testosterone measurements may be within the adult female range. During puberty, circulating testosterone increases more than 20-fold (Fig. 3). A small but significant increment in estradiol also occurs in the male, both as a result of testicular secretion and of the peripheral conversion of other hormones (e.g., testosterone) to estrogens.

The prepubertal testis may be easily stimulated when exposed to the appropriate tropic hormone. Human chorionic gonadotropin, a luteinizing hormone-like substance causes a prompt increase in measurable testosterone, and the administration of this material can aid in the assessment of testicular function even before the onset of puberty (29). The pubertal testis is highly responsive to HCG stimulation even within 24 to 48 hr. There are no data which suggest that testicular androgen secretion is a limiting factor in the onset of male puberty.

Pituitary Secretion

Prolactin measurements have been made during childhood and adolescence but do not show significant changes during this period. It has not been convincingly demonstrated in the human that prolactin plays a role in the onset of sexual maturation. The gonadotropins, of course, are the key hormones in this regard, and both follicle stimulating hormone (FSH) and luteinizing hormone (LH) have been quantified in blood and urine of prepubertal children (19).

There are no sex differences in gonadotropins during the major portion of childhood, although FSH levels do appear greater in girls than in boys in the first 2 years of life. Gonadotropin secretion may reach a nadir between 3 and 5 years of age, after which time the measurements steadily increase during the latter part of childhood. FSH appears to increase somewhat more rapidly than LH as puberty approaches, and attains adult levels before LH.

Plasma gonadotropin levels in the adult are generally only twofold to fourfold greater than in the child, with considerable variation between the results of cross-sectional studies. Data adapted from the longitudinal investigations of Faiman and Winter (10) are shown in Fig. 3. Striking increments in the urinary excretion of FSH and LH have been detected during puberty, e.g., adults excrete approximately 30 times as much LH and 10 times as much FSH as prepubertal children; with appropriate corrections for body size, this difference is reduced to eightfold for LH and threefold for FSH (21).

The hypothalamic factor-luteinizing hormone-releasing hormone (LRF), instrumental in the control of LH (and perhaps, to some extent, FSH), has now been synthesized and administered to children (12). The pituitary gland responds to this releasing factor with prompt secretion of LH and FSH, indicating that hypophyseal function is not a limiting factor in the onset of puberty.

Neural Control Mechanisms

The precise biochemical and anatomic processes leading to the onset of puberty remain unknown. Several phenomena relating to gonadotropin control do change during adolescence, presumably as a result of CNS contributions. The episodic nature of gonadotropin secretion (30) resulting from the pulsatile release of endogenous LRF exists during childhood as well as in later life. The magnitude of the pulses, however, changes as both peak and nadir levels rise in the course of sexual maturation; on the other hand, if pulse amplitude (nadir to peak) is expressed on a percentage basis no difference exists between mature and immature individuals (14).

Increased amounts of LH and testosterone during sleep have been detected in the blood (6) and urine of pubertal children (Fig. 4). Such circadian rhythms have also been described in prepubertal children (18) but not in adults. The increase in the absolute magnitude of sleep-associated LH secretion produces elevations in nocturnal testosterone levels in boys. These nocturnal elevations in testosterone may cause the first visible changes of puberty.

Feedback Relationships

Negative feedback is the homeostatic control mechanism which allows gonadal steroids to maintain a given level of FSH and/or LH. Elimination of the gonadal

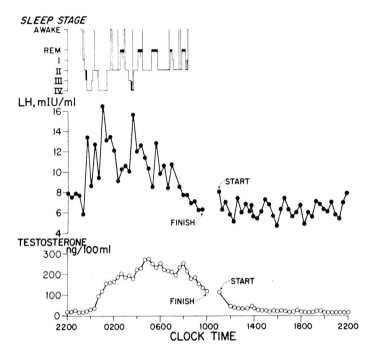

FIG. 4. Levels of LH and testosterone during sleep in a pubertal boy. (From ref. 6.)

product causes a release from negative feedback and a consequent increase in pituitary hormones; similarly, an increase in gonadal secretion suppresses FSH and LH.

There are several lines of evidence which suggest the existence of negative feedback in the prepubertal child. Most important is the fact that elevated levels of gonadotropins have been detected in children with absent gonads, a clinically useful finding in the evaluation of patients with suspected gonadal dysgenesis. Another interesting observation bearing on negative feedback is the fact that prepubertal boys with unilateral cryptorchidism have a larger scrotal testis than normal controls. This finding suggests that a decrease in gonadal secretory products in such individuals causes a secondary rise in gonadotropins and further stimulation of the remaining scrotal testis. Finally, estrogens have been administered to prepubertal children with the finding that a considerably lower dose is required for depression of gonadotropins in children than in adults. These observations indicate that negative feedback is present before puberty and operates at a highly sensitive level (17).

A change in the sensitivity of this negative feedback system occurs during sexual maturation in man (17,27). The adult-type interaction is attained only in mid-to-late puberty as levels of gonadotropins and gonadal steroids increase (Fig. 5). Interestingly, menopausal women may also display increased sensitivity

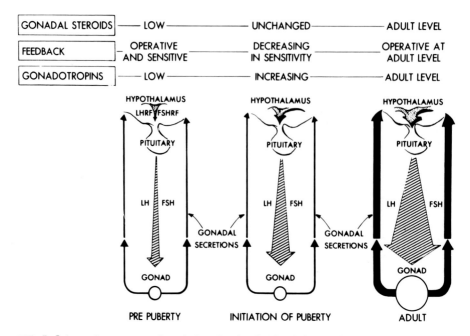

FIG. 5. Schematic representation of changing feedback relationship between hypothalamus, pituitary, and gonads from prepuberty until adulthood. Changes in negative feedback sensitivity (middle panel) are associated with the pubertal increment in gonadotropin secretion (From ref. 27.)

to negative feedback by estrogens and, thus, gonadal steroids themselves may play a role in the pubertal increase in resistance to this type of feedback. The site of negative feedback control is probably at hypothalamic and pituitary levels.

EVALUATION

Anatomic

Careful physical examination of the male reproductive tract is necessary to detect congenital anomalies and acquired defects of the various palpable or visible structures. In addition, useful information can be obtained for staging the degree of pubertal development (Fig. 1). Exact measurement of the length and width of the testes with a rule is easily accomplished and allows accurate assessment of testis size. Testis volume can also be determined by a technique which involves the comparison of a series of ellipsoids of increasing volume (the Prader orchidometer) with the patient's testes. Measurement of the length of the penis provides another useful parameter for following the progression of pubertal changes.

Quantitative assessment of prostate size is not sufficiently accurate for staging puberty but can serve as a marker of systemic androgen effects. The degree of scrotal rugation and color, the amount of axillary, pubic, and facial hair growth, and the presence or absence of gynecomastia may be quantitated accurately and are useful for staging pubertal changes. Finally, the sebaceous glands of the face are exquisitely sensitive to androgens, and the presence or absence of facial oiliness and acne provides a useful marker for the early effects of androgens.

Special procedures such as the radiologic determination of bone age are useful in evaluating a boy with delayed or precocious puberty, since this parameter correlates with the degree of hypothalamic pubertal maturation provided that growth hormone and thyroxine secretion are normal.

Testicular biopsy is a procedure with limited clinical usefulness. However, in the 16- to 20-year-old patient with delayed puberty, owing to primary testicular disorders, morphologic examination can provide additional information regarding the degree of stimulation by endogenous gonadotropins. Subjects with relative hypogonadotropism may be easily differentiated from those with primary testicular disorders such as Klinefelter's syndrome, but hormonal analysis will also allow distinction with ease.

Endocrine

While the measurement of basal hormone levels provides valuable information, assessment of the dynamic relationships which exist between hypothalamus, pituitary, and gonad are critically important in the evaluation of the patient with suspected abnormality of sexual development. The availability of the radioimmunoassay has now made the measurement of circulating levels of LH, FSH, prolactin, testosterone, estradiol, and DHAS relatively available to the specialist. However, the interpretation of these test results must be cautiously exercised since it is technically difficult to quantitate the low levels of these hormones found in children. Bioassays are rarely performed in endocrine evaluations, but they remain as the final method of determination of a given hormone effect. Sensitivity, expense, and the arduous nature of many bioassay procedures limit their usefulness and general availability.

Because the biologic effects of steroids are so dramatic, certain tests which reflect these changes directly may be clinically useful. For instance, an increase in sebum production may be one of the earliest reflections of an increment in adrenal androgen production (26). Urinary cytology can be used in the assessment of increased estrogen effects in boys with gynecomastia (8), revealing differences that even the radioimmunoassay may not detect. Nitrogen retention in a carefully controlled, balanced setting remains as a clinically useful bioassay for testosterone (25). Finally, in appropriate patients, a sperm count can provide useful information concerning the hormone level necessary for adult testicular function.

Radioimmunoassay techniques for measurement of LH and FSH deserve further comment. These hormones, particularly LH, are secreted in a pulsatile

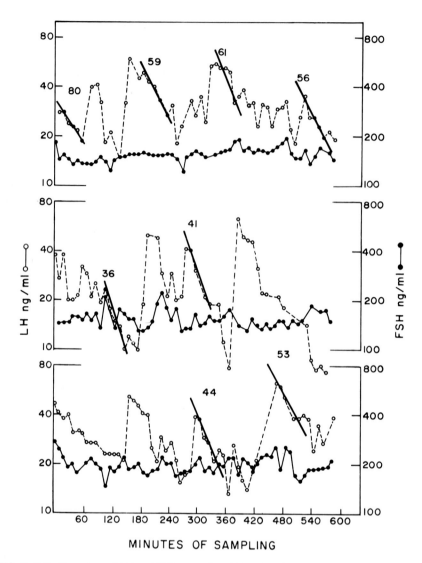

FIG. 6. Pulsatile nature of LH and FSH secretion. LH and, to lesser extent, FSH are secreted by a series of pulses which are characterized by varying amplitude and frequency. After an abrupt episode of LH secretion, levels of LH decline in a log linear fashion (solid lines) with half-lives (numbers above solid lines) approaching that of exogenously administered LH. (From ref. 30.)

fashion (30), which limits the value of a result obtained from a single blood specimen (Fig. 6). Consequently, multiple blood samples are needed to assess these hormones accurately. Furthermore, assays carried out in blood may not be sensitive enough to measure LH and/or FSH in some prepubertal children.

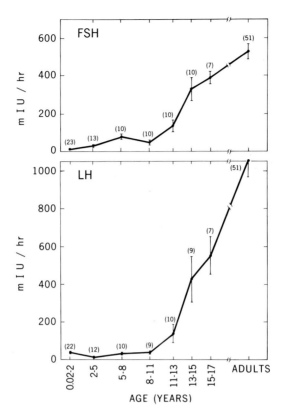

FIG. 7. Radioimmunoassay measurements of urine LH and FSH (mean ± SEM) made from acetone concentrates of timed urine collections in subjects of varying age. Numbers in parenthesis indicate number of subjects tested with each age group. (From ref. 21.)

Because urine specimens can be concentrated prior to radioimmunoassay, they lend themselves particularly well to gonadotropin measurements during childhood and adolescence (16) (Fig. 7). Irrespective of the biologic specimen chosen, repeated basal hormone measurements performed over several months may be among the most reassuring laboratory evidence of normal pubertal progression.

Dynamic tests of the hypothalamic-pituitary-gonadal axis are available to assess the functional reserve of each level of this circuit. Gonadal responsivity can be determined by administering 1,000 to 2,000 IU of HCG (human chorionic gonadotropin) for 2 to 3 days and determining testosterone levels basally and on days 3 and 4 (43). In fact, if the HCG is administered for 2 weeks, adult male levels of testosterone can be achieved even in the prepubertal boy (Fig. 8). With the onset of puberty the testis is particularly responsive to HCG; testosterone levels achieved in such boys occasionally exceed results obtained in adult men.

The pituitary gland also changes in its responsiveness to LRF during puberty

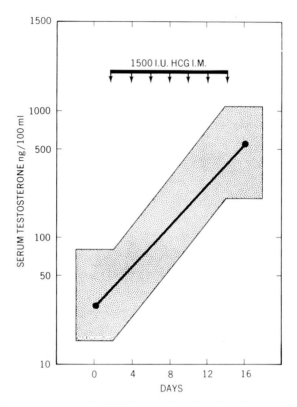

FIG. 8. Testosterone responses to HCG in prepubertal and early pubertal boys. Solid line reflects the mean and shaded area the absolute ranges. Testosterone is plotted on a log scale. (From ref. 29.)

(Fig. 9). This change is primarily in LH secretion, since FSH responses may be quantitatively similar in children and adults. The amount of gonadotropin released after the acute administration of LRF probably depends on the amount of LH stored in the pituitary, which in turn is reflective of the levels of endogenous releasing hormone. While the LRF test (12) may provide reassuring information about pituitary function (Fig. 9), a negative response may be difficult to interpret (33). Furthermore, the response parameters utilized have varied widely among different laboratories.

In adults, clomiphene citrate has been administered to test the integrity of the complete hypothalamic-pituitary-gonadal circuit. This material acts as an antisteroid at the hypothalamic-pituitary level to provoke gonadotropin release. Unfortunately, clomiphene has weak intrinsic estrogenic effects and will actually cause suppression of gonadotropins in prepubertal and early pubertal children. A stimulatory response to the drug occurs in late puberty, (20,34) and, in that setting, clomiphene test results may provide useful information regarding hypothalamic maturity (Fig. 10).

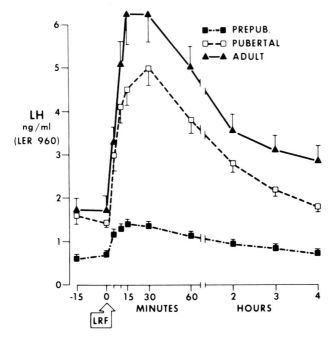

FIG. 9. Response to luteinizing hormone releasing factor (LRF) in prepubertal, pubertal, and adult subjects. (From ref. 12.)

Certain genetic tests may provide important information in a number of endocrine diseases, particularly those involving abnormalities of gonadal function. Analysis of the karyotype determined on blood lymphocytes, skin fibroblasts, buccal mucosal cells, or gondal tissue may be extremely useful in such conditions as gonadal dysgenesis and Klinefelter's syndrome. Patients who have mosaic forms of such conditions may not have all of the phenotypic manifestations of a given syndrome. In this situation, it is imperative that an adequate number of cells are counted and karyotyped for determination of the number and type of sex chromosomes. When properly performed, the buccal smear remains as a good indicator of the number of X chromosomes present. Attention should be paid to the size of the sex chromatin body and the precise percentages of cells which contain this chromatin material. A tool has been developed to aid in the identification of the Y chromosome on buccal smear. This method involves staining the cells with quinacrine mustard which results in specific fluorescence of the Y chromosome.

DELAYED PUBERTY

Delayed puberty and associated short stature are a common problem in boys. The major concerns voiced to the pediatrician are whether the boy will ultimately undergo pubertal changes, whether he will experience a growth spurt to allow

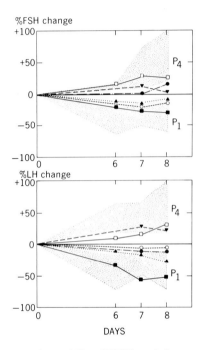

%FSH change

%LH change

DAYS

FIG. 10. Percentage changes of plasma LH and FSH in male hypogonadotropic hypogonadism compared with normal responses to clomiphene (100 mg/day from day 1 to day 7) in five control prepubertal (P_1) and five control pubertal boys (P_4). Shaded area is the normal range. (From ref. 34.)

him to reach adult height, and whether treatment is available or necessary. To answer these questions appropriately, it is first necessary to decide if the patient is actually outside the normal range of development for his age. As a practical guide, the earliest physical change of puberty, testicular enlargement, occurs in 95% of boys by age 13.5 years and the growth spurt peaks 1 to 2 years after this event (24). If no testicular enlargement is present by age 14, pubertal development is clearly delayed and evaluation should be undertaken to determine the etiology.

A useful classification of the disorders associated with delayed adolescence is based on the initial assessment of gonadotropin secretion either in blood or urine. With this test, patients can be divided into two general categories: (a) hypogonadotropic hypogonadism, a condition involving the hypothalamic-pituitary axis which results in decreased gonadotropin secretion and hypogonadism, and (b) hypergonadotropic hypogonadism, the existence of a primary testicular disorder and a secondary elevation of gonadotropins in response to deficient gonadal secretions. The various clinical entities found in these two categories, the means of making the appropriate diagnosis, and treatment will be discussed separately.

TABLE 2. *Classification of hypogonadotropic hypogonadism*

1. Multiple tropic hormone deficiencies (panhypopituitarism)
   A. Idiopathic
   B. Secondary to tumor
   C. Miscellaneous
      Histiocytosis X
      Hemochromatosis
      Granulomatous disease
         Tuberculosis
         Sarcoid
      Vascular disease

2. Isolated gonadotropin deficiency
   A. Hypogonadotropic eunuchoidism (Kallmann's syndrome)
   B. Classic form—decreased LH and FSH secretion
   C. Incomplete form—partial LH and FSH deficiency
   D. Variant form—isolated LH deficiency ("fertile eunuch")
   E. Prader-Labhart-Willi syndrome
   F. Hypogonadotropism associated with neurologic disorders

3. Chronic illness

4. Physiologic delayed puberty (constitutional delay in growth and adolescence)

Hypogonadotropic Hypogonadism

The presence of low gonadotropins in a patient with delayed puberty may be related to a number of causes (Table 2). Physiologic delayed puberty, the most common cause of hypogonadotropic hypogonadism, is a diagnosis which can be made with certainty only after excluding specific organic disorders. The clinical features which allow the diagnosis of organic hypogonadotropism are discussed first and then the more common entity of physiologic delayed puberty is described.

Multiple Tropic Hormone Deficiencies

Patients with multiple tropic hormone deficiencies (panhypopituitarism) may present with severe growth retardation as well as sexual infantilism. Careful examination of the growth records reveals a flattening of the growth curve as early as the second year of life in some instances or, more commonly, later in childhood. Height is usually retarded more than 3.5 standard deviations below the mean. The history may elicit symptoms suggesting deficient secretion of TSH and ACTH or symptoms of hypoglycemia. If a tumor, particularly a cranio-pharyngioma, is present, the patient may complain of progressive headache, visual disturbances, or symptoms of diabetes insipidus. Other specific manifestations may suggest that tuberculosis or other systemic diseases (e.g., sarcoidosis) are responsible for the anterior pituitary hormone deficiencies. With idiopathic panhypopituitarism, onset of growth retardation at an early age may be the only feature favoring this etiology.

A diagnosis of panhypopituitarism is made by demonstrating a decrease in secretion of growth hormone, LH, FSH, TSH, and ACTH with standard tests. Initial radiologic studies include an evaluation of the sella turcica. Computerized axial tomography (CAT scan), pneumoencephalogram, and arteriography are then performed if tumor is suspected and surgery is considered.

Mention should be made of the tests used to differentiate between the hypothalamus and pituitary as the site of the abnormality causing panhypopituitarism. The administration of thyrotropin releasing factor (TRF) and LRF serve as possible means of evaluating pituitary reserve directly. Theoretically, patients with hypothalamic disorders should respond to TRF and LRF whereas those with pituitary hypofunction should not. In actual practice, there is overlap and these tests may not always be definitive.

Isolated Gonadotropin Deficiency

Gonadotropin deficiency without loss of other anterior pituitary hormones results from a number of different genetic disorders. All of the subjects with these conditions present with sexual infantilism or incomplete sexual development (36). The specific diagnosis may be made easily if a family history is elicited or if the characteristic physical findings are demonstrated. The specific disorders and their associated anomalies are discussed below.

Hypogonadotropic eunuchoidism (Kallmann's syndrome) is the most common cause of isolated gonadotropin deficiency and is inherited as an autosomal dominant syndrome with relative sex limitation to males (32). It is thought that this disorder reflects a maturation arrest of the normal processes initiating puberty. Although the cause of this arrest is unknown, it probably results in a reduction in the secretion of LRF by the hypothalamus. Abnormalities observed in subjects with this condition are shown in Fig. 11 and include hyposmia or anosmia, cryptorchidism, harelip or cleft palate, and congenital deafness in addition to the hypogonadism. Most hypogonadal subjects of pubertal age have eunuchoid proportions, with long arms and legs relative to total height and delay in bone age. This somatic alteration results when the epiphyseal growth centers do not close under the influence of androgen at the appropriate age and long bone growth continues.

The degree of gonadotropin deficiency in patients with this disorder may be variable. In the classic form, both FSH and LH levels are low and no evidence of sexual maturation is apparent. In other patients, sexual maturation begins but fails to progress in a normal fashion and results in arrested sexual development. The relative degree of LH as opposed to FSH deficiency may be variable as well. If the defect of LH secretion is greater than that involving FSH, germinal cell maturation of the testis may proceed normally while testosterone secretion is negligible. These patients have been referred to as "fertile eunuchs" since spermatozoa may be present on testicular biopsy or in the ejaculate (31). In reality, few of these patients are actually fertile. The fertile eunuch syndrome

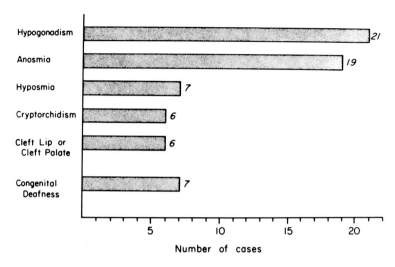

FIG. 11. Frequency of anomalies found in 97 adult family members from 6 kindred studied who had either hypogonadotropic eunuchoidism or were at risk because they were born to an affected or carrier parent.

is considered a variant of hypogonadotropic eunuchoidism since anosmia and other anomalies of the genetic disorder may be present.

The major problem in diagnosis is to differentiate between patients with hypogonadotropic eunuchoidism and those with physiologic delayed puberty. No definitive test is available to distinguish between these two groups of patients. The diagnosis of hypogonadotropic eunuchoidism is suspected in a boy with delayed sexual maturation if very low gonadotropin levels are demonstrable. The relative amount of LH and FSH secreted may be quantitated most precisely by radioimmunoassay of multiple blood samples or timed urine collections. Methods which concentrate the urine before assay are most useful since the sensitivity of measurements is markedly enhanced by this technique (22). Serial measurements of LH, FSH, or testosterone longitudinally over a period of several months can be used to exclude hypogonadotropic eunuchoidism if progressive increments in the levels of these hormones are observed (Fig. 12).

Demonstration of the clinical abnormalities associated with hypogonadotropic eunuchoidism (e.g., anosmia, harelip) provides the best means of excluding the diagnosis of physiologic delayed puberty. Approximately 80% of boys with hypogonadotropic eunuchoidism exhibit either anosmia or hyposmia; therefore, this clinical finding is useful. If no associated congenital anomalies are present, the only definitive means of making the diagnosis of hypogonadotropic eunuchoidism may be to wait until the patient is older than 18 to 20 years of age, when all boys with physiologic delay will have undergone pubertal changes.

It was originally hoped that the response to LRF might allow earlier differentiation between subjects with physiologic delay and those with isolated gonadotro-

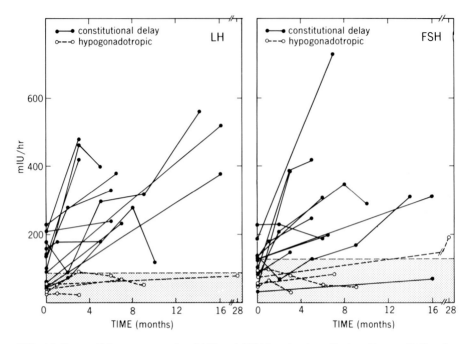

FIG. 12. Sequential measurements of LH and FSH in urine in patients with constitutionally delayed puberty and in boys with hypogonadotropic hypogonadism. The shaded area represents the range of LH and FSH levels observed in the urine of normal subjects prior to the onset of puberty.

pin deficiency. However, variable increments in LH and FSH have been observed after single injections of LRF in patients with hypogonadotropic eunuchoidism and particularly in those with the incomplete forms (5) (Fig. 13). Patients with physiologic delayed puberty, on the other hand, may exhibit diminished responses to LRF prior to the onset of testicular enlargement. When sexual maturation, as reflected by testicular enlargement, has progressed, the LH increments after LRF then may become normal (Fig. 14). Because of this variability, the overlap between normal boys and those with incomplete hypogonadotropic hypogonadism often makes the acute LRF test difficult to interpret. Under these circumstances, correlation with other clinical parameters and serial clinical and laboratory observations may be necessary.

Other methods of administering LRF, such as the constant infusion of this material over 4 hr, have also produced variable responses in hypogonadotropic eunuchoidism. Bremner et al. (7) observed definite increases in LH and FSH in some patients, but variable responses in others during LRF infusion (Fig. 15). The pattern of LH secretion was of interest in the boys with hypogonadotropic eunuchoidism. During the first 90 min, LH increments in the responders were similar to those of normal adult men. However, between 90 and 240 min, the values in normal subjects and patients with hypogonadotropic eunuchoidism

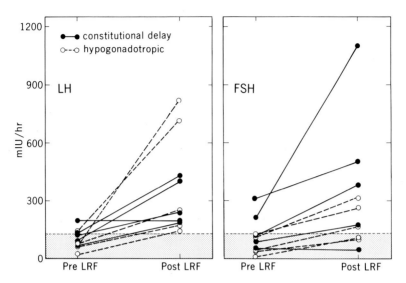

FIG. 13. Responses to LRF in boys with constitutionally delayed puberty and patients with hypogonadotropic hypogonadism. For measurement of LH and FSH in urine, 3-hr collections were obtained before and after 100 μg of LRF (Ayerst) was administered subcutaneously.

diverged. LH levels in the normal subjects exhibited progressive increments in LH over this time period, whereas stable or decreasing levels were observed in the patients with hypogonadotropic eunuchoidism. The lack of a late-phase rise in LH may reflect a pre-existing lack of exposure to LRF. This conclusion is supported by the observation that 4 days of treatment with exogenous LRF normalized the responses to LH-RH infusion in these patients.

While the LRF test may provide reassuring information about pituitary function and maturation, a negative or poor response may be difficult to interpret. Furthermore, the response parameters utilized have varied widely among different laboratories. In our estimation, gonadotropin measurements either in blood or urine following LRF have not allowed the reliable separation of boys with constitutionally delayed adolescence from those with hypogonadotropic eunuchoidism. Clearly, the best data have been provided by the infusion type technique (7).[1]

Stimulation of the hypothalamic pituitary axis with clomiphene has also been suggested to differentiate organic from functional disorders of sexual maturation. However, boys with delayed puberty, as well as those with hypogonadotropic eunuchoidism, respond to clomiphene similarly with a paradoxic suppression of LH and FSH (31). The fall in gonadotropin levels reflects their sensitivity to the minimally estrogenic properties of clomiphene.

---

[1] Since this chapter was prepared, an additional study of the LRF infusion test has been published. (See deLange et al., ref. 8a.)

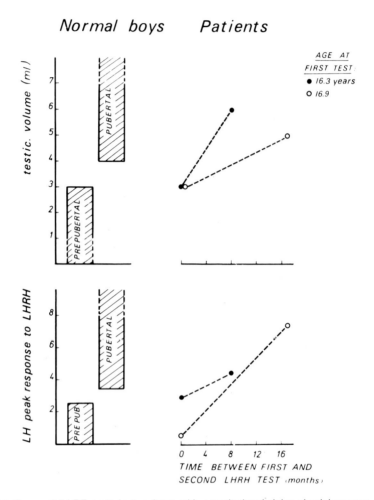

FIG. 14. Sequential LRF tests in two boys with constitutional delayed adolescence whose initial serum responses were prepubertal. (From ref. 9a.)

Patients in whom the diagnosis of hypogonadotropic eunuchoidism can be established because of associated congenital anomalies are treated early with long-term androgen replacement therapy. If a definitive diagnosis is not possible, intermittent treatment with androgen is considered on practical grounds.

Androgen replacement may be accomplished by administering HCG to stimulate the testes to produce testosterone. The dose required is 1,000 to 4,000 IU three times/week by i.m. injection. With gradually increasing doses of HCG (or human LH, which is available experimentally), testosterone increments and clinical changes can be induced in such a way as to duplicate normal puberty (Fig. 16). After Leydig cell function is adequately stimulated, FSH may be

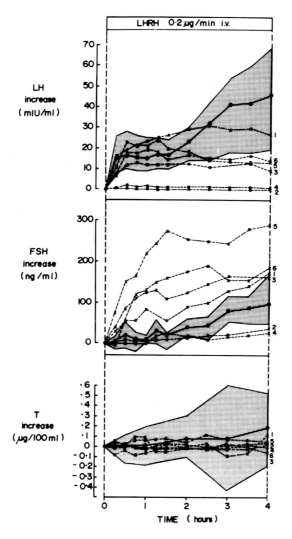

FIG. 15. Serum LH, FSH, and testosterone increases above basal values in six males with hypogonadotropic hypogonadism during their first exposure to exogenous LH-RH (0.2 μg/min for 4 hr i.v.). Numbers in the right hand margin refer to specific patients. Shaded areas and solid lines represent ranges and means of hormone increases during similar infusions in 5 normal men. (From ref. 7.)

given in the form of human menopausal gonadotropin (HMG). This aspect of therapy has been reviewed in chapter 6.

Bardin and co-workers (4) suggested that patients with hypogonadotropic eunuchoidism may have Leydig cells that are unresponsive to HCG and that this represents a "double effect." This concept has been controversial since the majority of patients in other series achieved normal testosterone levels if

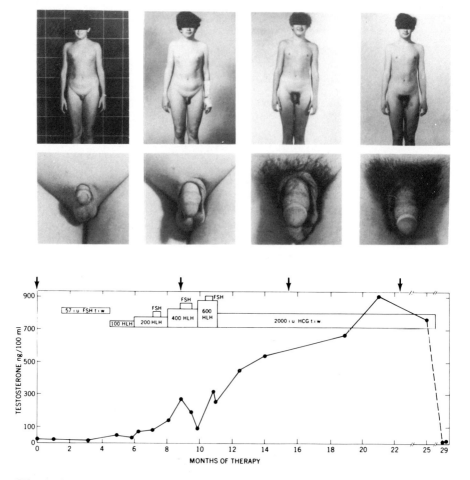

FIG. 16. A patient with hypogonadotropic eunuchoidism given gradually increasing amounts of human LH and then HCG. Small amounts of FSH were co-administered with HLH intermittently. The arrows above the data indicated the times that the photographs were taken.

sufficient amounts of HCG were given for greater than 6 weeks to 2 months (41). We believe that the "double effect" is limited to patients with bilateral cryptorchidism based on data from 7 patients with classical Kallmann's syndrome and bilateral cryptorchidism seen in our clinic. No patient in this group (Table 3) achieved normal testosterone levels after 3 to 8 weeks of treatment with 4,000 IU of HCG t.i.w.

It is unlikely that the impaired Leydig cell response results merely from the cryptorchid position of the testes since Walsh et al. (40) found testosterone levels of 206 ± 37 ng/100 ml were achieved after only 2 days of HCG administration to 8 boys with bilateral cryptorchidism without hypogonadotropism. Thus,

TABLE 3. *Response to HCG in patients with Kallmann's syndrome and bilateral cryptorchidism*

Patient	Age	Anosmia or hyposmia	Weeks of treatment with HCG, 4,000 IU t.i.w. Serum testosterone, ng/100 ml								
			Basal	1	2	3	4	5	6	7	8
A.P.	30	+	50			50					
F.H.	22	+	60			60					
D.E.	32	+	<50								80
L.J.	25	±	80								120
L.Z.	24	+	12				137				204
R.K.	13	+	<10				35				
K.K.	17	+	33				19				70

caution must be advised in treating patients who have hypogonadotropic eunuchoidism associated with bilateral cryptorchidism with HCG since they appear to have an additional testicular defect. This defect may be partial in some subjects. Sherins et al. *(personal communication)* studied one patient with hypogonadotropic eunuchoidism with bilateral cryptorchidism who did achieve normal testosterone levels after HCG. However, this patient was unable to develop normal spermatogenesis after HCG plus HMG and was the only one of 10 patients who did not produce sperm after this regimen.

Direct administration of long acting testosterone in the form of testosterone enanthate or testosterone cyclopentylpropionate, 200 mg every 2 to 3 weeks administered i.m., is more appropriate therapy in most cases of hypogonadotropic hypogonadism because it is less expensive. This form of treatment does not allow testicular enlargement. Methyltestosterone, 25 to 50 mg/day by linguet, or fluoxymesterone, 5 to 10 mg orally per day, has been advocated as well but does not appear as effective at these doses as injectable androgens.

The Laurence-Moon-Biedl syndrome is a rare form of hypogonadotropic hypogonadism and is characterized by retinitis pigmentosa, obesity, mental retardation, and polydactyly (28). The inheritance is autosomal recessive. Hypogonadotropic hypogonadism may also be associated with the multiple lentigenes syndrome (11), Moebius syndrome, congenital icthiosis (3), and cerebellar ataxia (39). Diagnosis of these disorders is made by recognizing the associated congenital anomalies. Treatment is with androgen replacement or HCG, if warranted by the clinical circumstances.

Another type of inherited disorder causing hypogonadism is the Prader-Labhart-Willi syndrome (38). Boys and, occasionally, girls with this disorder have hypotonia, especially in early childhood, obesity, mental retardation, short stature, and adult-onset diabetes mellitus in addition to hypogonadism. Other distinguishing features often present include acromicria, micrognathia, strabismus, fish-like mouth, clinodactyly, and absence of auricular cartilage. The degree of hypogonadotropism in this disorder is variable and ranges from partial to severe. Diagnosis is made by identifying the clinical stigmata of this syndrome and documenting the presence of reduced amounts of LH and FSH levels in blood or urine. Testosterone or HCG therapy in the same dosage recommended for patients with hypogonadotropic eunuchoidism is the preferred method of androgen replacement.

Chronic Illness

Systemic diseases such as regional enteritis or ulcerative colitis which are severe enough to reduce somatic growth will also cause delayed sexual maturation. The etiology of delayed puberty in these patients is usually identified by detecting evidence of the primary disease. Treatment with exogenous androgens for their anabolic or psychologic effects should be considered. The regimen used is identical to that described for the treatment of physiologic delayed puberty.

Physiologic Delayed Puberty (Constitutional Delay)

This common disorder often appears to be familial but may involve other genetic and constitutional factors. Characteristically, from an early age, boys with this disorder lag 1 to 2 years behind their peers in growth, with measurements in the third percentile on the growth chart. Bone age is usually retarded by 1 to 2 years. The diagnosis is suspected in a somewhat short, adolescent aged boy with no significant testicular enlargement whose father, brothers, or cousins initiated puberty between the ages of 14 and 18. In some instances, no family history can be elicited. The absence of hyposmia, anosmia, cryptorchidism, or other congenital anomalies supports the diagnosis of physiologic delay. Retardation in bone age and/or height of more than 3.5 standard deviations below the mean suggests the presence of an organic cause for delayed puberty. Additionally, evidence of thyroid-stimulating hormone (TSH) or ACTH deficiency by history or physical examination would point to organic rather than functional causes of delayed sexual maturation.

The major problem in diagnosis is the differentiation of boys with physiologic delayed puberty from those with complete or incomplete forms of hypogonadotropic eunuchoidism. There is no definitive means of establishing the diagnosis of delayed puberty other than prolonged observations. With physiologic delay the pubertal process may occasionally be initiated as late as age 18 to 20.

Since it is inappropriate to withhold treatment until late in the teen-age period, major efforts have been made to develop functional tests to identify the patients who will ultimately undergo sexual development. As discussed under hypogonadotropic eunuchoidism, basal gonadotropin titers quantitated with sensitive assays may be helpful. LH and FSH levels which approach those observed in early pubertal boys suggest a diagnosis of physiologic delayed puberty. Progressive increments in gonadotropin titers longitudinally over a period of months also point to physiologic delay. A clearly pubertal response to LRF favors this diagnosis, although caution must be advised regarding definitive conclusions from this test.

What, then, should be the approach to the 14- to 15-year-old boy with sexual infantilism and low gonadotropin levels in whom physiologic delayed puberty is suspected? The physician should be aware that severe psychologic effects may result from delay in adolescence (9). These include the following manifestations:

1. Symptoms of emotional tension, irritability, depression.
2. Psychosomatic complaints, e.g., abdominal pain.
3. Inferiority feelings in regard to masculinity.
4. Symptoms of over compensation, e.g., fighting or extreme competitiveness in sports.
5. Regression or withdrawal from peer contact.
6. Poor school performance.
7. Decreased sports activity.
8. Increase in school absenteeism.
9. Inadequate vocational and educational goals for age.
10. Increased parental dependence and parental overprotection.

Counseling will be adequate for a few minor symptoms, but marked impairment in several or all of the above areas indicates a need for hormone replacement therapy, regardless of the diagnostic quandaries. Intermittent androgen therapy is recommended using either HCG, 1,000 to 4,000 IU i.m. three times weekly,[2] or testosterone enanthate, 200 mg i.m. every 3 weeks. A course of therapy should be given for 3 months and then stopped for an additional 3 months. During this latter period the boy is observed for further pubertal changes and spontaneous increments in gonadotropin and serum testosterone levels. If no further progression is noted, the course is repeated for an additional 3 months. Continuous therapy may be recommended if no spontaneous sexual maturation occurs after several intermittent courses of exogenous androgens. The rationale for this regimen is that exogenous androgen initiates the somatic changes of puberty without retarding the spontaneous processes which control pubertal onset. As further support for this approach, it has been speculated that exogenous androgens might also accelerate hypothalamic maturation and hasten spontaneous puberty. The evidence for this is not conclusive. No harmful effects on the potential for full somatic growth or subsequent testicular function will result from this treatment regimen.

It has been observed that boys with isolated growth hormone deficiency go through puberty normally, but at the age of 14 to 17 (37). This condition is usually diagnosed by demonstrating absent growth hormone secretion in a boy with severe growth retardation.

---

[2] Editorial note added in proof: Recent findings suggest that once-weekly dosage may be adequate.

Hypergonadotropic Hypogonadism

Primary disorders of testicular function may also result in delayed sexual maturation. The detection of elevated gonadotropin secretion allows this group of patients to be differentiated from those with hypothalamic-pituitary disorders in whom gonadotropin secretion is diminished. Because the defect in testosterone secretion is partial in many cases, androgen-related somatic changes are experienced at the appropriate age but are incomplete. Whereas the normal progression through puberty is usually completed in 4 years, subjects with testicular disorders progress through two or three stages of genital development and then fail to proceed further. Testicular growth is retarded or nonexistent since this gland is defective. The gynecomastia which frequently develops during normal puberty is more severe than that observed in normal boys. While these disorders will be covered in chapter 15, special mention should be made of (bilateral) anorchia. In our own clinic setting we have found these individuals to constitute the largest group of patients presenting with delayed adolescence who have hypergonadotropin hypogonadism.

Functional Prepubertal Castrate Syndrome (Anorchia)

Individuals with this disorder (2) lack anatomically demonstrable or functioning testes. The appearance of the external genitalia, with the exception of an empty scrotum, is normal. Since testosterone is required for development of the external genitalia during the critical fetal development period of 8 to 14 weeks, it is assumed that testes were present at that time in fetal development. The cause of later testicular degeneration is unknown but has led to the clinical description of this disorder as the syndrome of "vanishing testes" (1). Patients with this condition present either with suspected bilateral cryptorchidism prior to the pubertal age or with sexual infantilism in the pubertal years. Palpation of the scrotum reveals the vas deferens or small masses of tissue consisting of Wolffian duct remnants. With gonadotropin assays, elevated levels for age may be documented even in childhood (42). In the pubertal years, the levels of LH and FSH increase and ultimately reach adult castrate levels in patients with anorchia. The finding of normal gonadotropin levels in a patient suspected of having anorchia would serve to exclude this condition.

A definitive diagnosis of anorchia can be made by demonstrating a lack of response to HCG in a boy without palpable testes (23). After 3 weeks of HCG, 1,000 to 4,000 IU three times weekly, boys with functioning testes, either scrotal or cryptorchid, reach adult male testosterone levels (Fig. 8), whereas those without testes exhibit little testosterone increment. Abdominal exploration may be avoided in boys with anorchia if gonadotropin levels are high and an absent response to HCG is demonstrated. Treatment consists of androgen replacement therapy and the insertion of prosthetic testes.

REFERENCES

1. Abeyaratne, M. R., Aherne, W. A., and Scott, J. E. (1969): The vanishing testis. *Lancet*, 2:822–824.
2. Aynsley-Green, A., Zachmann, M., Illig, R., Rampini, S., and Prader, A. (1976): Congenital bilateral anorchia in childhood: A clinical, endocrine and therapeutic evaluation of twenty-one cases. *Clin. Endocrinol.*, 5:381–391.
3. Bardin, C. W. (1971): Hypogonadotropic hypogonadism in patients with multiple congenital defects. In: *Birth Defects, Original Article Series*, Vol. VII, Part X, edited by D. Bergsma, pp. 175–178. Williams & Wilkins, Baltimore.
4. Bardin, C. W., Ross, G. T., Rifkind, A. B., Cargille, C. M., and Lipsett, M. B. (1969): Studies of the pituitary-Leydig cell axis in young men with hypogonadotropic hypogonadism and hyposmia: Comparison with normal men, prepubertal boys, and hypopituitary patients. *J. Clin. Invest.*, 48:2046–2056.
5. Bell, J., Spitz, I., Perlman, A., Segal, S., Palti, Z., and Rabinowitz, D. (1973): Heterogeneity of gondotropin response to LHRH in hypogonadotropic hypogonadism. *J. Clin. Endocrinol. Metab.*, 36:791–794.
6. Boyar, R. M., Rosenfeld, R. S., Kapen, S., Finkelstein, J. W., Roffwarg, H. P., Weitzman, E. D., and Hellman, L. (1974): Human puberty, *J. Clin. Invest.*, 54:609–618.
7. Bremner, W. J., Fernando, N. N., and Paulsen, C. A. (1977): The effect of luteinizing hormone-releasing hormone in hypogonadotrophic eunuchoidism. *Acta Endocrinol.*, 86:1–14.
8. Collett-Solberg, P. R., and Grumbach, M. M. (1965): A simplified procedure for evaluating estrogenic effects and the sex chromatin pattern in exfoliated cells in urine. *J. Pediatr.*, 66:883–890.
8a. de Lange, W. E., Snoep, M. G., and Doorenbos, H. (1978): The effect of LH-RH infusion on serum LH, FSH and testosterone in boys with advanced puberty and hypogonadotropic hypogonadism. *Acta Endocrinol.*, 89:209.
9. Ehrhardt, A. A., and Meyer-Bahlburg, H. F. L. (1975): Psychological correlates of abnormal pubertal development. *J. Clin. Endocrinol. Metab.*, 4:207–222.
9a. Ernould, C., Bourguignon, J. P., and Franchimont, P. (1979): Usefulness and limits of GnRH test in boys with lack of sexual maturation. *Acta Paediatr.*, 32:105–111.
10. Faiman, C., and Winter, J. S. D. (1974): Gonadotropins and sex hormone patterns in puberty. In: *The Control of the Onset of Puberty*, edited by M. M. Grumbach, G. D. Grave, and F. E. Mayer, pp. 32–55. Wiley, New York.
11. Gorlin, R. J., Anderson, R. C., and Blaw, M. (1969): Multiple lentigenes syndrome. *Amer. J. Dis. Child.*, 117:652–662.
12. Grumbach, M. M., Roth, J. C., Kaplan, S. L., and Kelch, R. P. (1974): Hypothalamic-pituitary regulation of puberty in man: Evidence and concepts derived from clinical research. In: *The Control of the Onset of Puberty*, edited by M. M. Grumbach, G. D. Grave, and F. E. Mayer, pp. 115–181. Wiley, New York.
13. Hopper, B. R., and Yen, S. S. C. (1975): Circulating concentrations of dehydroepiandrosterone and dehydroepiandrosterone sulfate during puberty. *J. Clin. Endocrinol. Metab.*, 40:458–461.
14. Johanson, A. (1974): Fluctuations of gonadotropin levels in children. *J. Clin. Endocrinol. Metab.*, 39:154–159.
15. Knorr, D., Bidlingmaier, F., Butenandt, O., Fendel, H., and Ehrt Wehle, R. (1974): Plasma testosterone in male puberty: I. Physiology of plasma testosterone. *Acta Endocrinol.*, 75:181–194.
16. Kulin, H. E., Bell, P. M., Santen, R. J., and Ferber, A. J. (1975): Integration of pulsatile gonadotropin secretion by timed urinary measurements: An accurate and sensitive 3-hour test. *J. Clin. Endocrinol. Metab.*, 40:783–789.
17. Kulin, H. E., Grumbach, M. M., and Kaplan, S. L. (1969): Changing sensitivity of the pubertal gonadal hypothalamic feedback mechanism in man. *Science*, 166:1012–1013.
18. Kulin, H. E., Moore, R. G., and Santner, S. J. (1976): Circadian rhythms in gonadotropin excretion in prepubertal children and pubertal children. *J. Clin. Endocrinol. Metab.*, 42:770–773.
19. Kulin, H. E., and Reiter, E. O. (1973): Gonadotropins during childhood and adolescence: A review. *Pediatrics*, 51:260–271.

20. Kulin, H. E., Reiter, E. O., and Bridson, W. E. (1971): Pubertal maturation of the gonadotropin stimulatory response to clomiphene. *J. Clin. Endocrinol. Metab.,* 33:551–557.
21. Kulin, H. E., and Santen, R. J. (1976): Endocrinology of puberty in man. In: *Regulatory Mechanisms of Male Reproductive Physiology,* edited by C. H. Spilman, T. J. Lobl, and K. T. Kirton, pp. 175–190. Excerpta Medica, Amsterdam.
22. Kulin, H. E., and Santner, S. J. (1977): Timed urinary gonadotropin measurements in normal infants, children, and adults, and in patients with disorders of sexual maturation. *J. Pediatr.,* 90:760–765.
23. Levine, L. S., and New, M. I. (1971): Preoperative detection of hidden testes. *Am. J. Dis. Child.,* 121:176–178.
23a. Marshall, W. A., and Tanner, J. M. (1969): Variations in the pattern of pubertal changes in girls. *Arch. Dis. Child.,* 44:291.
24. Marshall, W. A., and Tanner, J. M. (1970): Variations in the pattern of pubertal changes in boys. *Arch. Dis. Child.,* 45:13–23.
25. Prader, A. (1974): Male pseudohermaphroditism. *Helv. Paediatr. Acta,* (Suppl.) 34:79–86.
26. Ramasastry, P., Downing, D. T., Pochi, P. E., and Strauss, J. S. (1970): Chemical composition of human skin lipids from birth to puberty. *J. Invest. Dermatol.,* 54:139–144.
27. Reiter, E. O., and Kulin, H. E. (1972): Sexual maturation in the female, normal development and precocious puberty. *Pediatr. Clin. North. Am.,* 19:581–603.
28. Roth, A. A. (1947): Familial eunuchoidism: The Laurence-Moon-Biedl syndrome. *J. Urol.,* 57:427–445.
29. Saez, J. M., and Bertrand, J. (1968): Studies on testicular function in children: Plasma concentrations of testosterone, dehydroepiandrosterone and its sulfate before and after stimulation with human chorionic gonadotropins. *Steroids,* 12:749–761.
30. Santen, R. J., and Bardin, C. W. (1973): Episodic LH secretion in man: Pulse analysis, clinical interpretation, physiologic mechanisms. *J. Clin. Invest.,* 52:2617–2628.
31. Santen, R. J., Leonard, J. M., Sherins, R. J., Gandy, H. M., and Paulsen, C. A. (1971): Short- and long-term effects of clomiphene citrate on the pituitary-testicular axis. *J. Clin. Endocrinol. Metab.,* 33:970–979.
32. Santen, R. J., and Paulsen, C. A. (1973): Hypogonadotropic eunuchoidism: I. Clinical study of the mode of inheritance. *J. Clin. Endocrinol. Metab.,* 36:47–54.
33. Santner, S. J., Kulin, H. E., and Santen, R. J. (1977): Usefulness of urinary gonadotropin measurements to assess luteinizing hormone releasing factor (LRF) responsiveness in hypogonadotropic states. *J. Clin. Endocrinol. Metab.,* 44:313–321.
34. Sizonenko, P. C. (1975): Endocrine laboratory findings in pubertal disturbances. *Clin. Endocrinol. Metab.,* 4(1):173–206.
35. Sizonenko, P. C., and Paunier, L. (1975): Hormonal changes in puberty: III. Correlation of plasma dehydroepiandrosterone, testosterone, FSH, and LH with stages of puberty and bone age in normal boys and girls and in patients with Addison's disease or hypogonadism or with premature or late adrenarche. *J. Clin. Endocrinol.,* 41:894–904.
36. Spitz, I. M., Diamant, Y., Rosen, E., Bell, J., David, M. B., Polishuk, W., and Rabinowitz, D. (1974): Isolated gonadotropin deficiency. *N. Engl. J. Med.,* 290:10–15.
37. Tanner, J. M., and Whitehouse, R. H. (1975): A note on the bone age at which patients with true isolated growth hormone deficiency enter puberty. *J. Clin. Endocrinol. Metab.,* 41:788–790.
38. Tolis, G., Lewis, W., Verdy, M., Friesen, H. G., Solomon, S., Pagalis, G., Pavlatos, F., Fessas, P., and Rochefort, J. G. (1974): Anterior pituitary function in the Prader-Labhart-Willi (PLW) syndrome. *J. Clin. Endocrinol. Metab.,* 39:1061–1066.
39. Volpe, R., Metzler, W. S., and Johnston, M. W. (1963): Familial hypogonadotropic eunuchoidism with cerebellar ataxia. *J. Clin. Endocrinol. Metab.,* 23:107–115.
40. Walsh, P. C., Curry, N., Mills, R. C., and Siiteri, P. K. (1974): Plasma androgen response to HCG stimulation in prepubertal boys with hypospadias and cryptorchidism. *J. Clin. Endocrinol. Metab.,* 42:52–59.
41. Weinstein, R. L., and Reitz, R. E. (1974): Pituitary-testicular responsiveness in male hypogonadotropic hypogonadism. *J. Clin. Invest.,* 53:408–415.
42. Winter, J. S. D., and Faiman, C. (1972): Serum gonadotropin concentrations in agonadal children and adults. *J. Clin. Endocrinol. Metab.,* 35:561–564.
43. Winter, J. S. D., Taraska, S., and Faiman, C. (1972): The hormonal response to HCG stimulation in male children and adolescents. *J. Clin. Endocrinol. Metab.,* 34:348–353.

The Testis, edited by H. Burger and D. de Kretser.
Raven Press, New York © 1981.

15

Clinical Evaluation and Management of Testicular Disorders in the Adult

H. W. G. Baker

Howard Florey Institute of Experimental Physiology and Medicine, University of Melbourne, Parkville, Victoria 3052, Australia

Men with disorders of testicular function may consult the physician because of infertility, impotence, or gynecomastia. This chapter outlines an approach to the management of these problems. Related subjects are covered in other chapters: gonadotropin deficiency (chapter 14); semen analysis (chapter 16); cytogenetics (chapter 17); and varicocele (chapter 18). Because the diagnosis of most testicular disorders is usually obvious from the clinical features and can be confirmed by relevant investigations, general clinical and laboratory aspects are dealt with before infertility, impotence, and gynecomastia are considered separately.

CLINICAL EXAMINATION

Abnormalities of virility, genitalia, and breasts should receive particular attention in the assessment of men with testicular disorders but a general physical examination is also required.

Virility

General Features

Patients with hypogonadism which prevented puberty have a childlike face with smooth skin, no beard hair or temporal recession of scalp hair, and poor laryngeal development. In Caucasians, eunuchoidal proportions may indicate delayed fusion of the epiphyses of long bones because of androgen deficiency during adolescence. Facial pallor and fine wrinkling of the skin around the eyes and mouth, as well as reduced sebum production and beard growth, are features of androgen deficiency in adults. Poor musculature and feminine body contours: narrow shoulders, wide hips, flat ribcage, and fat hips, buttocks, and

357

lower abdomen may also occur but these signs are difficult to assess. Some symptoms are also in this category, for example, lethargy, night sweats, poor judgment, and vague aches and pains. However, some men with hypogonadism have hot flushes similar to those of menopausal women.

Pubertal Development

Delayed onset of puberty beyond 14 years, incomplete development, or requirement for hormone treatment during puberty may indicate gonadotropin deficiency or, rarely, severe primary testicular failure (chapter 14). Early puberty and somatic growth suggest congenital adrenal hyperplasia especially if there is short stature (chapter 13).

Hair Distribution

Beard and body hair varies in distribution, rate of development, and decline with age in different men. However, it is worth asking about the frequency of shaving and changes in hair growth because men who develop androgen deficiency after puberty may notice a decrease. Axillary and pubic hair is more constant in extent. Absence or, more often, incomplete development is seen with untreated prepubertal hypogonadism and in this situation it is useful to record the stage of pubic hair development according to the method of Tanner (chapter 14). Some loss of pubic and axillary hair occurs with prolonged androgen deficiency in adults. The assessment of pubic hair may be complicated by skin diseases such as alopecia areata and by shaving for surgical or religious purposes.

Sexual Function

Information about sexual function is required for the management of patients with infertility or impotence: frequency of spontaneous and sexually aroused erections and seminal emissions, adequacy of coitus including vaginal penetration, timing of ejaculation and orgasm, dyspareunia, vaginal dryness, or other problems in the partner, previous fertility, number of children, and time taken for each conception. Physical illness, surgery, drug treatment, and particularly emotional problems associated with a decline in sexual performance are important for understanding the causes of impotence and ejaculatory disturbances (30). Sensation of the muscular contractions of ejaculation without seminal emission indicates retrograde ejaculation.

Genitalia

Penis and Scrotum

The patient is questioned about urethritis and penile operations or injuries. The prepuce if present is retracted and the glans and urethral meatus examined for inflammation, hypospadias, or other abnormalities. The shaft of the penis, including the perineal portion is palpated for strictures. A small penis may result from prepubertal hypogonadism. The scrotal skin looses rugosity and color with androgen deficiency.

Testes

A history of changing size or involvement of the testes in any illness, injury, or operation should be noted as should the reason for excision of a testis. Undescended testes can be a feature of hypogonadotropic hypogonadism and other conditions in which androgen production or action is deficient in the fetus (40,54). Patients who had undescended testes frequently present with infertility although the disorder was unilateral and treated early in childhood (54). Bilateral testicular torsion or mumps orchitis may cause hypogonadism, and gonococcal epididymitis often produces obstruction. Syphilis, tuberculosis, leprosy, and schistosomiasis are important causes of testicular or epididymal destruction in some countries. Radiation, cytotoxic drugs, estrogens, and androgens produce transient or permanent testicular atrophy (22).

The position of the testes should be noted in patients with a history of undescended testes. Orchidopexy may have been only partially successful so that the testis is still in the line of descent or ectopic. An apparently absent testis may be palpated in the inguinal canal; alternatively the presence of vas and epididymis in the scrotum suggests the vanishing testis syndrome (1).

Testicular size is measured with an orchidometer—a set of ellipsoids with volumes of 1 to 25 ml. The testis is held lengthways between the thumb and index finger of one hand and matched with the appropriate ellipsoid held similarly in the other hand next to the testes. Healthy men have testes of greater than 15 ml and both are approximately equal in volume. Asymmetry, especially the left smaller than the right is a pointer to the presence of a varicocele. Tense hydroceles prevent measurement of the testes.

Testicular consistency and sensation are often mentioned but are very difficult to evaluate. Loss of sensation is said to be a sign of syphilis or neoplasia. Irregularities in consistency or shape of the testes are easy to detect and may signify a scar from previous orchitis or biopsy, or a tumor which is also suggested by an enlarged, hard, heavy testis.

Other Scrotal Contents

Questioning should reveal the known presence of lumps, past infections, and relevant surgery such as hernia repair and vasectomy. Large varicoceles may cause a dragging sensation in the scrotum. By holding the testis in one hand, the head, body, and tail of the epididymis can be palpated with the other. Normally, the vas is situated behind and separate from the muscles and blood vessels of the cord and can be followed from the tail of the epididymis to the neck of the scrotum.

The epididymal heads may be enlarged and slightly tender in obstructive azoospermia owing to congenital disorders of the distal parts of the ducts. Parts or all of the vasa are absent or abnormally thin with vasal agenesis. Induration or irregularities in the epididymides and vasa indicate scars or chronic infections such as tuberculosis. Small epididymides together with small testes occur with prepubertal androgen deficiency whereas relatively normal sized epididymides and small testes suggest postpubertal testicular atrophy or a germinal epithelial disorder with some androgen production, such as Klinefelter's syndrome.

When the patient stands, large varicoceles become obvious and both cords can be palpated simultaneously between the thumbs and index fingers for differences in size. A venous impulse in the cord during coughing, straining, or the Valsalva maneuver, indicates valvular incompetence of the internal spermatic veins (chapter 18). For this examination the most dilated part of the cord should be grasped and lifted towards the external inguinal ring to avoid confusing contraction of the cremaster with a venous impulse. Although varicoceles are usually larger on the left side they are often bilateral (chapter 18). Other abnormalities of the scrotal contents are shown in Fig. 1.

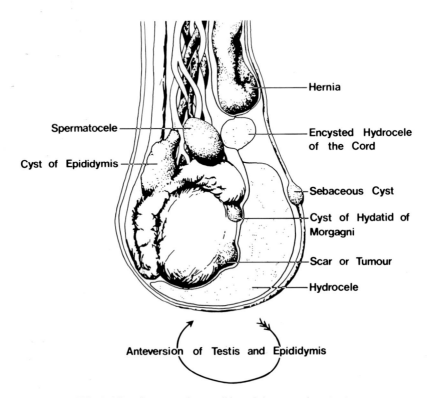

FIG. 1. Miscellaneous abnormalities of the scrotal contents.

Prostate and Adenexae

The prostate gland is often small with androgen deficiency. Chronic inflammation of the prostate, seminal vesicles, and urethra (adenexitis) is thought by some to cause infertility and impotence. Symptoms include painful erections and ejaculation, hematospermia, dysuria, and pain in the groin, pelvis, or sacral region which may be aggravated by sexual activity or abstinence. However chronic prostatitis is often symptomless and while signs—slight enlargement, tenderness, irregularities in consistency and bogginess—are described, they are subtle and their detection requires experience (27). The appearance of pus at the urethral meatus after palpation of the prostate indicates inflammation. Rarely, enlargement or induration of the seminal vesicles may be found on rectal examination.

Breasts

Examination of the male breast is difficult. Different examiners detect gynecomastia with variable frequencies (25,34). The obvious "breasts" of many obese men are composed of fat, and mammary tissue is hard to palpate, whereas in most thin men a few ducts are usually present beneath the nipples. Thus mild gynecomastia, especially as an incidental finding, is of little significance. Enlargement, pain, asymmetry, and pigmentation of the areola or discharge from the nipple bring the condition to the attention of the patient. Cysts, fibroadenosis, and carcinoma can occur in the male breast. Galactorrhea is rare in men and may or may not be accompanied by a palpable increase in breast tissue and enlargement of the nipples. Galactorrhea suggests hyperprolactinemia but is not pathognomonic.

General Physical Examination

Testicular function is impaired in many chronic diseases (e.g., hepatic cirrhosis) but patients rarely present with symptoms of the testicular disorder, these being incidental to the more serious features of the illness. Most men who seek help for infertility, impotence, or gynecomastia are otherwise in good health. However, details of general health and past treatments should be recorded and a full physical examination performed. Some uncommon but relevant factors may be discovered. For example, in the Melbourne clinics approximately 30% of patients with obstructive azoospermia not due to vasal agenesis have bronchiectasis. It is possible these men have a mild form of cystic fibrosis (50). Other rare disease associations are listed in Table 1. The combination of anosmia or hyposmia with hypogonadism strongly suggests Kallman's syndrome. Excessive alcohol consumption or drug addiction may interfere with testicular function without causing major damage to other organs. Extreme heat as with saunas may suppress spermatogenesis. Occupational exposure to estrogens, anabolic

TABLE 1. *Some uncommon associations or causes of testicular disorders*[a]

Testicular disorder	Association/cause
Hypogonadotropic hypogonadism	Craniofacial anomalies
	Congenital deafness
	Intellectual impairment
	Cerebellar ataxia
	Laurence-Moon-Biedl syndrome
	Prader-Willi syndrome
	Hemochromatosis
	Anorexia nervosa
Primary hypogonadism	Myotonic dystrophy
	Noonan's syndrome
	Reifenstein's syndrome
	Partial androgen resistance
Obstructive azoospermia	Cystic fibrosis
Zero motility (cilial defects)	Kartagener's syndrome
Varicocele	Renal carcinoma
	Renal malformations
Testicular infarction/orchitis	Polyarteritis nodosa
	Hemophilia
	Sickle cell anemia
	Brucellosis
	Gonorrhea

[a] From refs. 2,20,36,38,49–51.

steroids, pesticides, and radiation is also relevant (49,56). Epididymal cysts and poor semen quality have been found in a large number of a group of men whose mothers took stilbestrol during pregnancy (23).

Psychological Aspects

Abnormalities of masculinity and fertility are a severe psychological blow to most men. The engendered feeling of inadequacy may lead to serious mental illness, for example suicidal depression. Denial reactions are common and can cause disintegration of marriage, obstructiveness during investigation, and fruitless searching for magical cures. A rare degree of finesse may be required in dealing with these problems. The unavailability of rational and effective medical therapy for many of the disorders does not help the physician to be positive and encouraging but obviously sufficient time should be allowed for explanation of the condition and answering the patient's questions. Care should be exercised when advising changes in life style which are disruptive and not certainly helpful. Some infertile men find the following type of advice intolerable—stop smoking tobacco and drinking alcohol, wear shorts instead of brief underpants, take

TABLE 2. *Investigations of testicular disorders*

Semen evaluation
Semen analysis
Seminal fructose
Semen culture
Prostatic fluid cytology and bacteriology
Postcoital tests
Sperm-cervical mucus interaction *in vitro*
Hormone measurements
FSH
LH and testosterone
Estradiol
Prolactin
Stimulation tests (hCG, clomiphene)
Radiology
Pituitary fossa
Bone age
Miscellaneous
Karyotype
Sperm autoantibodies
Testicular biopsy

cold showers, vitamins and a special diet, avoid stress at work, and have sexual intercourse only at the time of the wife's ovulation using the split ejaculate withdrawal technique!

LABORATORY INVESTIGATIONS

Investigations used in the management of testicular disorders are listed in Table 2. Details are given in other chapters but some comments on their clinical application are necessary.

Evaluation of Semen

Semen Analysis

Semen analysis should be performed in a reliable laboratory, preferably one specializing in this investigation and having intramural facilities for collection of semen by masturbation. Generally several analyses are performed during the initial investigation of infertile men although a single specimen may be adequate in some situations, for example, if it is normal in all respects in a healthy man whose wife has an obvious reason for the infertility such as anovulation or bilateral tubal obstruction. Also a single azoospermic sample may be enough in a man with severe hypogonadism. Otherwise at least 3 semen analyses should be obtained at intervals of 2 or more weeks when some other abnormality is found or suspected. Multiple samples are required because of the variability in results. In 371 untreated infertile men in Melbourne clinics, with 3 or more semen analyses and at least 1 sperm concentration greater than 5×10^6/ml, the ratio of maximum to minimum sperm concentration was less than 2 in 36%, between 2 and 5 in 37%, and greater than 5 in 27%. That is, slightly more than one-quarter of the men had sperm concentrations which fluctuated more than fivefold. Such wide fluctuations may be caused by acute febrile illnesses, variations in the frequency of ejaculation, or poor ejaculation during collection of the specimen, but these factors probably only account for the variability in a small number of patients. Gross errors are possible if the prognosis or results of treatment are based on single semen analyses.

Seminal Fructose

Measurement of seminal fructose is helpful where obstructive azoospermia is a possibility. Very low levels occur with absence of the seminal vesicles which often accompanies vasal agenesis and also with a cyst of the veru montanum or postgonococcal strictures of the ejaculatory ducts. However, partial retrograde ejaculation may also produce azoospermia with low semen volume and fructose (3).

Semen and Prostatic Fluid Cultures

Some believe infection of the lower genital tract is a common and important contributor to infertility and recommend bacteriological examination of semen or expressed prostatic fluid in all infertile men (13,19). In our clinic no evidence of infection with pathogenic bacteria was found in the prostatic fluid of 24 men who had either symptoms of prostatitis or low sperm motility as an isolated abnormality (9). Further study of the value of these investigations is needed.

Sperm–Mucus Interaction Tests

Postcoital tests do not give quantitative information about fertility (28) but they may be useful as qualitative investigations when semen cannot be obtained for analysis, in couples with unexplained infertility and in testing the significance of low sperm motility. Failure of sperm to penetrate optimal midcycle or exogenous estrogen-induced cervical mucus may be further studied with donor sperm and cervical mucus *in vitro*. Lack of forward progression of sperm in wife's and donor cervical mucus, particularly if the sperm show the "shaking phenomenon," may be due to sperm immobilizing antibodies. The presence of immobilizing autoantibodies can be detected by mixing dilutions of serum with complement and suspensions of sperm and observing the decline in motility with time (16).

Hormone Measurements

FSH

Development of radioimmunoassays for serum FSH (follicle stimulating hormone) has constituted a major advance in the management of infertile men. This test has to a large extent replaced testicular biopsy as a method of investigation of the status of the germinal epithelium. A high FSH level in the presence of azoospermia indicates a severe and usually irreversible primary testicular disorder (6). Measurement of serum FSH is particularly useful in men with azoospermia and normal testicular size, who might have either obstruction or germinal epithelial damage. Elevated levels suggest the latter and that exploration and vasoepididymostomy would be useless.

LH and Testosterone

Measurements of LH (luteinizing hormone) and testosterone are indicated where androgen deficiency is suspected. Low testosterone and high LH levels occur with primary hypogonadism and low testosterone and low or normal LH levels with secondary hypogonadism. Because these hormones are secreted episodically, additional samples should be assayed if the first results are not clearly within the normal ranges. Stimulation tests with chorionic gonadotropin and clomiphene for investigation of gonadotropin deficiency are described in chapters 13 and 14.

Estradiol

Plasma estradiol should be measured in men with gynecomastia of sudden onset or if there are other reasons to suspect an estrogen producing tumor.

Prolactin

The value of measuring prolactin in men with testicular disorders is a contentious issue at present. Several groups have concluded that hyperprolactinemia is a significant association of both oligospermia and impotence (10,44). This is not everyone's experience (47). In the Melbourne clinics hyperprolactinemia is rare and high levels in single samples are usually not confirmed when the measurements are repeated. In addition, some men with pathological hyperprolactinemia from a pituitary adenoma are neither impotent nor infertile.

MANAGEMENT OF MALE INFERTILITY

Clinical examination and semen analyses usually permit allocation of the infertile man into one of three treatment groups: (a) no treatment; (b) rational

TABLE 3. *Male infertility—treatment categories*

Category	Frequency[a] (%)
No treatment	
Primary testicular failure	13.1
Vasal agenesis	0.4
Rare congenital disorders	1.1
Rational treatment	
Secondary testicular failure	0.8
Obstructive azoospermia	6.2
Coital disorders	0.7
Empirical treatment	
Oligospermia	43.9
Low sperm motility	33.6

[a] Percentages based on 708 patients attending clinics specializing in male infertility who, with the exception of those with coital disorders, had abnormal semen. Oligospermia: $<20 \times 10^6$ sperm/ml, low sperm motility: $<60\%$ motile sperm but sperm concentration $\geqslant 20 \times 10^6$/ml. Varicoceles were found in all groups but appeared to be more common with oligospermia and low sperm motility. The frequency overall was 37%.

treatment; and (c) empirical treatment. Table 3 shows the composition of these groups.

No Treatment

Primary Testicular Failure

Patients with severe primary testicular failure—azoospermia, small testes, and high FSH levels—are sterile, and at present there is no treatment that will make them fertile. About one-quarter have Klinefelter's syndrome and some others have histories of undescended testes, orchitis, testicular torsion or trauma, treatment with irradiation, and cytotoxic drugs, etc., but in about half the cause is unknown. Testicular biopsies may show severe hypospermatogenesis, germinal cell arrest, or aplasia, or tubular hyalinization but this information adds little to the management of the patient. Although there are reports of recovery of sperm production and fertility several years after depopulation of the germinal epithelium with irradiation or cytotoxic drugs (14,35), most of these disorders appear to be permanent.

Vasal Agenesis

Absence of vasa should be detected by palpation. Careful examination is necessary in men with features suggestive of obstruction: azoospermia, normal sized testes and FSH levels, especially if semen volume and fructose are low. In this condition, clinical diagnosis obviates an unnecessary surgical exploration of the scrotum.

Rare Congenital Disorders

It is also important to recognize total teratospermia and zero sperm motility for these cause sterility without azoospermia. Total teratospermia is a constant defect of *all* sperm such as pin heads, absent heads, absent acrosomes, or detached tails. Immotile sperm with normal morphology on light microscopy can result from inherited defects of the contractile mechanism. The defect may be generalized and affect all flagellae. Combinations of immotile sperm, bronchiectasis, sinusitis, and situs inversus are described (20,38,51). While these conditions are very uncommon, accurate diagnosis is necessary to prevent useless courses of therapy and additional psychological trauma.

With these untreatable conditions, the sterility and options of remaining childless, adopting, or the wife having artificial insemination with donor semen (AID) are discussed with the couple. General health is not compromised by most causes of sterility. However, exploration and excision of intraabdominal testes should be considered for cryptorchidism, and periodic examination to detect testicular tumors advised where there is a history of orchidopexy for undescended testes. Replacement therapy is indicated for androgen deficiency.

Rational Treatment

A small group of infertile men have disorders for which there are clearly defined methods of treatment.

Secondary Testicular Failure

Men with gonadotropin deficiency can be made fertile by injecting gonadotropins (chapter 14). Treatment with GnRH (gonadotropin releasing hormone) may also be effective (33). While most men with untreated congenital adrenal hyperplasia are not infertile some have secondary testicular failure which will recover after adrenal suppression with glucocorticoids (32,52).

Obstructive Azoospermia

Obstructive azoospermia not owing to vasal agenesis or blocks at the level of the rete testis can be treated surgically. The best results are for the rare congenital cyst of the veru montanum. Incision should produce normospermia.

Reanastomosis of the vasa after vasectomy is moderately successful. Patency, as assessed by reappearance of sperm in the ejaculate, is obtained in up to

70% of patients but possibly only half of these are fertile. Persisting infertility after an anatomically successful vasectomy reversal may be associated with the presence of sperm immobilizing antibodies (16,18). Perhaps a man requesting this operation should be tested for sperm antibodies, and if these are present in high titer he could be advised of the reduced chance of a successful outcome.

Results of vasoepididymostomy are generally unsatisfactory. Some surgeons claim fair results, especially with postinflammatory blocks in the cauda (18, 29,42). Our experience is poor, patency being established in less than 10% of operations and the appearance of sperm in the ejaculate is transient in some patients. Newer microsurgical techniques may improve the results in the future, alternatively implantable artificial spermatoceles may be developed from which sperm can be collected for artificial insemination. However, there remains the theoretical problem that if much of the epididymis is bypassed, sperm maturation and attainment of fertilizing ability may be inadequate.

An approach to men with persistent azoospermia and normal testicular size and FSH levels is to discuss the possibility of obstruction, the unlikelihood of a successful outcome from surgery and the alternatives of adoption or AID. The additional anesthetic risk in those patients with bronchiectasis is also evaluated. Where the man wants everything possible done and is prepared to accept the low chance of success, bilateral scrotal explorations and vasoepididymostomies are performed at the one operation. The testes are biopsied, the vasa injected with saline from below the level of anastomosis to demonstrate patency, and aspirates of the epididymal heads examined for sperm. If the vasa are patent and sperm are present in the epididymides, vasoepididyostomies are performed.

Coital Disorders

Minor sexual problems are common in infertile couples: infrequent or poorly timed coitus, transient and partial impotence, but these are rarely the only factors and they usually respond to counselling. Major sexual problems as a cause of the infertility are uncommon. These include permanent impotence, inability to ejaculate, and retrograde ejaculation. Behavioral therapy and other treatments aimed at cure are usually unsuccessful, but artificial insemination with husband's semen (AIH) can be used where semen of good quality is obtainable by masturbation, stimulation with a vibrator, collection of nocturnal emissions, or other methods. Semen has also been collected from men with paraplegia by electroejaculation, but semen quality is often poor and insemination rarely results in conception. Pregnancies have resulted from insemination of semen voided or recovered from the bladder after retrograde ejaculation. The bladder must be catheterized and washed out before ejaculation and as most of the patients with retrograde ejaculation seen in an infertility service are poorly controlled diabetics, there is a serious risk to health from urinary infection following repeated catheterizations (21). Occasionally retrograde ejaculation is corrected by drugs such as ephedrine and brompheniramine (4).

Empirical Treatment

The largest group of men seen for infertility have either low sperm motility as an isolated disorder or low concentrations of sperm usually combined with low motility and a high proportion of abnormal morphology. The etiology and nature of the conditions causing the low semen quality are not understood and treatments are empirical rather than clearly defined and logical (49).

General Management

Varicoceles are often present (Table 3) and varicocelectomy may improve semen quality and fertility (chapter 18) but this is not proved (41). Some patients have chromosomal variants and translocations said to be associated with infertility (chapter 17), histories of maldescended testes, orchitis, or other factors which may account for the disturbed spermatogenesis but many do not. Furthermore these associations do not appear to influence the outcome as regards fertility. The prognosis for fertility depends more on the severity of the semen abnormalities. Although it is suggested that sperm motility, morphology, or indices combining several measurements of semen quality are superior predictors of fertility (chapter 16; 31,45,46), mean sperm concentration is less complicated and gives some useful information. For example, a retrospective life table analysis of the pregnancy rates in the Melbourne clinics showed that approximately 18% of the wives of men with mean sperm concentrations of less than 5×10^6/ml became pregnant within 1 year of their first visit. The figure for men with mean sperm concentrations between 5 and 20×10^6/ml was 30% and for those with more than 20×10^6/ml but low sperm motility, 40%. About 75% of fertile couples conceive within 1 year of trying (31,48). These figures are useful for advising patients about their chances for fertility. Continued collection of data should extend the range of prediction beyond 1 year and may reveal other factors of prognostic significance.

One approach to these men is to explain the prognosis and the lack of clearly effective treatments to improve fertility. Details of the investigations of the woman should be reviewed and further tests and treatments arranged as necessary. The couple benefit from some understanding of the physiology of fertilization and this and the adequacy and timing of coitus can be discussed at several visits to maximize the chances of conception. The mucus symptoms described by Billings et al. (11) are detected by most women and are very helpful for timing coitus. Frequent intercourse, at least every 48 hr during the 8 to 10 days spanning the expected time of ovulation is advised. The other possibilities of adoption and AID should be mentioned at an early stage in management. In Australia, very few children are available for adoption, and most people wishing to adopt are unsuccessful. Thus for most couples the decision is whether to keep trying on their own and possibly end up childless, or have AID and at what stage. Those who would accept AID and have severe disorders of semen quality, for example severe oligospermia ($< 5 \times 10^6$/ml), might be advised to have it sooner than those with better semen quality.

This group of patients is often the most difficult to handle. The need to make such crucial decisions while the outcome is so uncertain adds to the psychological stress of the infertile couple. An alternative approach is to tell the men that there is virtually no chance of fertility and that if they want children they must either adopt or accept AID. This more straightforward approach may be better accepted in the long run by some of the patients who remain infertile, but there is a risk for the others that when a pregnancy occurs naturally there may be considerable suspicion on the part of the husband about the paternity of the child.

Medical Therapy

A variety of hormones and drugs have been recommended for treatment of oligospermia and low sperm motility (3). In general the reasons for their use are not very sound and they have not been properly investigated by controlled clinical trials. Despite this there are many reports claiming improvement in semen quality and fertility. As the men considered suitable for drug treatment are subfertile rather than sterile, the occurrence of 20 to 40% "pregnancy rates" during treatment does not prove the drug is valuable (24).

Treatments for Oligospermia

Testosterone Rebound.

Testosterone esters are injected in sufficient dosage (e.g., testosterone enanthate 250 mg every 2 weeks for 3 months) to suppress the secretion of gonadotropins and cause a temporary cessation of spermatogenesis. When sperm production resumes after 4 to 6 months, there is supposed to be a rebound rise in sperm concentrations above the pretreatment levels (15).

Antiestrogens.

Clomiphene, tamoxifen, and other antiestrogens will increase the levels of LH and FSH in men, and there are reports of improved sperm production after several months treatment with these drugs. The usual dosage is 25 to 50 mg/day for clomiphene and 20 mg/day for tamoxifen (37,53).

Mesterolone.

This weak androgen was recommended for oligospermia on the basis that it would not suppress gonadotropin secretion but might have some direct effect on the germinal epithelium (43).

Gonadotropin Releasing Hormone.

Injections of GnRH have been used in small groups of men with apparent improvements in oligospermia (5,33).

Gonadotropins.

Extracts of urinary or pituitary gonadotropins containing FSH and LH have been given alone or with hCG (human chorionic gonadotropin) to men without gonadotropin deficiency but the results are not clear (3).

Bromocriptine.

Bromocriptine blocks prolactin secretion and there are reports that it may increase sperm output in men with hyperprolactinemia and oligospermia (44).

Other.

Thyroxine, vitamin C, vitamin E, arginine, and glucocorticoids in low dosage are also given for oligospermia, but there is no reason to suspect they might be beneficial in the absence of a clearly defined deficiency state.

Treatments for Low Sperm Motility

Chorionic Gonadotropin.

HCG in doses of 2,500 to 4,000 U 2 or 3 times a week for about 3 months has been suggested as a method for improving sperm motility, possibly through increased androgen delivery to the epididymis and improved sperm maturation (3).

Androgens.

Low doses of androgens such as methyltestosterone 10 to 50 mg/day, mesterolone 200 mg/day or fluoxymesterone 5 to 20 mg/day have been given for 1 to 3 months also because this treatment might have a beneficial effect on epididymal function (3,12).

Antibiotics.

Antibacterial agents are commonly given to men with leucocytes and debris in their semen—the so-called "dirty semen." Some physicians reserve this treatment for men who have cytological or bacteriological evidence of chronic prostatitis (13,19). While there is some evidence that chronic lower genital tract inflammation may impair semen quality, the effect of treatment on fertility has not been studied appropriately. In our clinic a significant improvement in sperm motility was found in a small group of men with either low sperm motility as an isolated abnormality or symptoms of prostatitis although there was no evidence of infection with pathogenic bacteria (9). Because of this result a double blind placebo controlled trial of erythromycin for low sperm motility is in progress. If this trial confirms the beneficial effect of erythromycin on sperm motility the mechanism will be investigated.

Glucocorticoids.

Men with sperm autoantibodies have been treated with glucocorticoids in immunosuppressive doses. Reduced antibody titers, improved sperm motility and cervical mucus penetration and some pregnancies have resulted but, as usual, the trials lack controls (16). Side effects are considerable and potentially serious. Because the treatment can only be given for a few months, the transient improvement may not allow sufficient time for many pregnancies to occur. Possibly semen could be collected in the nonfertile phases of the wife's cycles and frozen for later artificial insemination.

Results of Medical Treatment

An experience of the use of some drugs for oligospermia or low sperm motility is summarized in Table 4. Comparison of results between groups is not justified because the patients were specially selected for the various treatments. It is possible that the drugs did improve or further impair fertility but this cannot be evaluated without random allocation to control and treatment groups. However, it is clear that none of the treatments was associated with a dramatic increase in fertility, there being no significant difference in the pregnancy rates in the wives of men either given a treatment or not treated. The effects on semen quality may be summarized. Sperm concentration was suppressed for 6 months after testosterone treatment, but this was not followed by a significant "rebound" above the pretreatment values. Sperm concentration was also suppressed for 6 months with hCG treatment without any significant improvement in sperm motility. Semen quality was not significantly changed by the other treatments. Overall, these results are disappointing but they highlight the need for controlled clinical trials of putative treatments for oligospermia and low sperm motility. Until such trials confirm the usefulness of these drugs, their indiscriminate use is illogical and probably not warranted.

Other Methods

Coital Techniques

Abstinence from ejaculation until the day of ovulation has been suggested on the basis that sperm concentration may fall with frequent ejaculation, but

TABLE 4. *Results of medical treatments of infertile men*[a]

	No. of patients in group	Observed no. of pregnancies (O)	Expected no. of pregnancies (E)	Relative pregnancy rate (O/E)
Mesterolone	48	5	9.6	0.52
T Rebound	25	4	3.8	1.06
hCG	9	1	2.7	0.37
Clomiphene	22	2	4.3	0.46
Bromocriptine	24	2	4.2	0.46
Antibiotics	41	8	7.7	1.04
None	115	33	22.6	1.46
All patients	284	55	55.0	1.00

[a] Pregnancy rates in wives of men with poor semen quality who were either treated with various drugs or not treated. These have been analyzed by the logrank test which takes into account both the number of pregnancies and the time at which they occurred (39). Patients with azoospermia or wives with persistent anovulation or bilateral tubal obstruction were excluded. Stratification on mean pretreatment sperm concentration ($<5 \times 10^6$/ml, 5–20×10^6/ml, and $>20 \times 10^6$/ml with motility $<60\%$) was used because some groups contained more men with a poorer prognosis than others. At 1 month intervals after the start of treatment or after the first visit to the clinic for the no treatment group, the total number of pregnancies was multiplied by the proportion of men in each treatment group and the figures summed to give the expected number of pregnancies. There was no significant difference between the groups ($X^2 = 10.64$, df $= 6$, $p > 0.1$). The relative pregnancy rate is an estimate of the ratio of the monthly pregnancy rate in each group to that of all groups combined.

many couples practising this technique appear to miss midcycle completely. Furthermore, MacLeod and Gold (31) found evidence of higher fertility in couples who had intercourse frequently although these authors were the main proponents of the reduction in sperm concentration with frequent ejaculation. Amelar and Dubin (3) recommended a split ejaculate withdrawal technique, whereby only the first part of the ejaculate containing higher concentrations of more motile sperm is deposited in the vagina. As with the medical treatments these methods have not been investigated to determine whether or not they improve fertility.

Artificial Insemination with Husband's Semen (AIH)

AIH with semen of good quality is useful when natural insemination is impossible because of anatomical defects, anejaculation, or impotence and where semen has been stored prior to vasectomy, orchidectomy, or cytotoxic therapy. However, the value of AIH with oligospermia or low sperm motility is uncertain. Pregnancies do occur but some also occur with natural insemination of such semen. Again controlled clinical research is necessary. Probably the most logical use of AIH is for low sperm motility, particularly if there is no forward progressive motility in estrogen primed cervical mucus. Intrauterine insemination may bypass a barrier. The rare patients with oligospermia but good sperm motility and morphology might also benefit from intrauterine AIH as sperm may reach the site of fertilization in greater numbers than with natural insemination. Methods for washing antibodies off sperm and for harvesting the better sperm from abnormal semen are being investigated and may be useful in the future (16).

INVESTIGATION OF IMPOTENCE

Impotence is a common problem. As serious underlying illnesses are rare, the physician must decide how much investigation is required for each patient. History and physical examination help distinguish the small numbers of patients who might have an organic cause for the impotence from the majority who do not.

Types of Impotence

Primary Impotence

A lifelong absence of erections and ejaculations is very rare, and usually psychological in origin although it might also occur with prepubertal hypogonadism.

Functional Impotence

The most common type of impotence is a secondary disorder with decreased sexual performance because of inadequate or absent erections. There may be a change in ejaculation, either early, delayed, or absent. Similarly, sexual urge may be unchanged or decreased. Most patients have no clear evidence of hormonal, vascular, or neurological diseases. Often psychological factors are important in aggravating and perpetuating the condition even if not as the whole cause. Other features may point away from a serious illness; these include fluctuations in severity and selectivity. Selective impotence with certain women, such as the wife, but normal sexual function with other women, and the combination of impotence with an unchanged frequency of spontaneous erections or successful masturbation is unlikely to have organic causes (30).

Organic Impotence

Impotence is frequent during debilitating illness and may be the presenting symptom of hepatic cirrhosis, chronic renal failure, peripheral neuropathy, diabetes, and temporal lobe tumors. However, the impotence is more often overshadowed by the other serious disturbances accompanying the illness. Alcoholism without gross liver or nervous system damage may cause transient impotence as may a variety of drugs: antihypertensives, tranquillizers, spironolactone, and estrogens. Estrogen producing tumors usually produce impotence with loss of sexual urge and evidence of feminization. Impotence of neurologic origin is progressive and absolute (21). In these situations the major problem is usually apparent on clinical examination. Vascular causes are more difficult to detect. Stenosis of the bifurcation of the aorta or common iliac arteries causes intermittent claudication and impotence. Atherosclerosis of smaller arteries is also said to cause impotence, however, angiography is required for diagnosis (26). There is a possibility that varicoceles may impair testosterone secretion and potency but this requires confirmation (17).

Androgen Deficiency

Patients with primary or secondary testicular failure may present in adult life with impotence. Usually there is progressive deterioration in all aspects of virility: impotence, loss of spontaneous erections, decreased beard and body hair, and reduced testicular size. Secondary impotence may be a feature of Klinefelter's syndrome, undescended testes, or other severe primary testicular disorders. The patient may be adequately androgenized in young adulthood but later develop impotence from declining androgen production in middle age. A deterioration in testicular function accompanies aging. Many men over the age of 70 years have reduced testicular size, clinical features of androgen deficiency, and elevated gonadotropin and low testosterone levels (8). This senescent testicular failure might also occur in middle aged men but most patients in this age group investigated for the so-called "male climacteric" do not have objective evidence of androgen deficiency.

Secondary testicular failure results from pituitary destruction by tumors, surgery, or trauma. Some patients with pituitary tumors have hyperprolactinemia and their impotence may improve following suppression of the prolactin levels with bromocriptine (10).

Disorders of Ejaculation

Ejaculatory disturbances may result from autonomic neuropathy, bladder neck damage, treatment with antihypertensive drugs, or acute intoxication with alcohol. However, anejaculation with normal erections is often psychogenic. Premature ejaculation is a functional disturbance which usually responds well to behavioral therapy.

Investigations

Laboratory investigations are not necessary if psychological factors are obvious, there are no abnormalities on physical examination, and no glycosuria. However, measurement of plasma testosterone may help reassure the patient that there is no hormonal cause. Sexual counselling or behavioral therapy by specialists in these techniques are often successful (30). Severe depression should be recognized and treated appropriately. When hypogonadism is incidental to serious illness or senescence and the man is unconcerned, investigations are also not warranted except where another problem, such as hypopituitarism, is a possibility.

In other patients with clinical evidence of hypogonadism, measurement of FSH, LH, and testosterone levels should differentiate primary from secondary testicular failure. If the basal levels of the gonadotropins are not elevated, dynamic tests of gonadotropin secretion, visual fields, radiography of the pituitary fossa, and tests of the other pituitary hormones should be performed at an appropriate stage in the management of the patient (chapter 14).

Patients with androgen deficiency usually regain potency with replacement therapy whereas those with other forms of organic impotence respond poorly. Some with psychogenic impotence may experience an increase in spontaneous erections and some improvement in sexual function initially, but this is usually transient. Injection of long acting testosterone esters (e.g., testosterone enanthate 250 mg) at intervals of 1 to 3 weeks depending on the response is recommended for replacement therapy. The currently available oral androgens probably should not be used for long term therapy because of their relatively low potency. Also, changes in the liver occur with methyltestosterone (55). Replacement therapy for androgen deficiency will produce normal sexual function and secondary sex hair growth. Muscle mass and strength often increase and there may be an improvement in mental outlook. The side effects include pain and nerve damage at the injection site, increased skin oiliness, acne, gynecomastia, sodium retention, and aggressive personality changes. The increases in erythrocyte mass and prostatic size could have deleterious effects in the long term but this has not been investigated. Obviously androgens should be used carefully in old men with cardiovascular and prostatic disorders.

INVESTIGATION OF GYNECOMASTIA

Clinical Aspects

Minor degrees of gynecomastia are common, particularly during puberty and old age (25,34). The majority of men are unaware of the presence of breast tissue in themselves, and most of those who present with gynecomastia do not have a serious illness. Often the breast development is first noticed during puberty or young adult life, virility is normal, and the gynecomastia may be unilateral or markedly asymmetrical. These patients are said to have "idiopathic" or "essential gynecomastia."

Gynecomastia is a well recognized feature of chronic liver, kidney and lung, or mediastinal diseases. It also occurs with thyrotoxicosis, paraplegia, immobilization, and during recovery from starvation. A variety of drugs may cause gynecomastia: estrogens, androgens, progestins, chorionic gonadotropin, spironolactone, digoxin, tranquillizers, amphetamines, and methyldopa. These associations are usually obvious and rarely present a diagnostic problem.

The combination of gynecomastia and hypogonadism as in Klinefelter's syndrome and hypogonadotropic hypogonadism should be suspected from the small testes and signs of androgen deficiency. Occasionally adolescents or young adults with mild types of male pseudohermaphroditism present with gynecomastia. Often hypospadias is present or was treated in childhood and there are relatives with the same condition (36). Estrogen or gonadotropin secreting tumors of the testes or adrenals cause gynecomastia, suppression of the secretion of the pituitary gonadotropins, and secondary testicular failure. Symptoms and androgen deficiency are usually marked. Other tumors, especially bronchial carcinomas, may also cause gynecomastia either by synthesis of hCG-like material or more often by unknown mechanisms.

Hormone Measurements

Very high levels of estrogens and low LH and FSH levels are found with estrogen producing tumors. The tumor gonadotropin may crossreact in LH radioimmunoassays and can be measured more specifically with hCG β-subunit assays. As described in the previous sections, measurements of sex steroids, gonadotropins, and prolactin are required for management of patients with hypogonadism but these investigations are of little help in diagnosis or understanding the pathogenesis of gynecomastia. Plasma estradiol levels are slightly elevated in some but not all patients (7). If the cause of gynecomastia is not obvious in middle aged or elderly men, periodic examinations (chest radiographs and sputum cytology) are warranted to detect bronchial carcinoma. In all age groups, thyrotoxicosis should be considered as a possible cause of gynecomastia.

ACKNOWLEDGMENTS

The author thanks the National Health and Medical Research Council of Australia for support, Dr. Bryan Hudson for criticizing the manuscript, colleagues in the Infertility Clinic of Prince Henry's Hospital and the Reproductive Biology Unit, Royal Women's Hospital for their interest and discussions, and Miss Betty Heginbothom for the typing.

REFERENCES

1. Abeyaratne, M. R., Aherne, W. A., and Scott, J. E. S. (1969): The vanishing testis. *Lancet,* 2:822–824.
2. Aiman, J., Griffin, J. E., Gazak, J. M., Wilson, J. D., and MacDonald, P. C. (1979): Androgen insensitivity as a cause of infertility in otherwise normal men. *N. Engl. J. Med.,* 300:223–227.
3. Amelar, R. D., and Dubin, L. (1977): The management of idiopathic male infertility. *J. Reprod. Med.,* 18:191–200.
4. Andaloro, V. A., and Dube, A. (1975): Treatment of retrograde ejaculation with brompheniramine. *Urology,* 5:520–522.
5. Aparicio, N. J., Schwarzstein, L., Turner, E. A., Turner, D., Mancini, R., and Schally, A. V. (1976): Treatment of idiopathic normogonadotropic oligoasthenospermia with synthetic luteinizing hormone-releasing hormone. *Fertil. Steril.,* 17:549–555.

6. Baker, H. W. G., Bremner, W. J., Burger, H. G., de Kretser, D. M., Dulmanis, A., Eddie, L. W., Hudson, B., Keogh, E. J., Lee, V. W. K., and Rennie, G. C. (1976): Testicular control of follicle-stimulating hormone secretion. *Recent Prog. Horm. Res.,* 32:429–469.
7. Baker, H. W. G., Burger, H. G., de Kretser, D. M., Dulmanis, A., Hudson, B., O'Connor, S., Paulsen, C. A., Purcell, N., Rennie, G. C., Seah, C. S., Taft, H. P., and Wang, C. (1978): A study of the endocrine manifestations of hepatic cirrhosis. *Q. J. Med.,* 45:145–178.
8. Baker, H. W. G., Burger, H. G., de Kretser, D. M., Hudson, B., O'Connor, S., Wang, C., Mirovics, A., Court, J., Dunlop, M., and Rennie, G. C. (1976): Changes in the pituitary-testicular system with age. *Clin. Endocrinol. (Oxford),* 5:349–372.
9. Baker, H. W. G., Straffon, W. G. E., Murphy, G., Davidson, A., Burger, H. G., and de Kretser, D. M. (1979): Prostatitis and male infertility: A pilot study. Possible increase in sperm motility with antibacterial chemotherapy. *Int. J. Androl.,* 2:193–201.
10. Besser, G. M., and Thorner, M. O. (1976): Bromocriptine in the treatment of the hyperprolacti-naemia-hypogonadism syndromes. *Postgrad. Med. J.,* 52(Suppl 1): 64–70.
11. Billings, E. L., Billings, J. J., Brown, J. B., and Burger, H. G. (1972): Symptoms and hormonal changes accompanying ovulation. *Lancet,* 1:282–284.
12. Brown, J. S. (1975): The effect of orally administered androgens on sperm motility. *Fertil. Steril.,* 26:305–308.
13. Caldamone, A. A., and Cockett, A. T. K. (1978): Infertility and genitourinary infection. *Urology,* 12:304–312.
14. Chapman, R. M., Rees, L. H., Sutcliffe, S. B., Edwards, C. R. W., and Malpas, J. S. (1979): Cyclical combination chemotherapy and gonadal function. Retrospective study in males. *Lancet,* 1:287–289.
15. Charny, C. W., and Gordon, J. A. (1978): Testosterone rebound therapy: A neglected modality. *Fertil. Steril.,* 29:64–68.
16. Cohen, J., and Hendry, W. F. (1978): *Spermatozoa, Antibodies and Infertility.* Blackwell Scientific Publications, London.
17. Comhaire, F., and Vermeulen, A. (1975): Plasma testosterone in patients with varicocele and sexual inadequacy. *J. Clin. Endocrinol. Metab.,* 40:824–829.
18. Dubin, L., and Amelar, R. D. (1977): Surgical therapy for male infertility. *J. Reprod. Med.,* 18:211–217.
19. Eliasson, R. (1976): Clinical examination of infertile men. In: *Human Semen and Fertility Regulation in Men,* edited by E. S. E. Hafez, pp. 321–331. Mosby, St. Louis.
20. Eliasson, R., Mossberg, B., Canmer, P., and Afzelius, B. (1977): The immotile-cilia syndrome. A congenital ciliary abnormality as an etiologic factor in chronic airway infections and male sterility. *N. Engl. J. Med.,* 297:1–6.
21. Ellenberg, M. (1976): Diabetic neuropathy: Clinical aspects. *Metabolism,* 25:1627–1655.
22. Fairley, K. F., Barrie, J., and Johnson, W. (1972): Sterility and testicular atrophy related to cyclophosphamide therapy. *Lancet,* 1:568–569.
23. Gill, W. B., Schumacher, G. F. B., and Bibbo, M. (1977): Pathological semen and anatomical abnormalities of the genital tract in human male subjects exposed to diethylstilbestrol in utero. *J. Urol.,* 117:477–480.
24. Glass, R. H., and Ericsson, R. J. (1979): Spontaneous cure of male infertility. *Fertil. Steril.,* 31:305–308.
25. Hall, P. F., (1959): *Gynaecomastia.* Australian Medical Publishing Co., Sydney.
26. Herman, A., Adar, R., and Rubenstein, Z. (1978): Vascular lesions associated with impotence in diabetic and nondiabetic arterial occlusive disease. *Diabetes,* 27:975–981.
27. Johannisson, E., and Eliasson, R. (1978): Cytological studies of prostatic fluids from men with and without abnormal palpatory findings of the prostate. *Int. J. Androl.,* 1:201–212.
28. Kovacs, G. T., Newman, G. B., and Henson, G. C. (1978): Postcoital tests: What is normal? *Br. Med. J.,* 1:818.
29. Lee, N. Y., (1978): Corrective surgery of obstructive azoospermia. *Arch. Androl.,* 1:115–121.
30. Levine, S. B. (1976): Marital sexual dysfunction: Erectile dysfunction. *Ann. Intern. Med.,* 85:342–350.
31. MacLeod, J., and Gold, R. Z. (1953): The male factor in fertility and infertility. VI. Semen quality and certain other factors in relation to ease of conception. *Fertil. Steril.,* 4:10–33.
32. Molitor, J. T., Chertow, B. S., and Fariss, B. L. (1973): Long-term follow-up of a patient with congenital adrenal hyperplasia and failure of testicular development. *Fertil. Steril.,* 24:319–323.

33. Mortimer, C. H. (1977): Clinical applications of the gonadotrophin releasing hormone. *Clin. Endocrinol. Metabol.,* 6:167–179.
34. Nuttall, F. Q. (1979): Gynecomastia as a physical finding in normal men. *J. Clin. Endocrinol. Metab.,* 48:338–340.
35. Oakberg, E. F. (1975): Effects of radiation on the testis. In: *Handbook of Physiology,* Section 7, Endocrinology, Vol. 5, Male Reproductive System, edited by D. W. Hamilton and R. O. Greep, pp. 233–243. American Physiological Society, Washington, D.C.
36. Odell, W. D., and Swerdloff, R. S. (1976): Male hypogonadism. *West. J. Med.,* 124:446–475.
37. Paulson, D. F. (1977): Clomiphene citrate in the management of male hypofertility: Predictors for treatment selection. *Fertil. Steril.,* 28:1226–1229.
38. Pedersen, H., and Rebbe, H. (1975): Absence of arms in the axoneme of immotile human spermatozoa. *Biol. Reprod.,* 12:541–544.
39. Peto, R., Pike, M. C., Armitage, P., Breslow, N. E., Cox, D. R., Howard, S. V., Mantel, N., McPherson, K., Peto, J., and Smith, P. G. (1977): Design and analysis of randomized clinical trials requiring prolonged observation of each patient. II. Analysis and examples. *Br. J. Cancer,* 35:1–39.
40. Rajfer, J., and Walsh, P. C. (1977): Hormonal regulation of testicular descent: Experimental and clinical observations. *J. Urol.,* 118:985–990.
41. Rodriguez-Rigau, L. J., Smith, K. D., and Steinberger, E. (1978): Relationship of varicocele to sperm output and fertility of male partners of infertile couples. *J. Urol.,* 120:691–694.
42. Schmidt, S. S., Schoysman, R., and Stewart, B. H. (1976): Surgical approaches to male infertility. In: *Human Semen and Fertility Regulation in Men,* edited by E. S. E. Hafez, pp. 476–493. Mosby, St. Louis.
43. Schnellen, T. M. C. M., and Beek, J. M. J. H. A. (1972): The influence of high doses of mesterolone on the spermiogram. *Fertil. Steril.,* 23:712–714.
44. Segal, S., Polishuk, W. Z., and Ben David, M. (1976): Hyperprolactinemic male infertility. *Fertil. Steril.,* 27:1425–1427.
45. Sherins, R. J., Brightwell, D., and Sternthal, P. M. (1977): Longitudinal analysis of semen in fertile and infertile men. In: *The Testis in Normal and Infertile Men,* edited by P. Troen and H. R. Nankin, pp. 473–488. Raven Press, New York.
46. Smith, K. D., Rodriguez-Rigau, L. J., and Steinberger, E. (1977): Relation between indices of semen analysis and pregnancy rate in infertile couples. *Fertil. Steril.,* 28:1314–1319.
47. Snyder, P. J., Bigdali, H., Gardner, D. F., Mihailovic, V., Rudenstein, R. S., Sterling, F. H., and Utiger, R. D. (1979): Gonadal function in fifty men with untreated pituitary adenomas. *J. Clin. Endocrinol. Metab.,* 48:309–314.
48. Southam, A. L. (1960): What to do with the "Normal" infertile couple. *Fertil. Steril.,* 11:543–549.
49. Steinberger, E., (1978): The etiology and pathophysiology of testicular dysfunction in man. *Fertil. Steril.,* 29:481–491.
50. Stern, R. C., Boat, T. F., Doershuk, C. F., Tucker, A. S., Miller, R. B., and Matthews, L. W. (1977): Cystic fibrosis diagnosed after age 13. Twenty-five teenage and adult patients including three asymptomatic men. *Ann. Intern. Med.,* 87:188–191.
51. Sturgess, J. M., Chao, J., Wong, J., Aspin, N., and Turner, J. A. P. (1979): Cilia with defective radial spokes. A cause of human respiratory disease. *N. Engl. J. Med.,* 300:53–56.
52. Urban, M. D., Lee, P. A., and Migeon, C. J. (1978): Adult height and fertility in men with congenital virilizing adrenal hyperplasia. *N. Engl. J. Med.,* 299:1392–1396.
53. Vermeulen, A., and Comhaire, F. (1978): Hormonal effects of an antiestrogen, tamoxifen, in normal and oligospermic men. *Fertil. Steril.,* 29:320–327.
54. Werder, E. A., Illig, R., Torresani, T., Zachmann, M., Baumann, P., Ott, F., and Prader, A. (1976): Gonadal function in young adults after surgical treatment of cryptorchidism. *Br. Med. J.,* 2:1357–1359.
55. Westaby, D., Ogle, S. J., Paradinas, F. J., Randell, J. B., and Murray-Lyon, I. M. (1977): Liver damage from long-term methyltestosterone. *Lancet,* 2:262–263.
56. Whorton, D., Krauss, R. M., Marshall, S., and Milby, T. H. (1977): Infertility in male pesticide workers. *Lancet,* 2:1259–1261.

The Testis, edited by H. Burger and D. de Kretser.
Raven Press, New York © 1981.

16

Analysis of Semen

Rune Eliasson

*Reproductive Physiology Unit, Faculty of Medicine, Karolinska Institute,
S-104 01 Stockholm, Sweden*

Analysis of semen can provide information on the testicular output of spermatozoa, the functional properties of the spermatozoa, and the secretory function of the accessory genital glands. Analysis of semen can, therefore, be of interest and value not only for those dealing with infertility problems but also for those interested in fertility regulation, and in the possible effects of diseases, drugs, chemicals, and environmental factors on the male reproductive system. However, like most clinical, chemical, and cytological analyses, the value of semen analysis depends upon several factors, e.g., the relevance of the test, the accuracy and precision of the methods, and an adequate knowledge of the "normal range." The "normal range" may be different for different problems, e.g., fertility versus infertility, and affected versus not affected (by a given drug) to give only two examples. Most investigators interested in the properties of human semen have neglected many of the problems associated with the determination of normal values. Among the reasons for this are, for example, the difficulties in obtaining semen samples from truly representative populations. On the other hand, such difficulties are not valid excuses for conclusions that actually have no solid basis. Unfortunately, certain conclusions and recommendations (e.g., related to sperm density or morphology) with reference to "normal" and/or "fertile" have been repeated so frequently that they are taken for granted and "true," despite the fact that they are often based on results from highly selected populations of semen samples. This has had a retarding effect on the development of andrology. In conclusion, semen analysis and the evaluation of the results must follow the same strict rules (technically and statistically) that we require for correctly performed and evaluated analyses of blood, urine, and other body fluids (see refs. 10,16,44).

Technical aspects of semen analysis have recently been published (e.g., 1,16,26) and therefore to avoid too much duplication this chapter deals not so much with simple technical problems but with some basic principles, differences of opinion, new aspects, and new results of importance for the evaluation of the laboratory report.

BASIC CONCEPTS

To assess a laboratory report one must know the "normal" values for a representative population. For most laboratory and domestic animals fertility can be objectively evaluated from serial matings or inseminations. We know that subfertile or sterile male animals can have "normal" semen qualities as assessed in the routine laboratory (28). The evaluation of human fertility is much more delicate and we have in most cases to use indirect methods. Objectivity is, however, necessary and any definition of male fertility that is based on semen characteristics (azoospermia being one exception) will automatically lead to fruitless and circular discussions. The definitions used in this article are presented in Table 1. Moreover, a semen sample is characterized as obtained from a "fertile" man only when the man has made a woman pregnant within 3 months before or after the examination of that sample. A man with a child is a father and should never be classified as a man of "proven fertility."

If the properties of semen samples from men with a barren union should be compared with semen from men whose wives are pregnant in the first trimester, the sample must be collected under similar conditions, e.g., similar period of abstinence, examined at the same time after ejaculation, and with comparable methods for which the methodological errors are known. This calls for strictly standardized conditions and the arguments given (e.g., 1,26) for a voluntary abstinence time cannot be accepted. On the other hand, the possible effect of a certain ejaculation frequency on the fertility of a given couple (or on the semen qualities) (16,29) can be of great interest but should then be studied as such and under controlled conditions. The standardization is also of importance for studies related to comparisons between populations other than "fertile" versus "infertile," e.g., Scandinavian versus South American or Japanese populations,

TABLE 1. *Definition related to human male fertility*

	Terminology	
Facts	Correct	Incorrect
One or more children	Father	Fertile
No children and not tried	Fertility unknown	
No children, tried > 1 year	Infertile	Subfertile
		Sterile
Wife has recently become pregnant	Fertile[a]	

Note: A semen sample should not be classified as fertile or infertile. These terms should be reserved for individuals or couples.

[a] Valid unless objective data prove that the man cannot be responsible for the pregnancy.

young versus old men, and smokers versus nonsmokers, to mention only a few examples.

The need for elaborate systems for the quality control of analyses performed in clinical chemistry laboratories is clear to most physicians. There is the same need for control systems for laboratories performing semen analyses. Each step in the procedures must be controlled: the instruments, the solutions, the recovery, etc. To emphasize these basic matters is unfortunately not superfluous!

The fact that patients frequently move from one area to another, the increased exchange of information between laboratories both directly and through scientific reports, and the need for more multicenter research projects make interlaboratory control an urgent matter. This is not easily arranged but is both possible (15) and necessary.

The value of a semen analysis will depend on each part of the Man-Laboratory-Physician unit. The man must understand why he is providing a semen sample and how his cooperation can influence the outcome. If he cannot provide a semen sample by masturbation after the requested time of abstinence, he must be informed how other methods of collection may influence the value of the analysis and why it is important that he gives correct information to the laboratory. The laboratory must provide information about the precision and accuracy of methods used. Material used for collection or storage of semen must not contain or leak substances that can interfere with the analyses (special care should be given to plastic material and rubber stoppers). The laboratory must provide reference values from relevant populations. The laboratory report should only contain facts, i.e., terms like "fertile," or "infertile," should not be used. The physician must be able to evaluate the laboratory report in relation to clinical information, medical history, indication(s) for the semen analysis, and—in cases of infertility—to the female partner.

COLLECTION

The semen should be collected by masturbation after 3 to 5 days of abstinence (acceptable limits 2–7 days). Shorter or longer periods of abstinence will influence different variables, e.g., volume, sperm count, and motility. It is important that the whole ejaculate is collected. Most men who report incomplete collection mean that part of the last portion (usually the last few drops) was not included. This has no influence on the results. However, if the first part is lost this will in most cases have a significant influence on the semen characteristics since during a normal ejaculation most of the spermatozoa and the fluid from the prostate are in the first portions (22). "Incomplete collection" must therefore be specified. Collection by interrupted intercourse involves a risk of incomplete sampling (loss of first portion!) and of contamination from the vagina (negative effect on motility and survival). Rubber condoms must not be used. (See also ref. 16).

PRELIMINARY EXAMINATIONS

The initial examination of the semen (within 30–60 min) should include viscosity, liquefaction, color, and volume. A normal semen sample will be fully liquefied within 30 to 60 min. The presence of nonliquefied material 60 min after ejaculation indicates a prostatic dysfunction (in some rare instances a secretory dysfunction of the seminal vesicles). Add 0.2 to 0.4 ml of "normal" seminal plasma or saliva to the sample and check if this will induce complete liquefaction or not (1,31). Sometimes liquefaction can be seen after a short (10–15 sec), hard mixing of the sample with a Vortex-mixer. The viscosity can be classified as low (like water), normal, or high. A scientifically correct determination of the viscosity requires special equipment, and relevant reference material for the evaluation is not yet available (14,16). The volume is assessed by weighing or by transferring the semen to a graduated cylinder or centrifuge tube. The latter method introduces a significant error (10% or more) if the viscosity is high.

The semen sample must be well mixed before the first microscopic examination is performed. It is not sufficient to "invert the tube" a few times. An automatic rotator or a gentle use of a Vortex-mixer (maximum 10 sec) is required if the subsequent assessments are to have an acceptable degree of precision and accuracy.

A standard drop (e.g., 2–3 μl if the cover glass is 18 $\times$ 18 mm) of the well-mixed semen is placed on a clean glass slide and covered with a thin cover glass. The thickness of the fluid is important and the size of the drop must therefore be standardized (42). The motility of the spermatozoa is assessed (see below), the number of spermatozoa is given a preliminary rating number to determine a suitable degree of the subsequent dilution, and the presence of other cells (e.g., RBC, WBC, epithelial cells) is preliminarily rated as none, single, moderate or abundant (see below). The degree and type of aggregation of the spermatozoa must also be assessed. For all these evaluations one should use a magnification of 400 to 600 $\times$, randomly selected microscopic fields and if possible a phase contrast microscope. Avoid areas near the edge of the cover glass since evaporation will influence the behavior of the spermatozoa.

ASSESSMENT OF MOTILITY AND VIABILITY

The motility of the spermatozoa is usually assessed by a subjective method, although objective methods are now available (37,42). Whatever method is used one must assess both the progressive (forward) motility and the percentage of motile spermatozoa. Motility is highest soon after ejaculation and decreases with time. The decrease in motility is very different for different semen samples and it is therefore required that the time of assessment in relation to ejaculation is given in the report. The motility decreases faster at 37°C than at 20°C. The percentage of motile spermatozoa can be rather accurately assessed by counting motile and nonmotile spermatozoa in randomly selected fields. The results should be given as the nearest 5% interval, since the precision of the method does not allow for higher accuracy. Various methods have been recommended for reporting the quality of sperm motility. One is to give the percentage of spermatozoa with different progressive motility, e.g., 30% with good, 50% with poor, and 20% with no progressive motility. This method has a low degree of precision and accuracy, particularly if the sperm concentration is high. The rating can also be given as mean progressive motility using the scores none, poor, medium, and good, respectively. The limitation of this method is that the disparate motility of the spermatozoa will be expressed in one term.

In our laboratory we use the second method. In a special study we examined two semen samples from each of 50 men selected because their wives were pregnant in the first trimester. Motility assessments were performed within 40 min and again after 4 hr. The results are presented in Tables 2 and 3. It can be concluded that it is highly unlikely that a man whose wife is in early pregnancy will provide a semen sample with a mean progressive motility score less than "medium" and with less than 40% motile spermatozoa. The possibility of making a fertility prognosis decreases with an increased time after ejaculation.

Live spermatozoa do not stain when exposed to a 0.5 to 1% Eosin Y solution (from Merck or Gurr Ltd.) but dead cells take up this dye. The viability of the spermatozoa can therefore be evaluated with this technique. One drop of semen (approximately 0.1 ml) is mixed with an equal volume of 0.5 to 1.0% Eosin Y in isotonic phosphate buffer, pH 7.5 in a glass tube or dish. After 1 to 2 min a smear is made, air dried, and assessed with a negative phase contrast microscope at 1,000 to 1,250 × magnification. A modification of the original Blom's Eosin-Nigrosin technique has recently been published. With this technique one drop of semen is mixed with two drops of Eosin Y (1% in distilled water). After 30 sec three drops of 10% Nigrosin solution (distilled water) is added. The drop is smeared, air-dried, and can then be evaluated with an ordinary light microscope (18). The supravital staining technique is helpful when the

TABLE 2. *Frequency distribution of percent motile spermatozoa in 100 semen samples*[a]

Interval (%)	Observ. 1	Observ. 2
<20	0	0
20–25	0	4.2
30–35	0	6.3
40–45	2.1	25.0
50–55	31.3	56.2
60–65	62.4	8.3
70–75	4.2	0

[a] One hundred semen samples from 50 men whose wives were in early pregnancy were assessed. Assessments were made 20 to 40 min after ejaculation (Observ. 1) and again 4 hr later (Observ. 2). The semen samples were kept at 37°C.

TABLE 3. *Frequency distribution of mean progressive motility scores in 100 semen samples[a]*

Mean progressive motility score	Observ. 1 (%)	Observ. 2 (%)
None	0	4
Poor	0	19
Medium	7	51
Good	93	36

[a] One hundred semen samples from 50 men whose wives were in early pregnancy were assessed. Assessments were made 20 to 40 min after ejaculation (Observ. 1) and again 4 hr later (Observ. 2). The semen samples were kept at 37°C.

percentage of motile spermatozoa is low (<40%), and is essential when most of the spermatozoa lack motility (23).

NUMBER OF SPERMATOZOA

Sperm count has been given too much attention from a clinical point of view and too little attention from a technical point of view. Most authors recommend a dilution of 1:20 with a white blood cell pipet. This technique has a low degree of precision (26). The semen sample must be fully liquefied and carefully mixed before an exact volume (e.g., 20, 50, 100, or 200 μl) is transferred to a glass tube with a diluting fluid. The dilution should be in proportion to the sperm density, i.e., from 1:1 to 1:100 and two different dilutions should be used. The mean value of the two determinations is to be used. As diluting fluid one can use 50 g $NaHCO_3$, 10 ml 35% formalin and distilled water up to 1,000 ml. If a phase contrast microscope is not used, it is helpful to the technician if methylene blue (final concentration 1%) or gentian violet (final concentration 5%) is added to the diluting fluid. The diluted semen must then be carefully mixed before a drop is transferred to the hemocytometer. Place the hemocytometer in a moist chamber for 15 to 20 min to allow all cells to sediment (see also 1,16,26).

If a dilution of 1:200 or higher (e.g., washed spermatozoa) is used, one must consider that the spermatozoa tend to adhere to the glass. This can introduce a significant error (approximately 50%), but can be counteracted by adding bovine serum albumin (final concentration 0.2–2%) to the fluid (19,21). Sperm density can also be determined with electronic particle counters, but one must be aware of the possible interference from debris at low sperm densities (8).

Should only a few or no spermatozoa be seen at the initial examination, the sample must be centrifuged and the sediment examined for spermatozoa. The term azoospermia can only be used if no spermatozoa have been found in the sediment.

The relationship between sperm density and fertility prognosis has been studied by comparing the frequency distribution of semen samples with regard to sperm concentration for two populations of men. One group included men whose wives were pregnant in the first trimester ($n = 75$), and the other, men with a barren union ($n = 860$). For both groups the requirement was that two semen samples had been delivered within three weeks, the time of abstinence had been 3 to 7 days, the collection was by masturbation and was reported as complete. The mean values for different variables were calculated and used in the analysis. Three men from the "fertile" group had a mean value of less than 5 million spermatozoa/ml. For obvious reasons there were many in the infertile group that had azoospermia (approximately 4%) or 0.1 to 1 million/ml (approximately 3%). An almost equal distribution in the 2 groups started from 5 million/ml and above. To avoid the common mistake of comparing groups that are not comparable, all samples from individuals with a mean value of less than 5 million spermatozoa/ml were excluded. The remaining samples were then used for the study and the cumulative frequency distribution with regard to sperm count is presented in Fig. 1. Statistically there is no difference at any point between the two curves. Consequently, semen samples with a sperm density of 5 million/ml or higher do not discriminate fertile from infertile men. This conclusion

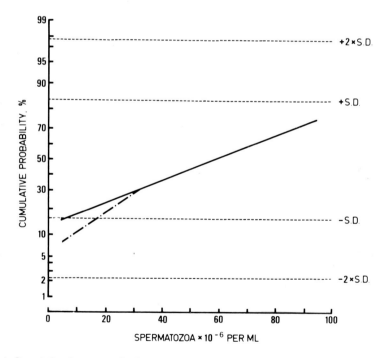

FIG. 1. Cumulative frequency distribution of spermatozoa (counts/milliliter) in semen samples from men whose wives were pregnant in the first trimester ($n = 75$) (—) and from men with a barren union ($n = 860$) (— — —).

conforms with statements in old and recent publications (e.g., 16,27,32,48,49, 50,54,55).

SEMEN MORPHOLOGY

Human semen contains not only spermatozoa but frequently also other cellular elements, e.g., spermatocytes, spermatids, leucocytes, erythrocytes, macrophages, epithelial cells, bacteria, fungi, and trichomonas. The possible importance of the presence of these other cells to male fertility is poorly understood and we cannot at the present time give values for "normal" limits. A major reason is that they have been given little attention and usually have not been assessed in a quantitative way and in relation to fertility as defined in Table 1.

The number of cellular elements other than spermatozoa can be presented in figures (e.g., million/ml) by recording the number of a given cell type seen per 100 spermatozoa in the stained smear. If, for example, 10 leukocytes are noted in the fields that contain 100 spermatozoa and the sperm density is known to be 125 million/ml, the concentration of leucocytes per ml is calculated from the formula

$$\text{WBC/ml} = \frac{10 \times 125}{100} = 12.5 \text{ million/ml}$$

More than occasional leucocytes are regarded by most authors as a sign of inflammation in the accessory genital glands. It must, however, be emphasized that the presence of leucocytes in semen is not always owing to pathogenic microorganisms, nor is the absence of leucocytes a guarantee that the man does not have prostatitis or vesiculitits (34). A significant number of macrophages has recently been identified by electron microscopy in semen samples from men with high titers of sperm-agglutinating antibodies in blood serum and seminal plasma *(unpublished)*. A major problem in the identification of many of the cellular elements in semen is that they have undergone different degrees of degeneration. An optimal technique for fixation, staining, and assessment is thus necessary.

The spermatozoa must be evaluated with regard to the whole cell, i.e., head, midpiece, and tail. A staining technique that visualizes these parts is a minimal requirement and therefore the commonly used Mayer's hematoxylin staining method is not acceptable. It is frequently forgotten that fixation is part of the staining technique. For Papanicolaou staining, the semen smears should be air-dried and fixed in ethanol (or methanol):ether (50:50). Formalin must not be used (30). Improved techniques for differentiating immature germ cells and leucocytes have recently been described (11,25). For those interested only in the shape of the spermatozoa, evaluation of the unstained smear under phase contrast microscopy can be acceptable. The modified technique for supravital staining described by Eliasson (18) is also very useful for the assessment of sperm morphology, provided that a 1% isotonic solution of Eosin Y is used *(to be published)*. In fact, the original Eosin-Nigrosin method by Blom (3) was introduced for assessment of bull sperm morphology and several interesting observations about sperm morphology and bull fertility were published by Blom (4). It seems highly relevant to perform similar studies on human spermatozoa.

The relationship between the configuration of a spermatozoon and its fertility cannot be objectively evaluated at the present time. We are therefore confined to a statistical approach and should thus use methods that are as reliable and reproducible as possible. The precision of the method must be known. The definition of fertility and infertility, respectively, must be objective. Methods that fulfil these requirements have been published (e.g., 12,16).

We have assessed spermatozoa in our unit since 1967 according to the guidelines given in Table 4. Blom (4) regards "pear shaped head" as a major sperm defect related to bull subfertility. It is possible that a high percentage of "pear shaped head" is also related to human male subfertility, which would be a motivation to include this as a special subgroup in the assessment. Data concerning a relationship between "pear shaped head" and human infertility has so far not been presented.

TABLE 4. *Principles for morphological assessment of human spermatozoa*

Classification	Length (μm)	Width (μm)	Remarks
Normal spermatozoa			
Head	3.0–5.0	2.0–3.0	Regular oval shape. Borderline forms are assessed as normal.
Midpiece	5.0–7.0	Approx. 1	
Tail	40–50		
Abnormal head			
Too large	>5.0	>3.0	As long as the shape approximates an oval, it is to be counted primarily according to its size (large, small, tapering).
Too small	<3.0	<2.0	
Tapering	>5.0 <5.0	<3.0 <2.0	Ratio length: width >1.8
Amorphous			Various irregular forms including those with a combination of irregular and elongated shape.
Duplicate			
Pear-shaped			Between oval and tapering, regular shape. Irregular forms are regarded as amorphous. Borderline as normal.
Abnormal midpiece	>8.0	>2.0	Missing or broken midpieces are also abnormal.
Abnormal cytoplasmic droplet			When larger than half of the sperm head
Abnormal tail			e.g., broken, coiled (not bent nor asymmetrical insertion), or short tails.

The reason for regarding a protoplasmic droplet which is larger than half the sperm head as abnormal needs clarification. During the maturation process, the spermatozoon will lose the protoplasmic droplet and a persistent protoplasmic droplet is regarded as a sign of "immaturity." However, everyone experienced in semen analysis knows that the size of these droplets can vary significantly. We have no real knowledge of the importance of small or large droplets in human male fertility. As an initial step in the assessment of this problem it was necessary to define the "abnormal" protoplasmic droplet, and as a working standard a group of European experts agreed to accept a size equal to or less than half of the head of the spermatozoon as normal (15). According to Blom (4), one should regard a proximal droplet as a major defect, but a distal droplet as a minor defect in the assessment of bull spermatozoa.

All definitions in Table 4 should be looked upon as working standards, the relevance of which are in the process of evaluation. The figures in Table 4 do not represent any scientifically proven truth with regard to "normal" and "abnormal." On the other hand, without defined standards which can be used with a certain degree of precision, an accurate evaluation would be impossible.

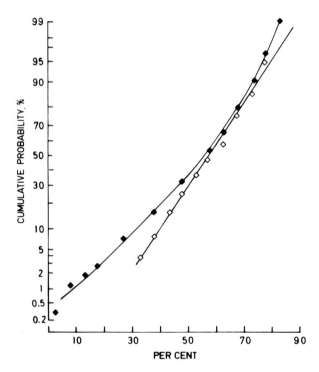

FIG. 2. Cumulative frequency distribution of spermatozoa with normal configuration in semen samples from men whose wives were pregnant in the first trimester ($n = 75$) (◇—◇) and from men with a barren union ($n = 1,250$) (◆—◆).

A spermatozoon can have several defects, e.g., an amorphous head, a defect midpiece, and a coiled tail. Each of these defects must be recorded separately and expressed in percent. As a consequence, the sum of the percentages for "normal" and the various "abnormal" forms will be more than 100. The true percentage of "abnormal" spermatozoa is: 100—the percentage of "normal" spermatozoa. Some authors have recommended that only the "main" defect should be considered. With such method the sum of all percentages for "abnormal" and "normal" will be 100 but subsequent statistical analysis will be impossible and the method must therefore not be used.

The frequency distributions of the percentage of spermatozoa with a "normal" configuration according to the classification in Table 4, are presented in Fig. 2 for semen samples from fertile and infertile men. The mean value for both populations is 57% and the value at −2 SD for the "fertile" group is 32%. Analyses of this nature form the basis for the limits given in Table 5. Only some of the defects in sperm morphology have been included, since for the other abnormalities (cf. Table 4) the frequency is almost always below 10%.

The importance of the coiled tail defect in human male fertility has been given little attention, although there is a known correlation between coiled tails and infertility in bulls and boars. Zinc seems to be one important factor in the development of coiled tails both in human and bull semen. An increased percentage of coiled tails can also be induced *in vivo*. (5,9,29,40,41).

It goes without saying that the limits given in Table 5 are valid only for assessments which conform with those in our laboratory. The limits are also

TABLE 5. *Guidelines for the evaluation of semen characteristics*

Variable	Normal	Doubtful	Not normal	Comments[a]
Volume (ml)	2–6	1.5–1.9	<1.5	
Sperm density (10^6/ml)	20–250	10–20	<10	a
Sperm count (10^6/ejacul.)	>80	20–80	<20	
Live spermatozoa (%)	>50	35–50	<35	b
Motile spermatozoa (%)	>50	35–45	<35	b
Mean progressive motility score	good	medium	poor	b
Spermatozoa with normal configuration (%)	>40	30–40	<30	
Amorphous heads (%)	<40	40–50	>50	
Defect midpieces (%)	<20	21–25	>25	c
Defect tails (%)	<20	21–25	>25	
Acid phosphatase (mkat/liter)	>6.9	4.2–6.9	<4.2	a,d
Zinc (mmol/liter)	1.2–3.8	0.8–1.2	<0.8	a
Magnesium (mmol/liter)	2.9–10.3	2.1–2.8	<2.1	a
Fructose (mmol/liter)	6.7–33	4.4–6.6	<4.4	a

[a] Comments: (a) Provided the volume is 2 to 6 ml. (b) Within 2 hr after ejaculation. (c) Includes also the cells with a protoplasmic droplet that is larger than half the head. (d) Assay according to Sigma Bulletin No. 104.

subject to change as our experience from different populations increases. General statements like "normal semen should have 60% normal spermatozoa" should not be used since they do not include the normal variation, nor the fact that various abnormalities can have a different importance in relation to fertility.

CHEMICAL ANALYSES

Chemical analyses are of interest with reference to the accessory genital glands and the spermatozoa. The spermatozoa will be briefly discussed in a separate section. The chemical analyses of the seminal plasma can give information on the secretory function of the accessory genital glands, provided that organ-specific factors are used as markers and due attention is given to the multiglandular origin of the seminal plasma.

Organ-specific factors for the prostate are citric acid, zinc, magnesium, and acid phosphatase, to mention some of the most commonly used. Fructose and prostaglandins are known to be secreted from the seminal vesicles (16,20,38). Glycerylphosphorylcholine and carnitine are possibly suitable markers for epididymides, but there are conflicting reports on their organ specificity (7,53). Normal limits for the markers used in our laboratory are presented in Table 5. Some of the more common pitfalls have been published elsewhere (16) and only a few remarks follow. One cannot rely on the organ content to trace the origin of a given factor, unless it is a factor unique for only one gland (e.g., fructose). Nor can one use the split-ejaculate technique unless the ejaculate is collected in at least three—preferably four to six—fractions and each of these fractions is analyzed for markers which are specific for the prostate and seminal vesicles (and epididymis when relevant). From a physiological point of view prostate and seminal vesicles (most likely also epididymis) are multiglandular organs. One can therefore find men with a very low prostaglandin content in the seminal plasma but with a normal content of fructose and vice versa. In most semen samples there is a close relationship between the concentrations of zinc and magnesium but clear exceptions are seen indicating that there are different parts or cells secreting these two ions.

Indications for chemical analyses are: (a) a semen volume below 2 ml; (b) a rapidly decreasing motility of the spermatozoa; and (c) assessment of the secretory function of the accessory genital glands. Some reasons for these indications will be briefly mentioned.

About two-thirds of the seminal plasma originates from the seminal vesicles. If a low volume is combined with a low level of fructose the reason is usually decreased secretory function of the seminal vesicles (a common result of an infection in these glands). A nondetectable level of fructose (and azoospermia) indicates that the patient either has an occlusion at the level of the ejaculatory ducts or a congenital absence of the glands (frequently combined with an absence of the vas deferens). In these cases, analyses of prostatic markers will give information on the secretory function of this gland only if the total amount of zinc, magnesium, etc., is considered. A "normal" concentration of zinc (i.e., 1.2–3.8 mmol/liter) (Table 5) in these semen samples is a clear indication of decreased prostatic function since there is no dilution with fluid from the seminal vesicles. A partially retrograde ejaculation can result in a low volume with a low number of spermatozoa but the chemical composition of the fluid is usually normal.

The effect of the seminal plasma on sperm motility and viability has been demonstrated by several authors (13,19,46). A rapidly decreasing motility is frequently associated with a prostatic dysfunction.

In patients with diagnosed or suspected diseases of the accessory genital glands (e.g., prostatitis, hemospermia, or unexplained ejaculatory pain), chemical analyses of the seminal plasma can give the physician information on the degree of secretory dysfunction which may be associated with the disease. By repeated analyses, it is possible to follow the effect of a given treatment with reference to the function of the accessory glands.

Chemical analyses of the seminal fluid are not widely used today but they will be in the future. Additional indications will most likely be prostatic cancer, prostatic hyperplasia, and epididymal dysfunction. Possible negative effects of drugs and potentially toxic compounds on the accessory genital glands will also be investigated by chemical analyses of the seminal plasma. It seems less likely that a man's fertility will be able to be evaluated from chemical analyses of the seminal plasma (e.g., 16,20,38), but examination of this fluid may very likely provide valuable information on the cause(s) of disturbed function of the spermatozoa which result in subfertility or sterility. The importance of this field in relationship to regulation of male fertility can hardly be overestimated. On the other hand, it is a field involving a tremendous number of problems and pitfalls.

FUNCTIONAL PROPERTIES OF THE SPERMATOZOA

The quality of the spermatozoa is of great importance for their fertilizing ability and it is therefore necessary to find methods which can properly assess their functional properties. Sperm motility is the only functional property related to fertility which is assessed in the routine analysis (Tables 2 and 3). Release of enzymes from the spermatozoa increases if the membranes are damaged. An increased leakage has been noted after freezing and thawing of spermatozoa and has also been found to correlate with the fertility (43,45,47). No difference has been noted in sperm respiration between semen samples from fertile and infertile men *(to be published)*. The zinc content of spermatozoa from fertile men was less than 10 μg per 100 million cells but a much higher content was frequently noted in specimens from men with a barren union, indicating that the amount of zinc in the spermatozoa is related to male fertility *(to be published)*. This is also of interest in view of the reported correlation between zinc content, coiled tails, and infertility (5,19,40).

There is a good correlation between fertility and sperm migration in normal cervical mucus but frequently an impaired migration is caused by immunological factors (6,24,33). The interaction between cervical mucus and spermatozoa and its importance for human fertility have been given too little attention in the past.

During their passage through the epididymis spermatozoa undergo several changes from a functional point of view (51,52). Bedford et al. (2) reported that ejaculated spermatozoa normally are resistant to sodium dodecyl sulphate (SDS), but the heads of spermatozoa taken from the caput epididymis swell significantly when exposed to a 1% SDS solution. An interesting observation was that ejaculated spermatozoa from infertile men frequently became swollen in this solution. The chromatin in the sperm heads will become more condensed during sperm transport through the epididymis. At the same time they gain a resistance to SDS. The stability of ejaculated spermatozoa to SDS could be a measure of their maturity (and/or degree of chromatin condensation), and thus indirectly reflect epididymal function. However, the stability of human spermatozoa to SDS is also significantly affected by factors in the seminal plasma, e.g., the zinc content (39). This is not the only functional property of human spermatozoa which can be influenced by factors in the seminal plasma. Other examples are the succinate-induced increase in sperm respiration, the formation of lipid peroxides, the oxygen consumption, and the release of enzymes (7,13,19,21, 35,36,46). The occurrence of agglutinating or immobilizing antibodies against the spermatozoa in seminal plasma from some men should also be recalled (6). The interaction between seminal plasma and spermatozoa has frequently been overlooked in the past. It is not a phenomenon related only to human spermatozoa. It should be given a lot of attention since it will not only affect many experimental results but may also open new ways to regulation of male fertility (17).

STATISTICAL EVALUATION

Statistics are frequently misused in reports on semen qualities. The mathematical aspects of a statistical analysis can be taken care of by professionals and computers. The problem is to use the appropriate statistical design, methods, and expressions. Three examples of common errors with relevance to semen analysis will be given.

The progressive motility is frequently presented in terms of "none," "poor," "medium," etc. The expressions can be replaced with figures like 0, 1, 2, etc. In this "ordered classification" there are not equal distances between each group; e.g., medium (2) is not twice as good as poor (1) and the figures 1, 2, 3, etc. are not numerical (measured) values. As a consequence one cannot calculate mean and variations (SD or SEM) on these variables, nor compare these incorrectly calculated means for different populations by using Student's *t*-test. For data grouped in classes as in this example one can present the frequency of samples in each group and apply for example the Chi-square test.

To calculate mean and standard deviation and to use Student's *t*-test for testing significance on data which have not an approximately normal distribution is another very common mistake. Most variables in semen analysis have a significant skewness and nonparametric methods should therefore be used. Transformation of the data (e.g., to logarithmic values) can sometimes give an approximately normal distribution and these transformed values can then be used in the calculations.

If different populations are compared, one must ensure that they are comparable. Violations of this basic rule are only too frequent in the literature related to semen analyses (and fertility in general). The differences between semen samples from men asking for voluntary sterilization and from men attending an infertility clinic can be described. But when the first group is classified as "fertile" and the second "infertile" and the results are presented as representative for "fertile" and "infertile" men and statistical methods are used to prove or disprove a difference between the two groups, this is a clear cut example of incorrect use of both terminology and statistics. Several examples can be found in recent publications.

Methods for laboratory control and for statistical evaluations have been published by several authors (e.g., 10,16,44). In work related to semen analysis it is also necessary to consider the time required for spermatogenesis and how the experimental conditions can influence the intra-individual variations for some variables. There are too few articles published which properly report (by fulfilling the elementary requirements with regard to experimental design and statistical evaluation) whether there has been a beneficial effect on the semen following treatment with drugs or operation.

TERMINOLOGY

A clear and distinct terminology should always be used. Sexology, fertility, and semen analysis are for many physicians and patients matters loaded with emotion. This makes it even more important to be objective and correct. A semen analysis that has been regarded as normal should be reported so—not with expressions related to fertility. If the man is classified as "fertile" it will automatically imply that the wife is infertile. An example related to this is presented in Table 6. The marriage had been infertile for 8 years. All semen samples delivered by the man had qualities that were well within normal limits. The wife had one extramarital affair and became pregnant. After a divorce she married a third man and was soon pregnant again. The first husband should not only be regarded as infertile (Table 1), but there is also reason to believe that he was the cause of the couple's infertility. The immunological properties of the semen have not been investigated in this case but the possibility that such a factor could be involved must be kept in mind.

In an objective report there is no place for terms like "oligozoospermia," "asthenozoospermia," or "teratozoospermia," not to mention various combinations of them. For example: What is the meaning of "asthenozoospermia"?

TABLE 6. *Properties of eight semen samples (1969–1975) from a man with "functional infertility"*

Variable	Mean	SD	Range
Sperm conc. $\times 10^{-6} \times ml^{-1}$	64	21.6	34–90
Total number of spermatozoa	388	131.6	224–588
Motile spermatozoa (%)	50	6.5	45–60
Normal spermatozoa (%)	54	8.2	40–75
Amorphous heads (%)	19	9.0	10–32
Tail defects (%)	14	4.3	10–21

Translated from the Greek it means that the "small animals in the semen are weak." But the physician should know whether it was the percentage of motile spermatozoa that was low or if it was the progressive motility that was decreased and also to what extent and how long after ejaculation. It makes a significant difference in the fertility prognosis if a semen sample contains 40% spermatozoa with coiled tails or 40% spermatozoa with amorphous heads. This information will not be revealed if the result is presented as "teratozoospermia." Note also the difference between "oligospermia" (small volume) and "oligozoospermia" (few animals in semen).

One word that frequently is used in an incorrect way is "parameter." In most cases it is used instead of "variable." In the equation:

$$Y = aX + b$$

Y and *X* are variables, *a* and *b* are parameters. This is also clear from the Greek meaning of the word parameter.

CONCLUSION

Indications for semen analysis today are infertility and diseases which can affect the secretory capacity of the accessory genital glands. In the future semen analysis will probably also be used to study the effects of chemicals and potential environmental hazards on the reproductive glands and on the spermatozoa.

The value of semen analysis depends not only upon the technical performance but also on the methods used for collection and evaluation. A meaningful evaluation is possible only if information is available on the normal range for different variables and for relevant populations.

Semen analysis should always be carried out with due attention to precision, accuracy, and reproducibility. In the evaluation one must also consider time for spermatogenesis and transport through epididymis, the influence of seminal plasma on the functional properties of the spermatozoa and time after ejaculation.

The need for an increased exchange of information and collaboration between laboratories calls for better standardization and for interlaboratory control as well as a uniformly accepted terminology that is not ambiguous.

Regarded as a cell population, spermatozoa are unique from many points of view, particularly the fact that they are so easily available without extensive isolation procedures. From a morphological point of view human spermatozoa are regarded as being very resistant to physical forces. On the other hand, recent experiments have revealed that not only the seminal plasma but also the composition of the suspending medium can influence many functional properties of the spermatozoa. They should therefore be treated with great care and respect.

There is a need for a rapid progress in our understanding of factors influencing male reproduction. However: "It's no good to do things in a hurry. Desire to have things done quickly prevents their being done thoroughly. The more the urging, the less the progress." (Teng Hsiao-Ping).

REFERENCES

1. Amelar, R. D., Dubin, L., and Schoenfeld, C. (1973): Semen analysis. *Urology*, II:605–611.
2. Bedford, J. M., Bent, M.-J., and Calvin, H. (1973): Variations in structural character and stability of the nuclear chromatin in morphologically normal human spermatozoa. *J. Reprod. Fertil.*, 33:19–29.
3. Blom, E. (1950): A one-minute live-dead sperm stain by means of eosin-nigrosin. *Fertil. Steril.*, 1:176–177.
4. Blom, E. (1973): The ultrastructure of some characteristic sperm defects and a proposal for a new classification of the bull spermiogram. *Nord. Vet. Med.*, 25:383–391.
5. Blom, E., and Wolstrup, C. (1976): Zinc as a possible causal factor in the sterilizing sperm tail defect, the 'Dag-defect,' in Jersey Bulls. *Nord. Vet. Med.*, 28:515–518.
6. Boettcher, B., (editor) (1977): *Immunological Influence on Human Fertility.* Proceedings from the Workshop on Fertility and Human Reproduction 1977. Academic Press, New York.
7. Bøhmer, T., and Johansen, L. (1978): Inhibition of sperm maturation through intervention of the carnitine system. In: *Endocrine Approach to Male Contraception,* edited by V. Hansson, M. Ritzén, K. Purvis, and F. S. French, pp. 565–573. Scriptor, Copenhagen.
8. Brotherton, J., and Barnard, G. (1974): Estimation of number, mean size and size distribution of human spermatozoa in oligospermia using a Coulter counter. *J. Reprod. Fert.*, 40:341–357.
9. Brown-Woodman, P. D. C., Mohri, H., Darin-Bennett, A., Shorey, C. D., and White, I. G. (1976): Metabolic and ultrastructural changes in ejaculated spermatozoa induced by heating the testes of rams. *J. Reprod. Fert.*, 46:501.
10. Colton, T. (1974): *Statistics in Medicine.* Little, Brown, Boston.
11. Couture, M., Ulstein, M., Leonard, J., and Paulsen, C. A. (1976): Improved staining method for differentiating immature germ cells from white blood cells in human seminal fluid. *Andrologia,* 8:61–66.
12. David, G., Bisson, J. P., Czyglik, F., Jouannet, P., and Gernigon, C. (1975): Anomalies morphologiques du spermatozoïde humain. 1. Propositions pour un système de classification. *J. Gynecol. Obstet. Biol. Reprod.*, 4, Suppl. 1:17–36.
13. Dott, H. M. (1972): Bibliography on effects of male accessory secretions on spermatozoa in man. *Bibliog. Reprod.*, 19:445–591.
14. Dunn, P. F., and Picologlou, B. F. (1977): Investigation of the rheological properties of human semen. *Biorheology,* 14:277–292.
15. Eliasson, R. (1971): Interlaboratory coordination and control in andrology. *Andrologia,* 3:113–115.
16. Eliasson, R. (1975): Analysis of semen. In: *Progress in Infertility,* II, edited by S. J. Behrman, and R. W. Kistner, pp. 691–713. Little, Brown, Boston.
17. Eliasson, R. (1976): Accessory glands and seminal plasma with special reference to infertility as a model for studies on induction of sterility in the male. *J. Reprod. Fert.*, (Suppl.)24:163–174.
18. Eliasson, R. (1977): Supravital staining of human spermatozoa. *Fertil. Steril.*, 28:1257.

19. Eliasson, R., Arver, S., Johnsen, Ø., Kvist, U., and Lindholmer, C. (1978): Some effects of human seminal plasma on the spermatozoa. In: *Recent Progress in Andrology,* edited by A. Fabbrini and E. Steinberger. Serono Symposium No. 14., pp. 215–220. Academic Press, London.
20. Eliasson, R., and Bygdeman, M. (1978): Prostaglandins and human reproduction. In: *Advances in Obstetrics and Gynecology,* edited by R. M. Caplan and W. J. Sweeney, pp. 387–393. Williams and Wilkens, Baltimore.
21. Eliasson, R., and Johnsen, Ø. (1978): Adhesiveness of spermatozoa to glass material as a source of error in sperm analysis. In: *International Andrology,* edited by R. Eliasson, D. M. de Kretser, J. M. Pomerol, and G. M. H. Waites, p. 174. Scriptor, Copenhagen.
22. Eliasson, R., and Lindholmer, C. (1972): Distribution and properties of spermatozoa in different fractions of split ejaculates. *Fertil. Steril.,* 23:252–256.
23. Eliasson, R., Mossberg, B., Camner, C. and Afzelius, B. (1977): The immotile cilia syndrome. *N. Engl. J. Med.,* 297:1–6.
24. Elstein, M. (1976): Non-immunological factors in infertility. In: *The Cervix,* edited by J. A. Jordan and A. Singer, pp. 175–184. Saunders, Philadelphia.
25. Franken, D. R. (1978): Letter to the Editor. *Andrologia,* 10:413.
26. Freund, M., and Peterson, R. N. (1976): Semen evaluation and fertility. In: *Human Semen and Fertility Regulation in Men,* edited by E. S. E. Hafez, pp. 344–354. St. Louis.
27. Froewis, J., and Leed, H. (1961): Konzeption bei hochgradiger Oligo Asthenospermie. *Wien. Klin. Wochenschr.,* 73:641–642.
28. Gledhill, B. L. (1970): Changes in nuclear stainability associated with spermateliosis, spermatozoal maturation, and male infertility. In: *Introduction to Quantitative Cytochemistry—II,* edited by G. L. Wied and G. F. Bahr, pp. 125–151. Academic Press, New York.
29. Gustafsson, B., Carbo, B., and Rao, A. R. (1972): Two cases of bovine epidymal dysfunction. *Cornell Vet.,* 62:392–402.
30. Hellinga, G., Ruward, R., and Oppers, V. M. (1973): The influence of fixation and staining on the morphology of spermatozoa. In: *Fertility and Sterility.* Proceedings from the VII World Congress 1971, edited by T. Hasegawa, M. Hayashi, F. J. G. Ebling, and I. W. Henderson, pp. 233–235. Excerpta Medica, Amsterdam.
31. Hirschhäuser, C., and Eliasson, R. (1972): Origin and possible function of muramidase (lysozyme). *Life Sci.,* 11, part II:149–154.
32. Hotchkiss, R. S., Brunner, E. K., and Grenley, P. (1938): Semen analysis of two hundred fertile men. *Am. J. Med. Sci.,* 196:362–384.
33. Insler, V., and Bettendorf, G., (editors) (1977): *The Uterine Cervix in Reproduction.* Georg Thieme, Stuttgart.
34. Johannisson, E., and Eliasson, R. (1978): Cytological studies of prostatic fluids from men with and without abnormal palpatory findings of the prostate. I. Methodological aspects. *Int. J. Androl.,* 1:201–212.
35. Johnsen, Ø., and Eliasson, R. (1978): Destabilization of human sperm membranes by albumin, EDTA and histidine. *Int. J. Androl.,* 1:485–488.
36. Jones, R., Mann, T., and Sherins, R. J. (1978): Adverse effects of peroxidized lipid on human spermatozoa. *Proc. R. Soc. (Lond)B.,* 201:413–417.
37. Jouannet, P., Volochine, B., Deguent, P., Serres, C., and David, G. (1977): Light scattering determination of various characteristic parameters of spermatozoa motility in a series of human sperm. *Andrologia,* 9:36–49.
38. Kelly, R. W. (1978): Prostaglandins in semen: Their occurrence and possible physiological significance. *Int. J. of Androl.,* 1:188–200.
39. Kvist, U., and Eliasson, R. (1978): Zinc dependent chromatin stability in the ejaculated spermatozoa. In: *International Andrology,* edited by R. Eliasson, D. M. de Kretser, J. M. Pomerol, and G. M. H. Waites, p. 178. Scriptor, Copenhagen.
40. Lindholmer, C. (1974): Toxicity of zinc ions to human spermatozoa and the influence of albumin. *Andrologia,* 6:7–16.
41. Lobl, T. J., and Mathews, J. (1978): Effect of 1-(2,4-dichlorobenzyl)-indazole-3-carboxylic acid on sperm tails in rhesus monkey. *J. Reprod. Fert.,* 52:275–278.
42. Makler, A. (1978): A new multiple exposure photography method for objective human spermatozoal motility determination. *Fertil. Steril.,* 30:192–199.
43. Mann, T. (1975): Trends in current research on the metabolism and storage of mammalian semen. *Perspect. Biol. Med.,* 19:59–67.

44. Martin, H. F., Gudzinowicz, B. J., and Fanger, H. (1975): *Normal Values in Clinical Chemistry.* Marcel Dekker, New York.
45. Pace, M. M., and Graham, E. F. (1970): The release of glutamic oxaloacetic transaminase from bovine spermatozoa as a test method of assessing semen quality and fertility. *Biol. Reprod.,* 3:140–146.
46. Müller, B., and Kirchner, C. (1978): Influence of seminal plasma proteins on motility of rabbit spermatozoa. *J. Reprod. Fert.,* 45:167–172.
47. Salisbury, G. W., and Hart, R. G. (1975): Functional integrity of spermatozoa after storage. *Bioscience,* 25:159–165.
48. Sherins, R. J., Brightwell, D., and Sternthal, Ph. M. (1977): Longitudinal analysis of semen of fertile and infertile men. In: *In Testis in Normal and Infertile Men,* edited by P. Troen and H. R. Nankin, pp. 473–488. Raven Press, New York.
49. Smith, K. D., Rodriguez-Rigau, L. J., and Steinberger, E. (1977): Relation between indices of semen analysis and pregnancy rate in infertile couples. *Fertil. Steril.,* 28:1314–1319.
50. Sobrero, A. J., and Naghma-E-Rehan (1975): The semen of fertile men. II. Semen characteristics of 100 fertile men. *Fertil. Steril.,* 26:1048–1056.
51. Voglmayr, J. K. (1975): Metabolic changes in spermatozoa during epididymal transit. In: *Handbook of Physiology,* Section 7, Vol. V, Male Reproductive System, edited by R. O. Greep and E. B. Astwood, pp. 437–451. American Physiological Society, Washington, D.C.
52. Waites, G. M. H. and Edwards, E. M. (1973): Bibliography on epididymal physiology in relation to sperm maturation. *Bibliog. Reprod.,* 22:729–738 and 915–922.
53. Wetterauer, U., and Heite H.-J. (1978): Carnitine in seminal fluid as parameter for the epididymal function. *Andrologia,* 10:203–210.
54. Zukerman, Z., Rodriguez-Rigau, L. J., Smith, K. D., and Steinberger, E. (1977): Frequency distribution of sperm counts in fertile and infertile males. *Fertil. Steril.,* 28:1310–1313.
55. van Zyl, J. A., Menkveld, R., van W. Kotze, T. J., Retief, A. E., and van Niekerk, W. A. (1975): Oligozoospermia: A seven-year survey of the incidence, chromosomal aberrations, treatment and pregnancy rate. *Int. J. Fertil.,* 20:129–132.

The Testis, edited by H. Burger and D. de Kretser.
Raven Press, New York © 1981.

17

Cytogenetics in Male Hypogonadism

Niels E. Skakkebæk

Laboratory of Reproductive Biology and Fertility Clinic, Department of Obstetrics and Gynecology, YA, Rigshospitalet, and Department of Obstetrics and Gynecology, Herlev Hospital, University of Copenhagen, DK-2100 Copenhagen, Denmark

Since Jacobs and Strong (36) in 1959 for the first time showed that a hypogonadal patient with Klinefelter's syndrome had an abnormal chromosome complement, numerous studies have contributed to our understanding of the role of cytogenetic factors in male hypogonadism.

In principle, chromosome abnormalities may cause testicular failure and/or infertility in several ways. A male fetus with an abnormal karyotype may develop into an individual with grossly abnormal genitalia. On the other hand, the effect of an abnormal karyotype on the reproductive system may not show until after birth with postnatal degeneration of germ cells in childhood or during puberty.

In the adult, a chromosome abnormality may be the etiologic factor in germ cell degeneration during all stages of spermatogenesis. An abnormal chromosome complement can also be transmitted through all stages of spermatogenesis and result in spermatozoa which are abnormal only in their genotype. This may result in gametes and fetuses with unbalanced chromosome complements. Thus the result of a chromosome abnormality in the male may also be spontaneous abortion, stillbirth, or birth of a child with a congenital malformation.

CHROMOSOME SURVEYS OF GROUPS OF INFERTILE MEN

In order to assess the contribution to male infertility made by chromosome abnormalities, several surveys of men attending infertility clinics have been conducted (14,22,38,39,43,50,54,64). The frequency of patients with abnormal karyotypes differs markedly in these studies, probably owing to differences in techniques and patient selection. Recently Chandley (14) in a systematic survey of 1,599 male patients attending a subfertility clinic found that 2.2% were chromosomally abnormal. The frequency was approximately 5 times higher than that of a control group. Almost half of the patients with abnormal karyotype had Klinefelter's syndrome. The remaining had Y-chromosome abnormalities, translocations, and extra marker chromosomes. Several investigators have found that the frequency of Klinefelter's syndrome among infertile males with azoospermia is as high as 10 to 20% (14,22,38).

It appears that most chromosome abnormalities exert their effect on male infertility through disturbance of spermatogenesis whereas the contribution made by chromosome abnormalities in men causing recurrent abortions in their female partners is very small (14).

It is interesting that some chromosome abnormalities which are associated with impairment of spermatogenesis in the male appear to have little or no effect on oogenesis in the female. This phenomenon has been demonstrated not only in human but in other mammals and Drosophila (6,14).

In the following pages some details are given on the function of the reproductive system in patients with chromosome abnormalities.

KLINEFELTER'S SYNDROME, 47 XXY

Several chromosome surveys have shown that approximately 1 per 1,000 newborn males have a 47, XXY chromosome constitution (46,58,66,70,83). Xg-blood group studies have demonstrated that the extra X-chromosome in patients with Klinefelter's syndrome can be of either paternal or maternal origin (25).

Clinical Findings

Klinefelter's syndrome was described in 1942 (42), 17 years before the etiological chromosome abnormality of the disease was revealed (36). In typical cases (Fig. 1), the syndrome includes small, firm testes (1–3 ml), gynecomastia, and eunuchoidal traits in the phenotype, including increased height (62). As pointed out already in 1945 by Heller and Nelson (28), one or more of the specific findings may not be present and some patients with Klinefelter's syndrome are phenotypically normal. Small testes appear to be the most constant finding, which may always be present in nonmosaic cases. Poor beard growth and feminine distribution of pubic hair are present in approximately 65 to 70% of the patients, while gynecomastia is seen in 30 to 60% of the cases (24). Some patients without gross gynecomastia have been found to have microscopic gynecomastia (60).

The association between the 47, XXY karyotype and subnormal IQ and mental disorders has often been discussed (see ref. 80). However, it remains to be seen how often such disorders are present in unselected men with 47, XXY karyotype in the general population. None or few of the symptoms of Klinefelter's syndrome may be present in childhood, although small prepubertal testes (45) and abnormal body proportions in childhood have been reported (69).

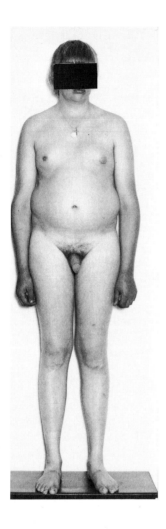

FIG. 1. A 20-year-old untreated male with Klinefelter's syndrome (47, XXY karyotype). Note eunuchoidal features including long arms and legs, female-like distribution of subcutaneus fat tissue, gynecomastia, absence of facial hair (the patient does not shave) and female-type pubic hair. Note also the normal-sized penis. The scrotum, which is not visible, is small, containing two small testes, each measuring 1 ml.

Laboratory Investigations

In most cases of Klinefelter's syndrome the seminal fluid contains no spermatozoa. However, several cases with a few spermatozoa in the ejaculate have been reported (22,27). These findings correlate well with the appearance of the testicular biopsy, which in typical cases demonstrates complete degeneration of the seminiferous tubules and hyalinization. A few preserved tubules are localized in or around Leydig cell-"clumps." The total Leydig cell volume appears to be normal or decreased (1). Some of the preserved tubules contain germ cells but the majority contain Sertoli cells only (Fig. 2). Skakkebæk (72) found preserved tubules in 32 of 37 testicular biopsies from consecutive cases of Klinefel-

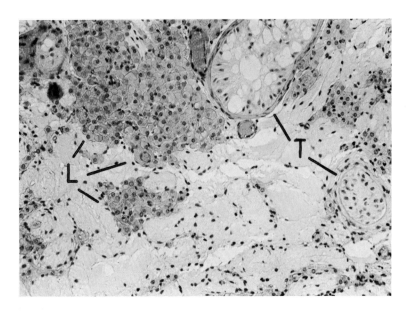

FIG. 2. Section of testicular biopsy from 47, XXY male with Klinefelter's syndrome. The pale, unstained areas are hyalinized tubules separated by a few fibroblast-like cells. T = tubules containing Sertoli cells only. L = Leydig cell-"clumps". ×175.

ter's syndrome with 47, XXY karyotype (nonmosaics). In 10 of these cases a few tubules with germ cells were present while the remaining 27 biopsies with preserved tubules contained Sertoli cells only. The Sertoli cells may be either undifferentiated or fully differentiated and both types may be present in the same biopsy.

The serum levels of follicle stimulating hormone (FSH) are increased in Klinefelter's syndrome and the level of luteinizing hormone (LH) is usually above the upper range of that of normal men. It remains to be seen if some patients with this syndrome pass through a period of normal gonadotropin levels during and after puberty until testicular degeneration has occurred. The testosterone levels in patients with Klinefelter's syndrome vary considerably and are often found in the lower range of that of normal men or lower. The Leydig cell reserve as defined by the HCG test may be reduced (60). These findings correspond to the poor virilization which is often seen at physical examination.

Although the vast majority of patients with Klinefelter's syndrome have a 47, XXY karyotype, several cases with 48, XXXY and 49, XXXXY karyotypes have been reported (24,59,60). Other patients with the syndrome have been demonstrated to have more than one stem cell line (24,59,60). Patients with 46, XY/47, XXY mosaicism demonstrate unpredictable clinical abnormalities and some of these individuals may be fertile (24,60,84). In rare instances, patients may exhibit all symptoms of Klinefelter's syndrome in spite of a normal chromosomal complement in all examined tissues (24,59).

An indirect evidence of 47, XXY karyotype may be obtained from analysis of nuclear chromatin in buccal smears (see ref. 12 for techniques). Supernumerary X-chromosomes are demonstrable as Barr bodies (X-chromatin) (5,67). It is interesting that X-chromatin cannot be demonstrated in fully differentiated Sertoli cells of 47, XXY men (26).

Treatment

It may seem logical to treat boys with Klinefelter's syndrome with testosterone, if they do not become adequately virilized during puberty. However, little is known about the effect of androgens on pubertal development in such patients (2,7,37,56). Androgen treatment is recommended in adults with Klinefelter's syndrome if they demonstrate androgen insufficiency (59). However, many adults with Klinefelter's syndrome have apparently normal serum testosterone levels and show no clinical signs of androgen insufficiency (60). No known treatment can prevent the degeneration of the seminiferous tubules during puberty. Patients with gross gynecomastia may need surgical extirpation of the glandular tissue for cosmetic reasons.

XX MALE

The incidence of the 46, XX karyotype in newborn males is approximately one in 10,000 to 20,000 (46,58,66,70,83). The general appearance and secondary sex characteristics resemble the features in Klinefelter's syndrome (Fig. 3). However, the mean height appears to be approximately 9 cm below the mean height in the 47, XXY male (16). It is not clear if there is a difference in intelligence, psychology, and gonadal structure between the XX male and the XXY male. Common features of testicular biopsies from XX males are hyalinization of the seminiferous tubules and polymorphism of the Leydig cells. The few preserved tubules which may exist usually contain Sertoli cells only, but a few germ cells may be present (16). This pattern may therefore not be distinguishable from the testicular histology in XXY males.

Several studies in humans and laboratory animals have shown that mammalian testicular differentiation only occurs in the presence of a Y-chromosome or part of a Y-chromosome. The XX male is an exception to this, and direct demonstration of fluorescent parts of the Y-chromosome has not been possible (63). However, serologic demonstration of a Y-linked gene in XX males (H-Y antigen) indicates that Y-chromosome material is present at least in some XX males (82). As in Klinefelter's syndrome, treatment should be directed towards androgen insufficiency if it is present.

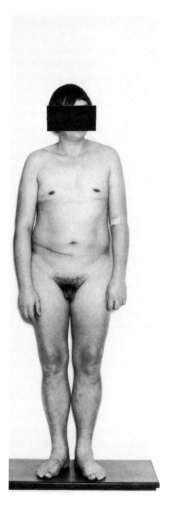

FIG. 3. A 40-year-old untreated man with 46, XX karyotype. Note the female-like distribution of subcutaneous fat. He was operated for bilateral gynecomastia at the age of 14. The penis and both testes are very small (0.5 ml each). Note absence of facial hair (the patient does not shave) and female-type pubic hair.

XYY MALE

Chromosome studies in series of neonates have shown that the 47, XYY karyotype occurs with a frequency of approximately 1/1,000 males (46,58,66, 70,83). The phenotypes of XYY males vary, although increased height is associated with this karyotype. Aggressive behavior has been suggested to be part of the "XYY-syndrome." However, a recent study by Witkin et al. (85) has shown that the elevated crime rate among XYY males is not associated with aggression but may be related to low intelligence.

Although the secondary sex characteristics and size of the testes are usually normal, there is little doubt that gametogenesis is impaired in the majority of XYY males. Testicular biopsies have revealed that spermatogenesis of XYY

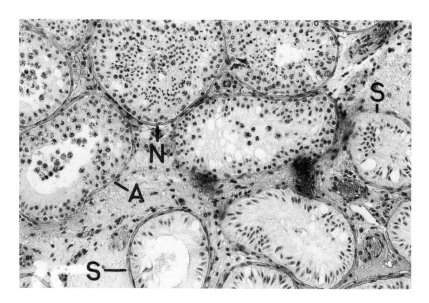

FIG. 4. Section of testicular biopsy from XYY male (47, XYY karyotype). Note the heterogenous pattern. S = tubules containing Sertoli cells only. A = tubles with complete arrest of spermatogenesis at spermatocyte level. N = tubule with normal spermatogenesis. (From ref. 74, ×175.)

males is normal in only a few cases and 80% of XYY males demonstrate severely damaged seminiferous tubules (74,76). The testicular histology does not have characteristics specific for the XYY karyotype. However, approximately 50% have tubules with arrest of spermatogenesis at the spermatocyte level and/or tubules containing Sertoli cells only (Fig. 4) (74,76). Serum testosterone is usually normal, whereas FSH may be raised owing to testicular failure (68,74). Results of seminal fluid analysis have correlated with the findings of testicular histology and vary from a normal spermiogram to azoospermia.

Meiotic chromosome studies have shown gonosomal XY/XYY mosaicism in germ cells of one individual without evidence of mosaicism in his somatic tissue (34). However, complete loss of the second Y-chromosome from the germ cell line prior to spermatocyte formation apparently occurs in most human XYY individuals (15,20,30,31,55,79,81). These findings correlate well with the reports of normal offspring of XYY males (17). In XYY mice the extra Y-chromosome can be traced in meiotic cells (18).

SPERMATOGENESIS IN MEN WITH BALANCED CHROMOSOME TRANSLOCATION AND OTHER AUTOSOMAL CHROMOSOME ABERRATIONS

Since Kjessler (40) in 1964 demonstrated abnormal spermatogenesis in a balanced D/D translocation carrier, spermatogenesis has been studied in several men with D/D, D/G, A/G and other translocations (13,44,75). No clear pattern has arisen. Some men with balanced translocations have been found to have normal spermatogenesis. However, men with autosomal translocations are found more frequently among infertile men than in control populations, which indicates that certain translocations are associated with failure of spermatogenesis. The most common feature of the testicular histology in these cases is a nonspecific reduction in the number of spermatids (75). The same pattern is, however, often seen in infertile men with a normal karyotype. The phenotype, including secondary sex characteristics and the size of the testes are usually normal in men with balanced translocation although small testes (<145 ml) have been described.

Also phenotypically normal men with an extra, small marker chromosome may be infertile due to impairment of spermatogenesis (Fig. 5) (33,75,77). The extra minute chromosome has been traced in both somatic and gonadal tissue (33).

Other rare chromosome abnormalities may or may not be associated with abnormal spermatogenesis (cf. 14,75).

Severe testicular atrophy is found in most cases of Down's syndrome (75), although a few cases with normal or near-normal spermatogenesis have been reported (41). It is noteworthy that several pregnancies in females with Down's

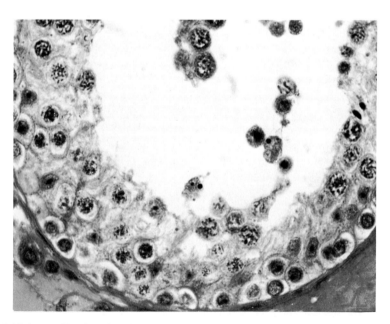

FIG. 5. High magnification of section of tubule from patient with an extra, small marker-chromosome. Note the severe reduction in number of spermatids and degenerated germ cells in the lumen. (From ref. 75, ×500.)

syndrome have been reported, although there is no report on a male patient with Down's syndrome who has fathered a child (52).

MEIOTIC CHROMOSOME ABNORMALITIES IN INFERTILE MEN WITH NORMAL KARYOTYPE

The etiology of male infertility is not known in a great proportion of cases (cf. chapter 15). Nelson (57) suggested in 1950 that meiotic chromosome abnormalities may be the cause of spermatogenic arrest at the spermatocyte level in some men with azoospermia. Twenty years later Hultén et al. (32) and Pearson et al. (61) clearly demonstrated abnormal meiotic chromosomes in infertile men with spermatogenic arrest who showed low chiasma counts, asymmetrical bivalents, multivalents, univalents, and fragments of chromosomes in primary spermatocytes (diakinesis) in spite of a normal karyotype in lymphocyte cultures. These authors found the same abnormality in all investigated cells of azoospermic men. Skakkebæk et al. (73) found a similar abnormality in a small proportion of cells in diakinesis in oligospermic, infertile men. An ultrastructural study indicated that the synaptenemal complex was abnormal in a patient with this abnormal meiotic chromosome pattern (35). The low chiasma frequency and other abnormalities may be owing to a primary defect in chromosome pairing in these cases. A high proportion of parental consanguinity indicates that the disorder may be caused by a recessive meiotic mutation (35).

So far, however, meiotic chromosome abnormalities in subjects with normal karyotype appear to be a relatively rare cause of male infertility (39,50,78). We (75) investigated meiotic chromosomes in diakinesis-metaphase I and metaphase II of 18 controls and 74 infertile men. The chiasma frequency was the same in the two groups except for three infertile men—including one with spermatogenic arrest—who showed a few cells with abnormally low chiasma frequency (Fig. 6). Three other men with spermatogenic arrest had normal chiasma frequency. The occurrence of nonpaired sex chromosomes and autosomes in diakinesis/metaphase I (Fig. 7) was also the same in the fertile and the infertile group, and the number of polyploid cells was increased among the infertile men. Few of the abnormalities observed may be owing to genetic disturbances. Other meiotic abnormalities may be secondary to impairment of spermatogenesis because of endocrine and other factors.

In conclusion, the present evidence does not indicate that meiotic chromosome abnormalities in men with normal karyotype play a major role in male infertility. However, the squash (39) and air-drying techniques (19) which have been used may not be suitable for detection of some chromosome abnormalities although the banding techniques make identification of chromosomes in pachytene and other stages of meiosis possible (9,47). It remains to be seen if sophisticated ultrastructural chromosome analyses will reveal meiotic abnormalities in infertile men with hitherto unexplained disruption of spermatogenesis (Fig. 8) (29).

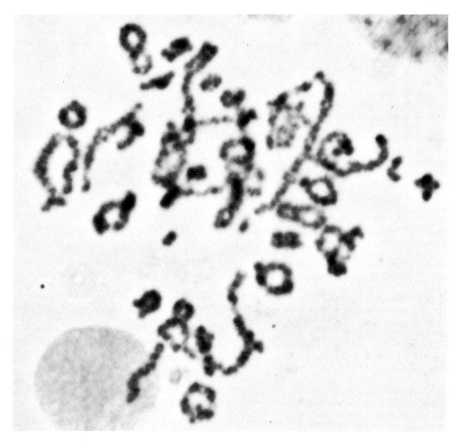

FIG. 6. A cell in diakinesis-metaphase I from an infertile male. Note the indistinct chromosomes with grossly fragmented chromosomes with extremely low chiasma frequency. (From ref. 73.)

THE PATHOGENESIS OF TESTICULAR FAILURE IN PATIENTS WITH CHROMOSOME ABNORMALITIES

Why do some chromosome abnormalities affect spermatogenesis and steroid production in the testis, while other chromosome abnormalities have apparently no effect on testicular function, including spermatogenesis? Why do some chromosome abnormalities affect spermatogenesis but not oogenesis? We can give no clear answers to these questions at the present time.

The extra X-chromosome in the karyotype of patients with Klinefelter's syndrome may exert its damaging effect on spermatogenesis directly on the germ cell population and/or via the Leydig cells or the Sertoli cells. Certainly Leydig cell function is impaired in some patients with Klinefelter's syndrome who may demonstrate a low degree of virilization and diminished Leydig cell reserve

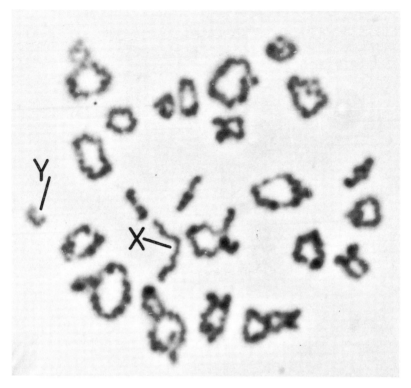

FIG. 7. A cell in diakinesis-metaphase I with normal chiasma formation. Note that the X- and Y-chromosomes are separated instead of being located end-to-end. Separation of the sex chromosomes is also often seen in individuals with normal spermatogenesis. (From ref. 73.)

capacity as demonstrated by the HCG test. There is no evidence that germ cell depletion itself can severely impair the function of the Leydig cells, although some patients with Sertoli-cell-only syndrome (10) have lower than normal serum testosterone levels (44). A minor Leydig cell failure may coexist with the germ cell depletion in such patients (51).

In boys with Klinefelter's syndrome the number of germ cells is reduced very considerably (21) and the size of the testes may be smaller than normal in some prepubertal boys with this syndrome (45). It is possible that the number of germ cells is normal early in fetal life, and a continuous germ cell loss may occur throughout the prenatal period and in childhood. This phenomenon is seen in females with Turner's syndrome which in typical cases (45, X karyotype) is associated with streak gonads in adults, although oocytes may be present at birth (8).

In spite of the finding that boys with Klinefelter's syndrome may have testes which contain up to 20% of the normal number of gonocytes (21), almost all

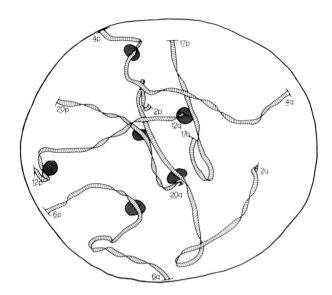

FIG. 8. Reconstruction of the synaptonemal complexes of six pachytene bivalents from a human spermatocyte nucleus. Testicular biopsies were fixed and embedded for electron micros- copy, serially sectioned and photographed in an electron microscope. The reconstruction was performed by tracing the synaptonemal complexes on transparent plastic sheets. The homolo- gous chromosomes are paired from telomere to telomere and all telomeres are anchored at the nuclear envelope. The cross-hatched areas denote the condensed chromatin of the cen- tromere region. The bivalents are classified on the basis of length measurements and the position of the centromere. The underlined numbers denote the number of the bivalents and p and q the short and the long arms, respectively, of the bivalents. (From ref. 29.)

germ cells are apparently lacking in adults with this syndrome. Lyon (48) sug- gested that both XX chromosomes of germ cells in XXY males are active, as in females, but the activity of more than one X chromosome is fatal to the germ cell. Short (71) also presented evidence for the theory that germ cells containing two X-chromosomes cannot survive in a testicular environment. An occasional tubule containing spermatogenesis may, however, be found in patients with a 47, XXY karyotype. Such germ cells may have lost the second X-chromo- some, allowing focal areas of normal spermatogenesis.

Several investigators have discussed the mechanisms by which Y-chromosome abnormalities cause disruption of spermatogenesis (3,11,18). Spontaneous univa- lence at male meiosis in the mouse has been associated with disruption of sperma- togenesis (4,65), and Miklos (53) has postulated a hypothesis which relates chromosome pairing and sterility in males. Ford (23) has suggested that interfer- ence with the normal development of the sex vesicle at early meiotic prophase may disturb spermatogenesis. The same author discussed the role of chromosome translocations in disruption of spermatogenesis. Cacheiro et al. (6) concluded that translocations, which cause sterility in the male mouse are those in which breaks occur close to one end of a chromosome.

Lyon and Meredith (49) found that translocations which caused sterility were often associated with a high frequency of chain quadrivalents and univalents at meiosis in the male mouse. An association between an extra marker chromosome and disruption of spermatogenesis (33,75,77) also supports the theory that univalence during meiotic prophase and metaphase is associated with disturbed spermatogenesis. Thus, although the mechanism of action is not clear, there is some evidence that univalence of both sex chromosomes and autosomes during meiotic prophase and metaphase is associated with an increased risk of disturbed spermatogenesis.

GENETIC COUNSELLING

Some chromosome abnormalities are compatible with fertility of the male carrier, who may need genetic counselling in regard to the desirability of attempting pregnancy. Most of the patients seeking genetic advice are phenotypically normal carriers of balanced structural chromosome abnormalities, especially translocations. Theoretically an individual with a balanced chromosome translocation may produce sperm with both normal complement and with abnormal chromosome complement in either balanced or unbalanced form; thus the result may be a fetus with abnormal phenotype. However, the present evidence suggests that a selection occurs against some gametes or zygotes with unbalanced chromosome complement. Some data on children of male D/D translocation carriers have shown a $1:1$ ratio of balanced heterozygotes to normals (13,27a), but other chromosome abnormalities may be associated with a risk of offspring with abnormal phenotype.

We offer advice from a clinical geneticist to all fertile patients with abnormal karyotype, although it may often be difficult to estimate the real risk of conception of a malformed child or a phenotypically normal child with balanced structural chromosome rearrangement. In addition, we offer prenatal chromosome analysis of amniotic fluid to all couples if one of the partners carries a chromosome abnormality. The prenatal chromosome analysis is relevant if the couple would consider induced abortion of a child with an abnormal karyotype. However, it must be borne in mind that ethical and religious attitudes vary from one country to another and each clinician must base his advice to patients on the traditions of his own community.

REFERENCES

1. Ahmad, K. N., Dykes, J. R. W., Ferguson-Smith, M. A., Lennox, B., and Mack, W. S. (1971): Leydig cell volume in chromatin-positive Klinefelter's syndrome. *J. Clin. Endocrinol.,* 33:517–520.
2. Annell, A. -L., and Gustavson, K. -H. (1969): Klinefelter's syndrom hos skolbarn (Klinefelter's syndrome in school children). *Läkartid.,* 66:577–585.
3. Baker, B. S., Carpenter, A. T. C., Esposito, M. S., Esposito, R. E., and Sandler, L. (1976): The genetic control of meiosis. *Annu. Rev. Genet.,* 10:53–134.

4. Beechey, C. V. (1973): X-Y chromosome dissociation and sterility in the mouse. *Cytogenet. Cell Genet.*, 12:60–67.
5. Bradbury, J. T., Bunge, R. G., and Boccabella, R. A. (1956): Chromatin test in Klinefelter's syndrome. *J. Clin. Endocrinol.*, 16:689.
6. Cacheiro, N. L. A., Russell, L. B., and Swartout, M. S. (1974): Translocations, the predominant cause of total sterility in sons of mice treated with mutagens. *Genetics*, 76:73–91.
7. Caldwell, P. D., and Smith, D. W. (1972): The XXY (Klinefelter's) syndrome in childhood: Detection and treatment. *J. Pediatr.*, 80:250–258.
8. Carr, D. H., Haggar, R. A., and Hart, A. G. (1967): Germ cells in the ovaries of XO female infants. *Am. J. Clin. Pathol.*, 49:521–526.
9. Caspersson, T., Hultén, M., Lindsten, J., and Zech, L. (1971): Identification of chromosome bivalents in human male meiosis by quinacrine mustard fluorescence analysis. *Hereditas*, 67:147–149.
10. del Castillo, E. B., Trabucco, A., and de la Balze, F. A. (1947): Syndrome produced by absence of the germinal epithelium without impairment of the Sertoli and Leydig cells. *J. Clin. Endocrinol.*, 7:493–502.
11. Cattanach, B. M., and Pollard, O. E. (1969): An XYY sex-chromosome constitution in the mouse. *Cytogenetics*, 8:80–86.
12. Chandley, A. C. (1977): Karyotyping of infertile men. In: *Techniques of Human Andrology,* edited by E. S. E. Hafez. Elsevier/North-Holland Biomedical Press, Amsterdam.
13. Chandley, A. C., Christie, S., Fletcher, J., Frackiewics, K., and Jacobs, P. A. (1972): Translocation heterozygosity and associated subfertility in man. *Cytogenetics*, 11:516–533.
14. Chandley, A. C., Edmond, P., Christie, S., Gowans, L., Fletcher, J., Frackiewics, A., and Newton, M. (1975): Cytogenetics and infertility in man. I. Karyotype and seminal analysis. *Ann. Hum. Genet. (Lond)*, 39:231–252.
15. Chandley, A. C., Fletcher, J., and Robinson, J. A. (1976): Normal meiosis in two 47,XYY men. *Hum. Genet.*, 33:231–240.
16. Chapelle, A. de la (1972): Analytic review: Nature and origin of males with XX sex-chromosomes. *Am. J. Hum. Genet.*, 24:71–105.
17. Court Brown, W. M. (1968): Males with an XYY sex-chromosome complement. *J. Med. Genet.*, 5:341–359.
18. Evans, E. P., Beechey, C. V., and Burtenshaw, M. D. (1978): Meiosis and fertility in XYY mice. *Cytogenet. Cell Genet.*, 20:249–263.
19. Evans, E. P., Breckon, G., and Ford, C. E. (1964): An air-drying method for meiotic preparation from mammalian testes. *Cytogenetics*, 3:289–294.
20. Evans, E. P., Ford, C. E., Chaganti, R. S. K., Blank, C. E., and Hunter, H. (1970): XY spermatocytes in an XYY male. *Lancet*, 1:719–720.
21. Ferguson-Smith, M. A. (1959): The prepubertal testicular lesion in chromatin-positive Klinefelter's syndrome (primary micro-orchidism) as seen in mentally handicapped children. *Lancet*, 1:219–222.
22. Ferguson-Smith, M. A., Lennox, B., Mack, N. S., and Stewart, J. S. S. (1957): Klinefelter's syndrome: frequency and testicular morphology in relation to nuclear sex. *Lancet*, 2:167–169.
23. Ford, C. E. (1970): The cytogenetics of the male germ cells and the testis in mammals. In: *Advances in Experimental Medicine and Biology,* Vol. 10: The Human Testis, edited by E. Rosemberg and C. A. Paulsen. Plenum Press, New York.
24. Frøland, A. (1969): Klinefelter's syndrome. *Dan. Med. Bull.*, Suppl. 16, no. 6:1–108.
25. Frøland, A., Sanger, R., and Race, R. R. (1968): Xg blood groups of 78 patients with Klinefelter's syndrome and of some of their parents. *J. Med. Genet.*, 5:161–164.
26. Frøland, A., and Skakkebæk, N. E. (1971): Dimorphism in sex chromatin pattern of Sertoli cells in adults with Klinefelter's syndrome: correlation with two types of "Sertoli-cell-only" tubules. *J. Clin. Endocrinol. Metab.*, 33:683–687.
27. Futterweit, W. (1967): Spermatozoa in seminal fluid of a patient with Klinefelter's syndrome. *Fertil. Steril.*, 18:492–496.
27a. Hamerton, J. L. (1968): Robertsonian translocations in man: evidence for prezygotic selection. *Cytogenetics*, 7:260–276.
28. Heller, C. G., and Nelson, W. O. (1945): Hyalinization of the seminiferous tubules associated with normal or failing Leydig-cell function. Discussion of relationship to eunuchoidism, gynecomastia, elevated gonadotrophins, depressed 17-ketosteroids and estrogens. *J. Clin. Endocrinol.*, 5:1–12.

29. Holm, P. B., and Rasmussen, S. W. (1977): Human meiosis I. The human pachytene karyotype analyzed by three dimensional reconstruction of the synaptonemal complex. *Carlsberg Res. Commun.,* 42:283–323.
30. Hsu, L. Y., Shapiro, L. R., and Hirschhorn, K. (1970): Meiosis in an XYY male. *Lancet,* 1:1173–1174.
31. Hultén, M. (1970): Meiosis in XYY men. *Lancet,* 1:717–718.
32. Hultén, M., Eliasson, R., and Tillinger, K. G. (1970): Low chiasma count and other meiotic irregularities in two infertile 46,XY men with spermatogenic arrest. *Hereditas,* 65:285–290.
33. Hultén, M., Lindsten, J., Fraccaro, M., Mannini, A., and Tiepolo, L. (1966): Extra minute chromosome in somatic and germline cells of the same person. *Lancet,* 2:22–24.
34. Hultén, M., and Pearson, P. L. (1971): Fluorescent evidence for spermatocytes with two Y chromosomes in an XYY male. *Ann. Hum. Genet.,* 34:273–276.
35. Hultén, M., Solari, A. J., and Skakkebaek, N. E. (1974): Abnormal synaptonemal complex in an oligochiasmatic man with spermatogenic arrest. *Hereditas,* 78:105–116.
36. Jacobs, P. A., and Strong, J. A. (1959): A case of human intersexuality having a possible XXY sex-determining mechanism. *Nature,* 183:302–303.
37. Johnson, H. R., Myhre, S. A., Ruvalcaba, R. H. A., Thuline, H. C., and Kelley, V. C. (1970): Effects of testosterone on body image and behavior in Klinefelter's syndrome: A pilot study. *Dev. Med. Child Neurol.,* 12:454–460.
38. Kjessler, B. (1972): Facteurs génétiques dans la subfertilité male humaine. In: *Fécondité et Stérilité du Male Acquisitions Recentes,* edited by C. Thibault. Masson, Paris.
39. Kjessler, B. (1966): Karyotype, meiosis and spermatogenesis in a sample of men attending an infertility clinic. In: *Monographs in Human Genetics,* edited by L. Beckman and M. Hauge. S. Karger, Basel.
40. Kjessler, B. (1964): Meiosis in a man with a D/D translocation and clinical sterility. *Lancet,* 18:1421–1423.
41. Kjessler, B., and de la Chapelle, A. (1971): Meiosis and spermatogenesis in two postpubertal males with Down's syndrome: 47,XY, G+. *Clin. Genet.,* 2:50–57.
42. Klinefelter, H. F., Reifenstein, E. C., and Albright, F. (1942): Syndrome characterized by gynecomastia, aspermatogenesis without a-Leydigism, and increased excretion of follicle-stimulating hormone. *J. Clin. Endocrinol.,* 2:615–627.
43. Koulisher, L., and Schoysman, R. (1974): Chromosomes and human infertility. I. Mitotic and meiotic chromosome studies in 202 consecutive male patients. *Clin. Genet.,* 5:116–126.
44. de Kretser, D. M., Burger, H. G., Fortune, D., Hudson, B., Long, A. R., Panesen, C. A., and Taft, H. P. (1972): Hormonal, histological and chromosomal studies in adult males with testicular disorders. *J. Clin. Endocrinol. Metab.,* 35:392–401.
45. Laron, Z., and Hochman, I. H. (1971): Small testes in prepubertal boys with Klinefelter's syndrome. *J. Clin. Endocrinol.,* 32:671–672.
46. Lubs, H. A., and Ruddle, F. H. (1970): Chromosomal abnormalities in the human population: Estimation of rates based on New Haven newborn study. *Science,* 169:495–497.
47. Luciani, J. M., Morazzani, M. R., and Stahl, A. (1975): Identification of pachytene bivalents in human male meiosis using G-banding technique. *Chromosoma (Berlin),* 52:275–282.
48. Lyon, M. F. (1974): Mechanisms and evolutionary origins of variable X-chromosome activity in mammals. *Proc. R. Soc. (Lond) B.,* 187:243–268.
49. Lyon, M. F., and Meredith, R. (1966): Autosomal translocations causing male sterility and viable aneuploidy in the mouse. *Cytogenetics,* 5:335–354.
50. McIlree, E., Price, W. H., Court Brown, W. M., Tulloch, W. S., Newsam, J. E., and Maclean, N. (1966): Chromosome studies on testicular cells from 50 subfertile men. *Lancet,* 2:69–71.
51. Mecklenburg, R. S., and Sherins, R. J. (1974): Gonadotropin response to luteinizing hormone-releasing hormone in men with germinal aplasia. *J. Clin. Endocrinol. Metab.,* 38:1005–1008.
52. Mikkelsen, M. (1971): Down's syndrome. Current stage of research. *Humangenetik,* 12:1–28.
53. Miklos, G. L. G. (1974): Sex-chromosome pairing and male fertility. *Cytogenet. Cell Genet.,* 13:558–577.
54. Millet, D., Plachot, M., Netter, A., and de Grouchy, J. (1972): Le caryotype dans la stérilité masculine. In: *Fécondité et Stérilité du Male,* edited by C. Thibault. Masson, Paris.
55. Melnyk, J., Thompson, H., Rucci, A. J., Vanasek, F., and Hayes, S. (1969): Failure of transmission of the extra chromosome in subjects with 47,XYY karyotype. *Lancet,* 2:797–798.
56. Myhre, S. A., Ruvalcaba, R. H. A., Johnson, H. R., Thuline, H. C., and Kelley, V. C. (1970): The effects of testosterone treatment in Klinefelter's syndrome. *J. Pediatr.,* 76:267–276.

57. Nelson, W. O. (1950): Testicular morphology in eunuchoidal and infertile men. *Fertil. Steril.,* 1:477–488.
58. Nielsen, J., and Sillesen, I. (1975): Incidence of chromosome aberrations among 11148 newborn children. *Humangenetik,* 30:1–12.
59. Paulsen, C. A. (1974): The testis. In: *Textbook of Endocrinology,* edited by R. H. Williams. Saunders, Philadelphia.
60. Paulsen, C. A., Gordon, D. L., Carpenter, R. W., Gandy, H. M., and Drucker, W. D. (1968): Klinefelter's syndrome and its variants: A hormonal and chromosomal study. *Recent Prog. Horm. Res.,* 24:321–363.
61. Pearson, P. L., Ellis, J. D., and Evans, H. J. (1970): A gross reduction in chiasma formation during meiotic prophase and a defective DNA repair mechanism associated with a case of human male infertility. *Cytogenetics,* 9:460–467.
62. Philip, J., Lundsteen, C., Owen, D., and Hinschhorn, K. (1976): The frequency of chromosome aberrations in tall men with special reference to 47,XYY and 47,XXY. *Am. J. Hum. Genet.,* 28:404–411.
63. Philip, J., Nielsen, H., Skakkebæk, N. E., and Boczkowski, K. (1971): Testing the hypothesis of Y translocation in XX males by fluorescence microscopy after quinacrine-dihydrochloride staining. *Lancet,* 1:298.
64. Philip, J., Skakkebæk, N. E., Hammen, R., Johnsen, S. G., and Rebbe, H. (1970): Cytogenetic investigations in male infertility. *Acta Obstet. Gynecol. Scand.,* 49:235–239.
65. Purnell, D. J. (1973): Spontaneous univalence at male meiosis in the mouse. *Cytogenet. Cell Genet.,* 12:327–335.
66. Ratcliffe, S. G., Stewart, A. L., Melville, M. M., and Jacobs, P. A. (1970): Chromosome studies on 3500 newborn male infants. *Lancet,* 1:121–122.
67. Riis, P., Johnsen, S. G., and Mosbech, J. (1956): Nuclear sex in Klinefelter's syndrome. *Lancet,* 1:962–963.
68. Santen, R. J., de Kretser, D. M., Paulsen, C. A., and Vorhees, J. (1970): Gonadotrophins and testosterone in the XYY syndrome. *Lancet,* 2:371.
69. Schibler, D., Brook, C. G. D., Kind, H. P., Zachmann, M., and Prader, A. (1974): Growth and body proportions in 54 boys and men with Klinefelter's syndrome. *Helv. Paediatr. Acta,* 29:325–333.
70. Sergovich, F., Valentine, G. H., Chen, A. T. L., Kingh, R. A. H., and Smout, M. S. (1969): Chromosome aberrations in 2159 consecutive newborn babies. *N. Engl. J. Med.,* 280:851–855.
71. Short, R. V. (1978): Sex determination and differentiation of the mammalian gonad. *Int. J. Androl.,* (Suppl. 2), *(in press).*
72. Skakkebæk, N. E. (1969): Two types of tubules containing only Sertoli cells in adults with Klinefelter's syndrome. *Nature,* 223:643–645.
73. Skakkebæk, N. E., Bryant, J. I., and Philip, J. (1973): Studies on meiotic chromosomes in infertile men and controls with normal karyotypes. *J. Reprod. Fertil.,* 35:23–36.
74. Skakkebæk, N. E., Hultén, M., Jacobsen, P., and Mikkelsen, M. (1973): Quantification of human seminiferous epithelium. II. Histological studies in eight 47,XYY men. *J. Reprod. Fertil.,* 32:391–401.
75. Skakkebæk, N. E., Hultén, M., and Philip, J. (1973): Quantification of human seminiferous epithelium. IV. Histological studies in 17 men with numerical and structural autosomal aberrations. *Acta Pathol. Microbiol. Scand.,* Section A. 81:112–124.
76. Skakkebæk, N. E., Zeuthen, E., Nielsen, J., and Yde, H. (1973): Abnormal spermatogenesis in XYY males: A report on 4 cases ascertained through a population study. *Fertil. Steril.,* 24:390–395.
77. Smith, K. D., Steinberger, E., Steinberger, A. and Perloff, W. H. (1965): A familial centric chromosome fragment. *Cytogenetics,* 4:219–226.
78. Templado, C., Marina, S., and Egozcwe, J. (1976): Three cases of low chiasma frequency associated with infertility in man. *Andrologia,* 8:285–289.
79. Tettenborn, U., Schwinger, E., and Gropp, A. (1970): Zur Hodenfunktion bei Männern mit XYY-Konstitution. *Dtsch. Med. Wochenschr.,* 95:158–161.
80. Theilgaard, A., Nielsen, J., Sørensen, A., Frøland, A., and Johnsen, S. G. (1971): *A Psychological Psychiatric Study of Patients with Klinefelter's Syndrome, 47,XXY.* Universitetsforlaget i Aarhus, Aarhus.
81. Thompson, H., Melnyk, J., and Hecht, F. (1967): Reproduction and meiosis in XYY. *Lancet,* 2:831.

82. Wachtel, S. S., Koo, G. C., Breg, W. R., Thaler, H. T., Dillard, G. M., Rosenthal, I. M., Dosik, H., Gerald, P. S., Saenger, P., New, M., Lieber, E., and Miller, O. J. (1976): Serologic detection of a Y-linked gene in XX males and XX true hermaphrodites. *N. Engl. J. Med.,* 295:750–754.
83. Walzer, S., Breau, G., and Gerald, P. S. (1969): A chromosome survey of 2400 normal newborn infants. *J. Pediatr.,* 74:438–449.
84. Warburg, E. (1974): A fertile patient with Klinefelter's syndrome. *Acta Endocrinol.,* 43:12–26.
85. Witkin, H. A., Mednick, S. A., Schulsinger, F., Bakkestrøm, E., Christiansen, K. O., Goodenough, D. R., Hirschhorn, K., Lundsteen, C., Owen, D. R., Philip, J., Rubin, D. B., and Stocking, M. (1976): Criminality in XYY and XXY men. *Science,* 193:547–555.

The Testis, edited by H. Burger and D. de Kretser.
Raven Press, New York © 1981.

18

Vasculature of the Testis: Assessment and Management of Varicocele

F. Comhaire

Department of Internal Medicine, Section of Endocrinology and Metabolic Diseases, Academisch Ziekenhuis, State University of Ghent, De Pintelaan 135, B-9000-Ghent, Belgium

VASCULATURE OF THE TESTIS

The blood supply of the testis depends mainly on the testicular artery which originates in the aorta, passes through the inguinal canal and is situated in the middle of the pampiniform plexus. In the scrotum this artery first reaches the rete testis and upper-anterior pole of the testis, it runs over the anterior aspect, inferior pole, and posterior aspect to the upper posterior pole of the testis. The deferential artery provides supplementary blood supply, this artery originates from the hypogastric artery and runs along with the deferential duct. Finally, some small arterial branches coming from the iliac artery are situated within the tunica vaginalis surrounding the spermatic cord.

The venous blood from the testicle and epididymal head drains into the pampiniform plexus. This plexus is build up of a variable number of intercommunicating veins running along with, and closely applied to, the spermatic artery. The number of venous branches decreases gradually and the plexus is reduced to a single or two internal spermatic veins in the retroperitoneal region. The left internal spermatic vein enters the renal vein and the right one normally opens into the inferior caval vein.

The veins from the epididymal corpus and tail join the deferential vein to accompany the vas deferens. This vein drains into the plexus around the prostate and urinary bladder which finally enters the hypogastric vein.

The superficial scrotal and cremasteric veins drain via the external spermatic vein into the saphenous vein. After their passage through the inguinal canal, the scrotal and testicular veins separate into three directions: the deferential vein curves toward the midline together with the vas deferens; the internal spermatic vein bends backwards to take its retroperitoneal course; and the external spermatic vein curves laterally towards the saphenous vein.

VARICOCELE

Pathology

Varicocele is a common cause of epididymal and testicular dysfunction in men resulting in subfertility (9,18) and/or deficient sexual adequacy (4). This affection is caused by insufficiency or congenital absence of the valves in the internal spermatic vein with inversion of the blood flow in this vessel (5). The reflux may cause varix-like distension of the pampiniform plexus, however reflux may be present without clinically detectable distension of the scrotal plexus in the so-called subclinical varicocele. There is no correlation between the volume of the varicocele and either the degree of testicular damage (11) or the fertility outcome after surgery (8,14,21).

Diagnosis

The clinical diagnosis is simple if the distension of the plexus is palpable and if care is taken always to examine the patient in upright position. Indeed, reflux disappears as soon as the patient is recumbent. However, in one out of five cases with reflux, varicocele cannot be palpated and the diagnosis can be made only by means of special techniques such as scrotal thermography and/ or retrograde venography of the internal spermatic vein.

Scrotal Thermography

Contact thermography uses cholesterol crystal covered plates applied directly against the scrotal skin. This technique is cheap and has been applied with good results by some authors (20). We perform telethermography using an Aga Thermovision 680 infrared camera system (5).

The patient first has to adapt to room temperature during 15 min by standing upright with the under part of the body uncovered and the penis fixed against the abdomen.

In normal men, the temperature of the scrotal skin is between three and four degrees lower than that of the inner-upper thigh and temperature distribution is symmetrical (Fig. 1). In the presence of spermatic venous reflux, blood at body temperature refluxes into the pampiniform plexus so that the scrotal skin overlying this plexus is warmer than normal (7). Such a warmer zone can be recognized as a hot spot in the upper quadrant of the affected hemiscrotum (Fig. 2). The temperature difference with the symmetrical point of the contra-lateral hemiscrotum is between 1.5 and 3°C. The warmer zone may extend over the whole affected hemiscrotum, the temperature difference then mostly exceeds 2.5°C (Fig. 3). Finally the whole scrotum or both lateral aspects of the scrotum may be warm, indicating either the presence of a large unilateral varicocele, or bilateral varicoceles (Fig. 4).

The accuracy of thermographical diagnosis is, in our hands, excellent. A

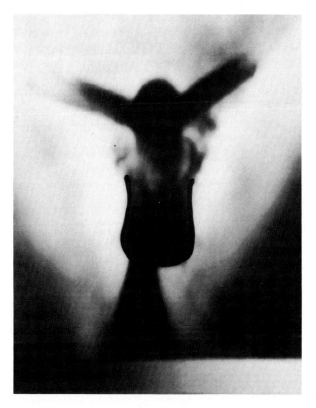

FIG. 1. Scrotal telethermogram in a man without varicocele. The scrotal skin presents a symmetrical dark appearance corresponding to a temperature which is ± 4° below that of the white zones over the inner-upper thigh.

normal thermogram in the presence of reflux, therefore falsely negative, is found in a few cases with associated atrophy of the testis at the varicocele side. This atrophy is owing to either torsion of the cord or to hernia operation (13).

An abnormal thermogram in the absence of reflux i.e., falsely positive, occurs in 2% of cases. In these patients the zone of increased temperature is restricted to the upper part of the affected hemiscrotum and the temperature difference generally does not exceed 1.5°C. Possibly skin folds or inflammatory conditions of the epididymis are responsible for the observed hyperthermia.

Scrotal thermography, therefore, is a highly reliable, rapid, and easy screening method which should be applied to all patients with unexplained subfertility.

Retrograde Venography of the Internal Spermatic Vein

Retrograde venography is practised using the Seldinger technique (1,3). Under local anesthesia a preformed cobra catheter is introduced into the femoral vein

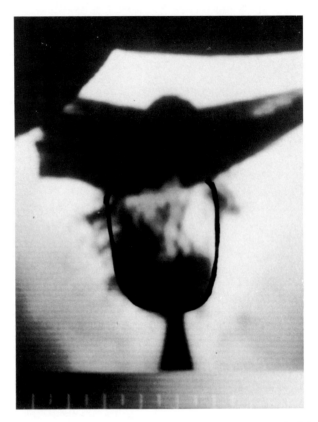

FIG. 2. Scrotal telethermogram in a patient with impalpable, so-called subclinical, varicocele. The skin of the upper quadrant of the left hemiscrotum is warm as can be recognized by the white zone, contrasting with the dark, cool skin covering the lower left quadrant and the right hemiscrotum.

and pushed via the iliac and inferior caval vein far lateral into the left renal vein. The patient is moved into half erect position using a tilting table, and while he practices a Valsalva maneuver, contrast medium is injected into the renal vein.

In normal men the spermatic venous outlet in the renal vein can be recognized, but no reflux opacification occurs owing to the presence of competent valves near the spermatic venous outlet (Fig. 5). In patients with varicocele reflux, opacification of the spermatic vein occurs readily after contrast medium injection in the renal vein (Fig. 6). In these patients the spermatic vein is selectively catheterized and injected. Now every detail of the traject taken by the refluxing blood is clearly depicted (Fig. 7) (6).

In many cases the spermatic vein presents peculiar anatomical variations. In one out of three cases the spermatic venous outlet and/or paravertebral

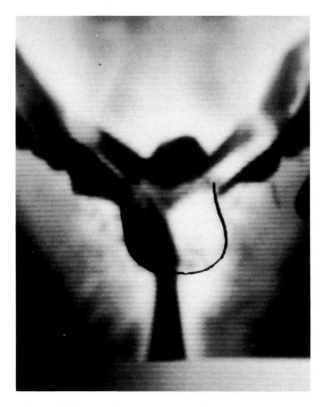

FIG. 3. Patient with grade II varicocele at the left side. The skin of the whole left hemiscrotum is warm.

traject is double or even triple. The distance between the venous branches may be important and amount to 5 cm. In 10% of the patients, the main spermatic vein presents no reflux and competent valves are found close to the outlet; however, reflux occurs under the valves which are by-passed by one or several collateral veins, communicating between the renal vein and the spermatic vein.

At the level of the inguinal canal, reflux passes through more than one vein in one-third of cases, however the venous branches are always close to each other.

Left to right shunts are observed in 20% of the venograms, in general they occur at the level of the ramus pubis and involve a clearly dilated vein along the vas deferens. Sometimes, shunting makes use of perineal or scrotal collateral circulation.

After left side exploration, catheterization of the right renal vein should always be performed. Indeed, reflux in the right internal spermatic vein, aberrantly entering the right renal vein, occurs in about 10% of cases with left side varicocele.

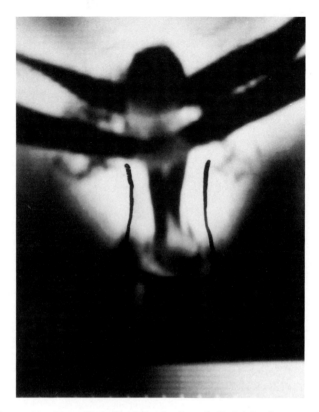

FIG. 4. Telethermogram in a patient with bilateral varicocele. Both lateral aspects of the scrotum are warm since the skin is depicted white, similar to the skin of the inner upper thigh.

Management of Varicocele

If varicocele is palpable, bilateral retrograde venography of the internal spermatic veins is indicated in order to detect possible bilateral reflux and to visualize the traject taken by the refluxing blood. Based on the radiological findings, complete surgical interruption of reflux can be performed more securely.

In all cases with either doubtful clinical palpation, or unexplained asymmetrical testicular development and turgor, or unexplained subfertility without palpable abnormalities, scrotal thermography should be performed.

If temperature disturbance of the scrotal skin is detected, retrograde venography should be performed in order to decide conclusively if spermatic venous reflux is present or not. If the thermogram is normal, no retrograde venography should be performed.

Surgical correction is aimed at the complete interruption of spermatic venous reflux. The spermatic vein(s) should be ligated cranial to the bifurcation of the vena vasa deferentia, near the internal inguinal ring (Ivanessewich procedure

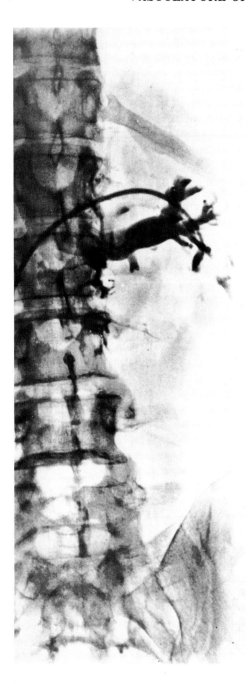

FIG. 5. Venogram of the left renal vein of a normal person standing in half erect position and performing a Valsalva maneuver. The spermatic venous outlet can be recognized. No reflux opacification occurs under competent valves which are localized near this outlet.

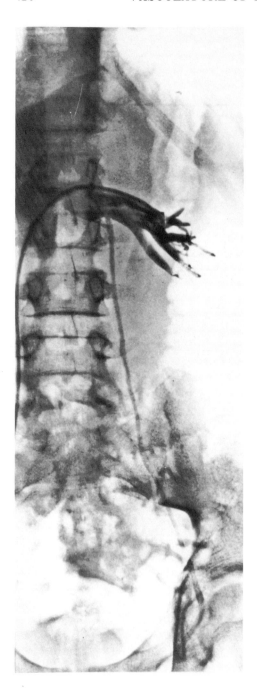

FIG. 6. Retrograde venogram of the renal and spermatic vein in a patient with subclinical varicocele. Reflux opacification of the spermatic vein already occurs during unselective injection into the distal branches of the renal vein. The spermatic vein is not clearly distended despite the presence of retrograde blood flow.

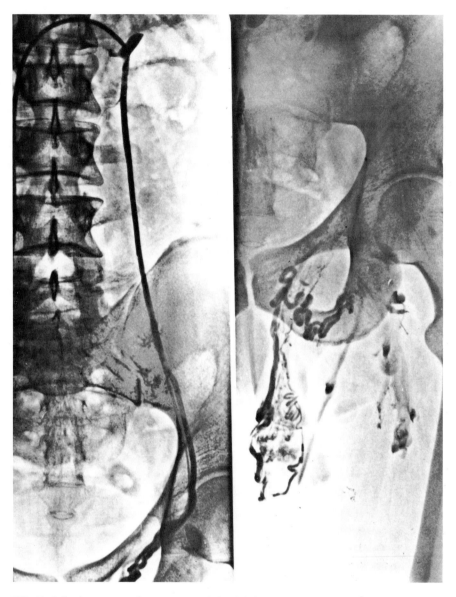

FIG. 7. Selective retrograde venogram of the left internal spermatic vein in a patient with grade II varicocele. The traject taken by the refluxing blood is clearly visualized. Notice opacification of collateral venous circulation between the pampiniform plexus and the superficial as well as deep femoral veins.

modified by Amelar and Dubin) (2). Care should be taken to preserve the lymphatic channels in order to prevent postoperative hydrocele formation. It is probably preferable not to ligate the spermatic artery, although this has been advocated by Palomo (19).

Whenever bilateral reflux is suspected from clinical examination or scrotal thermography, bilateral retrograde venography should be performed followed by bilateral operation if reflux is present. In patients with azoospermia the testicle(s) should simultaneously be biopsied in order to evaluate fertility prognosis.

Patients suffering from sexual inadequacy and varicocele, should be operated if there are any hormonal and/or seminal changes indicating testicular dysfunction. After surgical cure, the scrotal thermogram rapidly normalizes. Persistence of evident hyperthermia indicates that retrograde flow has not been interrupted completely and that operation was a failure.

Prognosis

Improvement of sperm quality may be expected in 70 to 80% of correctly operated cases (10,18) Complete recovery of fertility resulting in pregnancy depends on the degree of epididymo/testicular damage prior to operation. The selection of patients included in the statistics therefore greatly influences the pregnancy rate. Patients suffering from azoospermia or extreme oligozoospermia stand less chance to recover normal spermatogenesis, particularly if serum FSH concentration is clearly increased. Nevertheless some of these cases may benefit from surgery, and individual prognosis is hard to predict without testicular biopsy (12,16,21). Fertility outcome is better in cases with normal sperm morphology whereas patients with severe abnormalities of the sperm heads (amorphous forms, irregular outline), mid-piece (abnormal implantation or kinked) or tail (split or short) have a poor prognosis. As far as hormonogenesis is concerned, normalization of testosterone production may be expected if preoperative LH serum concentration is normal or slightly increased (4). Patients with severe testicular atrophy and/or highly elevated LH levels, mostly men over 45 years of age, will probably not benefit from surgical correction of the varicocele.

New Techniques in Management

Although distension of the external scrotal and cremasteric veins certainly is the result of reflux in the internal spermatic vein, dilatation of the former may persist after interruption of reflux in the latter. Some authors assume that the persistent dilatation of the superficial veins may encourage blood stasis in the testis and therefore should be corrected as well.

A new method to cure varicocele is to interrupt spermatic venous reflux by thrombosing the interal spermatic vein during catheterization for retrograde venography. This nonsurgical management has been successfully applied by a few groups and preliminary results are highly encouraging (7).

REFERENCES

1. Ahlberg, N. E., Bartley, O., Chidekel, N., and Fritjofson, A. (1966): Phlebography in varicocele scroti. *Acta Radiol.,* 4:517–528.
2. Amelar, R. D., Dubin, L., and Walsh, P. C. (1977): In: *Male Infertility,* pp. 65–67. Saunders, Philadelphia.
3. Charny, C. W., and Baum, S. (1968): Varicocele and infertility. *JAMA,* 204:1165–1168.
4. Comhaire, F., and Vermeulen, A. (1975): Plasmatestosterone in patients with varicocele and sexual inadequacy. *J. Clin. Endocrinol. Metab.,* 40:824–829.
5. Comhaire, F., Monteyne, R., and Kunnen, M. (1976): The value of scrotal thermography as compared with selective retrograde venography of the internal spermatic vein for the diagnosis of subclinical varicocele. *Fertil. Steril.,* 27:694–698.
6. Comhaire, F., and Kunnen, M. (1976): Selective retrograde venography of the internal spermatic vein: A conclusive approach to the diagnosis of varicocele. *Andrologia,* 8:11–24.
7. de Castro, M. P., and Santos Lima, S. (1977): Nonsurgical treatment of varicocele. *Fertil. Steril.,* 28:330–331 (Abstract).
8. Dubin, L., and Amelar, R. D. (1970): Varicocele size and results of varicocelectomy in selected subfertile men with varicocele. *Fertil. Steril.,* 21:606–609.
9. Dubin, L., and Amelar, R. D. (1975): Varicocelectomy as therapy in male infertility: A study of 405 cases. *Fertil. Steril.,* 26:217–221.
10. Dubin, L., and Amelar, R. (1977): Surgical treatment of varicocele. *Fertil. Steril.,* 28:331 (Abstract).
11. Etriby, A., Girgis, S. M., Hefnawy, H., and Ibrahim, A. A. (1967): Testicular changes in subfertile males with varicocele. *Fertil. Steril.,* 18:666–671.
12. Fernando, N., Leonard, J. M., and Paulsen, C. A. (1976): The role of varicocele in male infertility. *Andrologia,* 8:1–6.
13. Gasser, G., Strassl, R., and Pokieser, H. (1973): Thermogramm des Hodens und Spermiogramm. *Andrologie,* 5:127–131.
14. Glezerman, M., Bakowszczyk, M., Lunenfeld, B., Beer, R., and Goldman, B. (1976): Varicocele in oligospermic patients: Pathophysiology and results after ligation and division of the internal spermatic vein. *J. Urol.,* 115:562–565.
15. Gösfay, S. (1959): Untersuchungen der Vena spermatica interna durch retrograde Phlebographie bei Kranken mit Varikozele. *Z. Urol.,* 52:105–115.
16. Guillon, G., and Milhiet, H. (1976): Effets du traitement des varicocèles sur la stérilité masculine. *Nouv. Presse Med.,* 92:885–888.
17. Kormano, M., Kahanpää, K., Svinhufvud, U., and Tähti, E. (1970): Thermography of varicocele. *Fertil. Steril.,* 21:558–564.
18. MacLeod, J. (1965): Seminal cytology in the presence of varicocele. *Fertil. Steril.,* 16:735–753.
19. Palomo, A. (1949): Radical cure of varicocele by a new technique. *J. Urol.,* 61:604–609.
20. Salat-Baroux, J., Rotman, J., and Lelorier, G. (1977): Thermographie et stérilité masculine. In: *Spermatogénèse et Stérilité Masculine,* pp. 58–64. Institut Schering.
21. Stewart, B. H. (1974): Varicocele infertility: Incidence and results of surgical therapy. *J. Urol.,* 112:222–223.

Subject Index